'Everyday health', embodiment, and selfhood since 1950

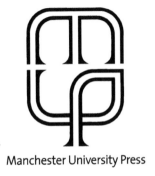

Manchester University Press

SOCIAL HISTORIES OF MEDICINE

Series Editors
David Cantor, Anne Hanley and Elaine Leong

Editorial Board
Diego Armus, Swarthmore College, PA, USA
Rana Hogarth, University of Illinois, Urbana-Champaign, USA
Angela Ki Che Leung, University of Hong Kong, China
Ian Miller, Ulster University, Northern Ireland

Social Histories of Medicine is concerned with all aspects of health, illness and medicine, from prehistory to the present, in every part of the world. The series covers the circumstances that promote health or illness, the ways in which people experience and explain such conditions, and what, practically, they do about them. Practitioners of all approaches to health and healing come within its scope, as do their ideas, beliefs, and practices, and the social, economic and cultural contexts in which they operate. Methodologically, the series welcomes relevant studies in social, economic, cultural, and intellectual history, as well as approaches derived from other disciplines in the arts, sciences, social sciences and humanities. The series is a collaboration between Manchester University Press and the Society for the Social History of Medicine.

To buy or to find out more about the books currently available in this series, please go to: https://manchesteruniversitypress.co.uk/series/social-histories-of-medicine/

'Everyday health', embodiment, and selfhood since 1950

Edited by

Hannah Froom, Tracey Loughran, Kate Mahoney, and Daisy Payling

MANCHESTER UNIVERSITY PRESS

Copyright © Manchester University Press 2024

While copyright in the volume as a whole is vested in Manchester University Press, copyright in individual chapters belongs to their respective authors, and no chapter may be reproduced wholly or in part without the express permission in writing of both author and publisher.

An electronic version of the Introduction, Chapter 5, Chapter 7, Chapter 8, Chapter 9, Chapter 11, Chapter 13, Chapter 15, and Chapter 16 has been made freely available under a Creative Commons (CC BY-NC-ND) licence, thanks to the support of the Wellcome Trust and Canada Research Chairs Program, which permits non-commercial use, distribution and reproduction provided the author(s) and Manchester University Press are fully cited and no modifications or adaptations are made. Details of the licence can be viewed at https://creativecommons.org/licenses/by-nc-nd/4.0/

Published by Manchester University Press
Oxford Road, Manchester, M13 9PL

www.manchesteruniversitypress.co.uk

British Library Cataloguing-in-Publication Data
A catalogue record for this book is available from the British Library

ISBN   978 1 5261 7065 1   hardback

First published 2024

The publisher has no responsibility for the persistence or accuracy of URLs for any external or third-party internet websites referred to in this book, and does not guarantee that any content on such websites is, or will remain, accurate or appropriate.

Typeset by New Best-set Typesetters Ltd

For our grandmothers, with love
Frances Vickers Davis (1928–2017)
Eleanor Froom (1929–2022)
Ella Ilott (1929–)
Georgina Johnson (1924–2021)
June Loughran (1930–2006)
Jean Payling (1929–2020)
Sally Thomas (1933–2003)
Marion Williams (1930–2019)

Contents

List of figures	*page* x
Notes on contributors	xii
Preface and acknowledgements	xviii
Abbreviations	xxi

Introduction: 'Everyday health', embodiment, and
selfhood since 1950   1
*Hannah Froom, Tracey Loughran, Kate Mahoney,
and Daisy Payling*

Part I: Experiential expertise

Part I: Introduction   31
Hannah Froom and Tracey Loughran

1 Alex Comfort's *The Joy of Sex* and the tensions of
liberal sexpertise   39
Ben Mechen

2 'Two more calls, one in tears ...': emotion, labour,
and ethics of care at the Calgary Birth Control
Association, 1970–79   60
Karissa Robyn Patton

3 Expertise and experience in the Greek feminist birth
control movement, c. 1974–86   82
Evangelia Chordaki

4 Migration, kinship, and 'everyday theorising': Black
British women's narratives of genetic diagnosis in
the postwar National Health Service   103
Grace Redhead

viii   *Contents*

Part II: Sites and spaces

Part II: Introduction   127
  Tracey Loughran
  5 Writing everyday life into law: the 'household duties
     test', disabled women, social security, and assumed
     normality   134
     Gareth Millward
  6 Friendship, mutual aid, and activism in British
     transfeminine spaces, 1968–85   154
     Fleur MacInnes
  7 A private matter? The Brook Advisory Centre and
     young people's everyday sexual and reproductive
     health in the 1960s–80s   176
     Caroline Rusterholz
  8 Queering the agony aunt: reusing and adapting
     a public engagement activity for different
     audiences   198
     Daisy Payling

Part III: Mass media and networks of communication

Part III: Introduction   221
  Daisy Payling and Tracey Loughran
  9 'Thirty years behind England'? Framing 'natural'
     childbirth in postwar Canada   230
     Whitney Wood
 10 'I started a new life when I joined Gemma': disability,
     community, and sexuality in Gemma newsletters,
     1978–2000   251
     Beckie Rutherford
 11 Talk shows and 'tanorexia': motherhood and 'sunbed
     addiction' on British television in the 1990s   272
     Fabiola Creed
 12 'Having been there … I know how hard it is':
     relatability and ordinariness in twenty-first-century
     British clean eating   294
     Louise Morgan

Contents

ix

Part IV: Subjectivity and intersubjectivity

Part IV: Introduction *Kate Mahoney and Tracey Loughran*	317
13 Girlhood menstrual management and the 'culture of concealment' in postwar Britain *Hannah Froom*	325
14 Is sex good for you? Risk, reward, and responsibility for young women in the late 1980s *Rosie Gahnstrom, Lucy Robinson, and Rachel Thomson*	345
15 'What your generation probably don't understand is …': exploring intergenerational dynamics in oral history *Kate Mahoney*	367
16 Cultivating vulnerability: power and the emotional ethics of oral history practice beyond the interview *Tracey Loughran*	386
17 … and breathe: style narratives at home, March 2020–March 2021 *Carol Tulloch*	408
Index	430

Figures

All rights reserved and permission to use the figures must be obtained from the copyright holder.

0.1 Cover illustration of 1970 Pelican edition of Hannah Gavron, *The Captive Wife: Conflicts of Housebound Mothers* (first published by Routledge & Kegan Paul, 1966). Original cover design and photograph by Graham Bishop. This photograph by Tracey Loughran. *page* 7

1.1 One of Charles Raymond's watercolours for the original edition of *The Joy of Sex* on display at the Wellcome Collection, London. Courtesy of Nils Jorgensen/Shutterstock. 44

2.1 'CBCA volunteer, Jean Phillips, gives birth control advice', *Calgary Herald*, 15 January 1973. Courtesy of Glenbow Archives, Archives and Special Collections, University of Calgary. 69

6.1 Final page of Tanya S1828's letter to the *Beaumont Bulletin*, May 1979, including cartoons. Photograph courtesy of Special Collections and Archives, Bishopsgate Institute. All attempts have been made to contact the copyright holders of cartoons. 160

8.1 'Dear agony aunt' activity from the 'Bodies, hearts, and minds: using the past to empower the future' toolkit. Courtesy of Tracey Loughran, Kate Mahoney, and Daisy Payling. 213

Figures

10.1 'Gemmas at Gay Pride', in Gemma anthology, *Silver Leaves* (June 2001). Courtesy of Special Collections and Archives, Bishopsgate Institute.   261

11.1 Esther Rantzen on the set of her talk show, 1998. Courtesy of Michael Stephens/Alamy Stock Photo.   280

14.1 Poster for 'Reanimating Data: Experiments with People, Places and Archives' (artist Mitchi Mathias). Courtesy of Rachel Thomson.   346

Notes on contributors

Evangelia Chordaki (she/her) is a post-doctoral research fellow at the Seeger Center for Hellenic Studies at Princeton University. She has published in national and international journals, edited volumes, and participated in numerous international conferences, workshops, and research groups. She is a historian of science and holds a PhD in Science Communication and Gender Studies (2022), funded by the Hellenic Foundation for Research and Innovation. Her research interest includes feminist epistemologies, the intertwinement between gender, technoscience, and digitality, emphasising cyberfeminism and xenofeminism. Her first monograph, *Making* Sense *of Knowledge: Feminist Epistemologies in the Greek Birth Control Movement (1974–1986)*, is forthcoming with Cambridge University Press.

Fabiola Creed (she/her) is a health and beauty historian specialising in the history of industry, mass media, and stigma in twentieth-century Britain. She is a research fellow on Professor Hilary Marland's Wellcome-funded project 'The Last Taboo of Motherhood? Postnatal Mental Disorders in Twentieth-Century Britain' (2021–24) at the University of Warwick. She has also converted her PhD research on the sunbed industry into several publications. These focus on the fake tan industry (*Technology and Health in the Age of Patient Consumerism*, Manchester University Press edited collection) and sunbed 'addicts' (*Social History of Medicine*, 35:3). Her first monograph is on *The Rise and Fall of the Sunbed: Tanning Culture from Fad to Fear* (forthcoming).

Hannah Froom (she/her) is an early-career researcher with interests in the relationship of girls and women to mass culture. Her doctoral

Notes on contributors

xiii

thesis 'Menstruation, Subjectivity and Constructions of Girlhood in Britain, 1960–1980' (University of Essex, 2022) used the topic of menstruation as a lens to explore the everyday experiences of female adolescents, the influence of psy disciplines on teen magazines, and the relationships between teen girls and magazines.

Rosie Gahnstrom (she/her) wrote her chapter while a PhD candidate in Childhood and Youth at the University of Sussex and research assistant for the 'Reanimating Data' project. She is an experienced social researcher and works in sexual health and youth work settings. Her research has focused on youth sexual cultures, relationships and sex education, and creative research methods.

Tracey Loughran (she/her) is Professor of History at the University of Essex. Her current research aims to create an intersectional history of women's 'everyday health' from the ground up, drawing on oral history interviews, Mass Observation directives, and mass-market magazines. She is the author of *Shell-Shock and Medical Culture in First World War Britain* (2017), and co-editor of *The Palgrave Handbook of Infertility in History: Approaches, Contexts and Perspectives* (2017; with Gayle Davis) and *Emotion and the Researcher: Sites, Subjectivities and Relationships* (2018; with Dawn Mannay). Her research interests centre on how knowledge is constructed, 'translated', and transformed across different disciplines and contexts, and the interaction of representation and experience in shaping selfhood.

Fleur MacInnes (they/them) is a trans feminist historian and DPhil candidate at the University of Oxford. They are funded by the Arts and Humanities Research Council and their thesis is titled 'A Trans-feminist Reconceptualization? Transfeminine Experiences of the Women's Liberation Movement in Britain, 1968–1985'. Fleur's doctoral research explores the interactions between transfeminine communities and feminist organisations, and it aims to establish a 'trans-feminist reconceptualization' of women's history in postwar Britain. Fleur holds a Master of Studies degree in Modern British History from the University of Oxford, which they completed in 2020, and expects to finish their DPhil in Autumn 2024.

Kate Mahoney (she/her) is Research Manager at Healthwatch Essex and a visiting associate professor at the Faculty of Health, Medicine and Social Care at Anglia Ruskin University. Kate has published on women's health, feminist politics, oral history, and researchers' xiv *Notes on contributors*

emotions. Her first sole-authored book, *Feminist Mental Health Activism in England, c. 1968–1995*, was published by Manchester University Press in 2023.

Ben Mechen (he/him) is a historian of culture and society in modern Britain at University College London. He is currently working on his first book, a study of sexual liberation in late twentieth-century Britain to be published by University of California Press. He is co-editor, with Matt Houlbrook and Katie Jones, of *Men and Masculinities in Modern Britain: A History for the Present* (Manchester University Press, 2024). He is also co-editor, with Laura Cofield and Matthew Worley, of a special issue of *Contemporary British History* on the cultural politics of sex in postwar Britain (2022).

Gareth Millward (he/him) is Assistant Professor in the Department of Culture and Language and the Danish Institute for Advanced Study at the University of Southern Denmark. His work focuses on the interaction between the welfare state and its citizens. In particular, his research has investigated public reactions to, and role in developing, policies around medicine and social security, analysing policy communities, professional organisations, the voluntary sector, and cultural attitudes towards the welfare state. The research presented in this volume was conducted at the London School of Hygiene and Tropical Medicine and the University of Warwick. His publications have covered disability, vaccination, and sick leave policy, including his recent monograph *Sick Note Britain: A History of the British Welfare State*.

Louise Morgan (she/her) is a historian of food and medicine, specialising in the history of nutrition, dieting, eating disorders, social media, and contemporary Britain. She is particularly interested in interdisciplinary methodologies and approaches to new media sources, as well as the use of religious metaphor and moralism in both contemporary and historical discussions about food and health. She held an early career fellowship at the University of Warwick's Institute of Advanced Study between 2023 and 2024. Most recently, she was a research assistant at the University of Nottingham's Business School, working on an interdisciplinary project researching the history of milk safety in Britain. She is currently working on developing her thesis, which examined the contemporary history of clean eating and orthorexia nervosa, into a monograph.

Notes on contributors xv

Karissa Robyn Patton (she/her) is a historian of gender, sexuality, health, and activism. She works as an interdisciplinary research fellow at the Centre for Biomedicine, Self, and Society at the University of Edinburgh, where she studies the history of feminist healthcare and activism in the United Kingdom and Canada. Her doctoral work at the University of Saskatchewan examined the history of local birth control centres in Southern Alberta. Some of this work is featured in her co-edited collection, *Bucking Conservatism: Alternative Stories of Alberta from the 1960s and 1970s* (open access: www.aupress.ca/books/120286-bucking-conservatism/). Her other work can be found in the *Canadian Journal for Health History*, the *Canadian Historical Review*, and *Compelled to Act*.

Daisy Payling (she/her) is a Research Development and Impact Manager in the Faculty of Arts and Humanities at University College London. Daisy has published on women's magazines, oral history, local government and activism, the latter of which is explored in her 2023 monograph, *Socialist Republic: Remaking the British Left in 1980s Sheffield*, published by Manchester University Press.

Grace Redhead (she/her) is a historian interested in the postcolonial welfare state, oral history, and health inequalities. She completed her PhD at University College London in 2019, titled 'Histories of Sickle Cell Anaemia in Postcolonial Britain, 1948–1997'. She is currently a postdoctoral fellow at the Wellcome Centre for Cultures and Environments of Health at the University of Exeter, where she is researching histories of regional health inequality in England. She is co-editor, with Saffron East and Theo Williams, of *Anti-racism in Britain: Traditions, Histories and Trajectories, c. 1880–present* (forthcoming, Manchester University Press).

Lucy Robinson (she/her) is Professor of Collaborative History at the University of Sussex. She writes on popular music, politics and identity, feminism, and subcultural pedagogy. Her book *Gay Men and the Left in Post-War Britain: How the Personal Became Political* was first published by Manchester University Press in 2007. Since then she has worked on the Falklands War, charity singles, music videos, zine cultures, digital memory, protest, and the politics of popular culture. As well as coordinating the Subcultures Network, and the open access digital project 'Observing the 1980s', during lockdown she curated Vivienne Westwood's Intellectual Unite online book club. Her new monograph, *Now That's What I Call a*

xvi *Notes on contributors*

History of the 1980s, is published by Manchester University Press (2023).

Caroline Rusterholz (she/her) is Assistant Professor at the Department of International History and Politics at the Graduate Institute in Geneva. Her research focuses on the transnational history of sexual and reproductive health, population, and family in the twentieth century. Her first book, *Deux enfants c'est déjà pas mal: famille et fécondité en Suisse*, explores why Swiss parents limited the size of their families in the 1960s. Her second monograph, *Women's Medicine, Sex, Family Planning and British Female Doctors in Transnational Perspective (1920–70)* (Manchester University Press, 2020), traces the key roles played by British women doctors in the production and circulation of contraceptive knowledge from a transnational perspective. Her new monograph, *Responsible Pleasure: The Brook Advisory Centres and Youth Sexuality in Postwar Britain*, is forthcoming with Oxford University Press.

Beckie Rutherford (she/her) is a historian of gender, sexuality, and disability in modern Britain with a particular interest in the politicisation of disability from 1970 to the present day. Beckie completed her PhD at the University of Warwick in 2023 and was the Royal Historical Society Centenary Fellow at the Institute of Historical Research 2022–23. She is currently an editorial fellow at History Workshop.

Rachel Thomson (she/her) is Professor of Childhood and Youth Studies at the University of Sussex. She is a sociologist with an interest in time, sexuality, and gendered biography. Her co-authored books include *Making Modern Mothers* (Policy Press, 2011), *Researching Social Change* (Sage, 2009) and *Researching Everyday Childhoods: Time, Technology and Documentation* (Bloomsbury, 2018).

Carol Tulloch (she/her) is a writer, curator, maker, and Professor of Dress, Diaspora and Transnationalism at Chelsea College of Arts, University of the Arts London. She is an honorary senior research fellow at the Victoria and Albert Museum. Her research studies how Black people negotiate their sense of self, through their styled body, within different cultural and social contexts alongside the lived experiences of other social groups for an expanded understanding of being and belonging to a place. She incorporates difference, style narratives, cultural and familial heritage, auto/biography, personal archives, activism, agency and making, and more recently personal narratives. Her publications include *The Persistence of Taste: Art, Museums and Everyday Life after Bourdieu* (2018; co-editor), *The Birth of Cool: Style Narratives of the African Diaspora* (2016), the exhibitions *Jessica Ogden: Still* (2017), *Rock against Racism* (2015; co-curator), *Handmade Tales: Women and Domestic Crafts* (2010).

Whitney Wood (she/her) is Canada Research Chair in the Historical Dimensions of Women's Health at Vancouver Island University. Her research interests include histories of gender, health, and the body, and cultural and medical representations of obstetric and gynaecological pain. Wood is currently working on a study entitled *Changing Childbirth in Postwar Canada, 1945–2000*, funded by a Social Sciences and Humanities Research Council of Canada Insight Development Grant, and is principal investigator of a new multi-year collaborative study, 'Pelvic Health and Public Health in Twentieth Century Canada', funded by the Canadian Institutes of Health Research.

Preface and acknowledgements

At the beginning of March 2020, we were looking forward to hosting a two-day conference on 'Gender, Subjectivity, and "Everyday Health" in the Post-1945 World' six weeks later. The conference had been in the works for some time, a long-planned outcome of our project on women's 'everyday health' in late twentieth-century Britain. Abstracts were in, programme drafted, and rooms booked. With much seriousness we had researched good inclusive practice, and with much more laughter had planned to book a mixologist to craft conference-themed cocktails. Would participants have enjoyed 'The Mooncup', a tequila sunrise-inspired libation featuring a red mist of grenadine rising upwards through the glass? We will never know. In mid-March, hanging on till the last possible moment amid reports of rising numbers of coronavirus cases, we decided to postpone the conference. Perhaps, we thought, it could be rescheduled for the late summer – or would that clash with annual conferences that our speakers and participants might want to attend? We decided to put off announcing a new date until we had looked into the roster of potentially competing events. A week later the United Kingdom entered its first lockdown.

An over-full academic calendar was the least of our, or anyone else's, problems that summer. Fast forward to January 2021, and we finally got to hear the first panel – over Zoom, in our respective living rooms/bedrooms/whatever working spaces we had managed to carve out in our homes. The conference became a seminar series that ran fortnightly over a six-month period. We weren't able to provide cocktails for participants; mostly we didn't know what they

Preface and acknowledgements

xix

looked like, or sometimes even their real names, as they silently logged on, and we wrestled with learning how to assign hosts and co-hosts, turn off microphones, and avoid the much-publicised phenomenon of Zoom hackers. But we did try to capture something of the conference spirit for our speakers, posting each person an individualised badge, laminated card relating to their research paper topic, and mug commemorating the seminar series (most did not survive the journey unbroken), and hosting an online zine-making workshop to conclude the programme. In turn, our speakers helped to keep our faith in the project at a time when it was sometimes difficult to see how, or even why, to keep going with plans from 'the before times'.

In 'the after times', which is to say now, this edited collection provides a lasting record of that seminar series. We have enjoyed working with the contributors over the past two years, and we're grateful for their persistence and belief in this volume in the face of the many upheavals of the pandemic and post-pandemic world. We are also thankful to those scholars who participated in the seminar series but were unable for different reasons to contribute to this book. Mark Anderson, Holly Ashford, Hannah Charnock, Teri Chettiar, Peder Clark, Hannah Elizabeth, Georgia Grainger, Richard Hall, Jessica Hammett, Yuliya Hilevych, Katherine Jones, Jill Kirby, Christina Lee, Katrina Louise-Moseley, Martin Moore, Chelsea Saxby, Stephanie Snow, and Angela Whitecross: thank you. Your papers were crucial in creating the intellectual environment out of which this book emerged.

As the Social Histories of Medicine series editor at Manchester University Press (MUP), David Cantor provided encouragement for the volume from the first announcement of the conference. Meredith Carroll, senior commissioning editor at MUP, has been extremely patient and supportive throughout the long process. In finalising the book for publication, we are also grateful to Stefan Dickers, the Special Collections and Archives Manager at the Bishopsgate Institute, for support with images. And, of course, neither the seminar series nor our individual chapters would have existed without the Wellcome Trust's generosity in funding an Investigator Award in the Humanities and Social Sciences, 'Body, Self and Family: Women's Psychological, Emotional and Bodily Health in Britain, c. 1960–1990' (ref: 208080/Z/17/Z), and especially in extending

xx   *Preface and acknowledgements*

that grant to compensate for research time lost during the global pandemic.

Finally, enormous thanks to Georgie Randall, the 'Body, Self, and Family' project officer, who did most of the organisational work for the conference that never happened – including workshopping ideas for creative uses of grenadine in cocktails to celebrate the history of 'everyday health', embodiment, and selfhood.

Hannah Froom
Tracey Loughran
Kate Mahoney
Daisy Payling

Abbreviations

A&E	Accident and Emergency Department
AIDS	acquired immunodeficiency syndrome
BAC	Brook Advisory Centre
BFI	British Film Institute
CBCA	Calgary Birth Control Association
CWF	Childbirth without Fear
DHSS	Department of Health and Social Security
ERDWC	Equal Rights for Disabled Women Campaign
FPA	Family Planning Association
GLM	Gay Liberation Movement
GP	general practitioner
HCA	Hall-Carpenter Archives
HIV	human immunodeficiency virus
HNCIP	Housewife's Non-Contributory Invalidity Pension
LGBTQ+	lesbian, gay, bi, trans, queer, questioning and ace
LSE	London School of Economics
MLW	Movement for the Liberation of Women
MOA	Mass Observation Archive
MOP	Mass Observation Project
NCIP	non-contributory invalidity pension
NHS	National Health Service
OED	*Oxford English Dictionary*
PoTS	postural tachycardia syndrome
SCD	sickle cell disease
SDA	Severe Disablement Allowance
STS	science and technology studies

xxii   *Abbreviations*

TAG   Transsexual Action Group
TNA   The National Archives
TSA   The Sunbed Association
TV/TS Group   Transvestite/Transsexual Group
UV   ultraviolet
VD   venereal disease
WGD   Women's Group in Denmark
WL   Wellcome Library
WLM   Women's Liberation Movement
WRAP   Women, Risk and AIDS Project

Introduction: 'Everyday health', embodiment, and selfhood since 1950

Hannah Froom, Tracey Loughran, Kate Mahoney, and Daisy Payling

What is 'everyday health'?

In 2017, Bodyform became the first UK brand to show menstrual pads stained with red liquid, rather than blue, in its adverts. The company's video campaign, accompanied by the #bloodnormal, also showed a woman in the shower with blood running down her thigh and a man buying menstrual products. Response to the campaign was largely positive, with many welcoming Bodyform's decision to challenge menstrual taboos. The campaign won the Grand Prix award in the 2018 Marketing Week's Masters Awards.[1] This positive response contrasts with previous storms over companies' attempts to push boundaries in menstrual advertising, including complaints in 1972 over the earliest foray into television advertising (a brief trial that was quickly pulled), in 1993 in response to the Vespre Silhouette ad featuring agony aunt Claire Rayner, and in 2003 when Lil-lets included a demonstration of the benefits of tampons in an ad filmed in the style of a 1970s children's television show.[2] If the Bodyform ad itself harnesses feminist celebration of menstruation to capitalist aims, the response to it demonstrates at least the partial success of menstrual activists in shifting public opinion.[3]

We could view this shift as an unambiguous advancement in attitudes towards menstruation – an everyday, normal health experience for millions of people, but one hidden and stigmatised for much of modern history. Yet, looking beyond public forms such as advertising, into private experiences of bodily and household management, challenges easy assumptions of unilinear progress towards

2 'Everyday health', embodiment and selfhood

greater comfort with our bodies and their functions. When we interviewed Tricia (b. 1958), she told us that when she was a teenager, the fireplace in their spare bedroom was used solely for burning menstrual products.[4] For Tricia, this allocation of household space was mundane; to listeners nowadays, it might seem bizarre, or cause an almost-instinctive recoil. The boundaries of the 'everyday' can shift in unexpected ways over time, and our understanding of what *was* 'everyday' in the past might well depend on where we fix our gaze: on public forms or private behaviours.

What do we mean when we talk about the 'everyday' and 'everyday health'? The 'everyday' has been the implicit and explicit focus of many scholarly traditions, from social histories that assumed the primacy of economic materialism, through the cultural studies of the 1980s onwards, to more recent historiographical debates on 'expertise' and 'ordinariness'.[5] The extent of this scholarship reflects the changing nature and importance of the 'everyday' in politics, society, and culture since 1950, spurred by multiple developments including the reshaping of democratic politics and the institution of welfare states,[6] the reconceptualisation of responsible citizenship in the aftermath of the Second World War,[7] the expansion of consumerism and its insistence on happiness in every aspect of life,[8] and the rise of identity-based political movements that broke down the boundaries between the public sphere and personal life.[9] These developments had momentous consequences for understandings of health. Welfarism reframed notions of health in relation to citizenship.[10] The flourishing of individualism, affluence, and consumerism meant the proliferation of privatised therapies for maladies of body and mind.[11] Liberationist activism tore open the ideological underpinnings and oppressive functions of traditional medical systems, throwing open the question of what good health really meant – accommodation to an unjust system or the flourishing of the entire self?[12] The concept of health that emerged out of these transformations was newly expansive, especially in its more recent association with terms like wellbeing, wellness, and self-care.[13]

The term 'everyday health' brings together multitudinous understandings of the 'everyday' and of 'health' and places them in historical and historicised contexts. We define 'everyday health' as the emotional, psychological, and bodily state-of-being in individuals' day-to-day lives, and the strategies they pursue (or do not) to maintain

Introduction: 'Everyday health' 3

equilibrium in this state-of-being.[14] More than a descriptive term or a neatly bounded concept, 'everyday health' is a lens. Histories of 'everyday health' centre on the experiences of 'ordinary' people in their daily lives, as they work, socialise, and pursue relationships, and the resources they draw on to make sense of the thoughts, feelings, and sensations that make up their sense of 'health'. The perspective of 'everyday health' exists in contrast to histories that focus on states, medical professionals, and other experts, and extends the work of existing social histories of health that have partially supplanted top-down medical narratives.

Because it works outwards from experience, 'everyday health' is an inclusive concept that requires an intersectional perspective, considering how multiple aspects of identity (gender, sexuality, 'race', class, disability, and age) influence experiences of health and well-being.[15] The concept therefore highlights embodiment and selfhood. This approach unites social history's attention to lived experience with the sweep of more recent cultural histories of emotion and subjectivity.[16] It also fractures the assumed 'everyday' experience (white, male, working-class) of traditional social histories. The history of 'everyday health' is a political project.

Locating 'everyday health', embodiment, and selfhood since 1950

The aim of this volume is to establish 'everyday health' as a lens through which to re-examine the history of health and medicine in different times and places. The majority of chapters examine case studies from the United Kingdom (UK). However, we also include material on Europe and North America to illuminate the interrelation of major political, social, economic, and cultural transformations across the globe in the decades after the Second World War. In the UK, the story went something like this: The rise of the welfare state led to improved health across the lifespan, albeit differentiated by class and 'race', and subsequent greater attention to mind as well as body, as seen in the rise of notions of 'wellbeing'.[17] These new psychological discourses, consequent upon improved bodily health, led to both a more expansive conception of 'health' and greater attention to interiority. This shift was evident in the mainstreaming

4   'Everyday health', embodiment and selfhood

of therapeutic approaches once perceived as part of the counterculture, and in the infiltration of medicalised concepts such as 'stress' into everyday arenas such as working life.[18] At the same time, the reshaping of citizenship, partially consequent on migration and changes to the ethnic composition of the UK, and eventually intersecting with the rise of the patient-consumer and liberatory activism, generated an altered discourse of rights and responsibilities.[19] By the end of the twentieth century, patient groups and activist campaigns proliferated, demonstrating the consolidation of 'ordinary' people's belief that they had a right to speak up and to organise around matters of importance to their own lives and wellbeing.[20]

At the same time, patterns of life were altering for young and old, partly in response to the wider changes ushered in by welfarism, and partly as an outcome of consumerism. Changes to the school leaving age, shifting parental expectations, and the further entrench-ment of the 'teenager' as a distinctive life stage meant that, for many, adolescence became a time of youthful 'freedom'.[21] The provision of old age pensions coupled with increased life expectancy democ-ratised the experience of a similar period of 'freedom' in older age.[22] These shifts coincided with revolutions in family life as changing patterns of marriage, divorce, and childbearing, as well as the assertion of LGBTQ+ rights, remodelled family forms and fractured the ideal of the nuclear family.[23] In turn, these transformations could not have happened without access to technologies that altered multiple aspects of life, from the influence of the Pill on bodily management and sexual autonomy,[24] to new household appliances that changed experiences of household labour and management,[25] through to the explosion of mass communication in magazines, television, and the internet that created new ways to understand health.[26] Because of these sweeping changes in technology and communication, it was difficult to remain entirely unaware of what was happening elsewhere in the world. As a result, new 'imagined communities' with shared expectations of the ideal body and mind formed across national boundaries – and new contests arose over which visions of healthy body, self, and society would achieve cultural domination.[27]

This volume explores 'everyday health', embodiment, and selfhood against this historical backdrop. It is divided into four parts that foreground prominent aspects of representations, experiences, and modes of understanding 'everyday health': experiential expertise;

Introduction: 'Everyday health'   5

sites and spaces; mass media and networks of communication; and subjectivity and intersubjectivity. We open with Part I, 'Experiential expertise' as a statement of intent: instead of starting from the position of formal expertise and working down to how this affects people and practice on the ground, we centre experience and throw open the question of what constitutes 'expertise'. We then move on in Part II to consider the diverse 'Sites and spaces' where 'everyday health' was lived and made, leaving behind institutional sites and instead roaming across spaces including schools, community organisations, birth control clinics, cultural venues, and the home. Part III, 'Mass media and networks of communication', zooms in on crucial forums for the articulation, dissemination, and shaping of body, self, and 'everyday health' in the interconnected twentieth- and twenty-first-century world: print culture, mass-market magazines, television, and social media. Finally, in Part IV we turn inwards to 'Subjectivity and intersubjectivity', thinking about sources and approaches that place embodied selfhood at the heart of 'everyday health'. We discuss the context and content of each part more fully in our part introductions. Here, we highlight cross-cutting themes that further illuminate 'everyday health', embodiment, and selfhood since 1950: agency, power, and resistance; visibility, invisibility, and hypervisibility; and the local, national, and global.

Agency, power, and resistance

Hannah Gavron's *The Captive Wife: Conflicts of Housebound Mothers*, published in 1966, explained how and why motherhood stripped women of their independence. It compared the experiences of working-class and middle-class women and detailed the political, social, and cultural causes of young mothers' unhappiness. Gavron excoriated myths of romantic love extolled by 'the pop song, the advertisement, the magazine', arguing that the 'ordinary woman persists in the belief that in marriage one ounce of perfume is still worth a peck of legal rights and her dreams of power still feature the *femme fatale* rather than the administrative grade of the Civil Service'.[28] Gavron herself had graduated from the Royal Academy of Dramatic Arts shortly after her marriage. Her children were born in 1959 and 1961, while she studied sociology at Bedford College,

6   *'Everyday health', embodiment and selfhood*

University of London (the book was based on her doctoral thesis). In retrospect, *The Captive Wife* established her as one of the pioneering female social scientists who 'helped to entrench new understandings of married women's employment as a fundamental feature of advanced industrial societies, and one that solved the dilemmas of "modern" woman across social classes'.[29] If this was the whole story, Gavron would be remembered as a liberated woman, the anatomist and antithesis of the captive wife; but, of course, it is not. She died by suicide in 1965.

Gavron did not accept many limitations in life. Beyond her extraordinary educational endeavours – embarking on a second undergraduate degree, motherhood, and doctorate at the same time – she seized on other opportunities, big and small, to change her life, change her self. Although she condemned women's magazines in print, a friend remembers the adolescent Hannah writing to *Woman's Own* for information about birth control, taking the matter of reproductive control into her own hands; her son writes about finding among her papers a 1964 clipping from a women's magazine showing the Mary Quant bob she adopted that autumn.[30] But within patriarchal culture, a woman's drive for research and her experimentation with appearance could leave her equally open to attack. Her family believed that she was let down by 'masculine sloth' when her supervisor kept her thesis in a drawer for six months, holding up award of her doctorate and the contract for *The Captive Wife*. Male malice was also suspected; the reference of another lecturer may have described her as a 'lightweight', presumably because he did not approve of her woman-centred research. Perhaps most devastating is the reported comment of Richard Titmuss, sociological behemoth, who chaired one of the London School of Economics interview boards that refused her a post: 'too much green eye make-up'.[31]

Hannah Gavron could stand outside the confines of women's roles and coolly analyse them, backed up by scholarly footnotes detailing qualitative and quantitative evidence. But these men could not see her as other than the archetypal young mother with children on the cover of *The Captive Wife*, trapped by the encircling golden ring, looking out but unable to escape (Figure 0.1). We always exercise our agentic capacities in relation to structures that we can work within, resist, or fight to change, but that we cannot control. Gavron's story reminds us of the potential for power and resistance,

Introduction: 'Everyday health' 7

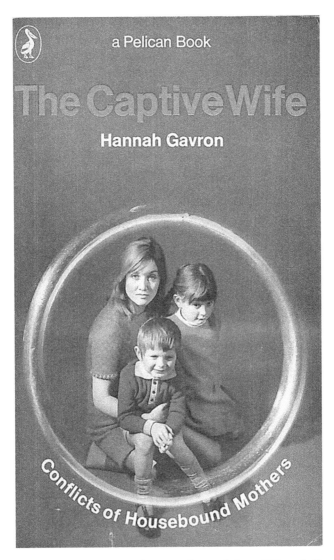

Figure 0.1 Cover illustration of 1970 Pelican edition of Hannah Gavron, *The Captive Wife: Conflicts of Housebound Mothers* (first published by Routledge & Kegan Paul, 1966). Original cover design and photograph by Graham Bishop. This photograph by Tracey Loughran. All rights reserved and permission to use the figure must be obtained from the copyright holder.

8   *'Everyday health', embodiment and selfhood*

its limitations under certain circumstances, and the importance of the long-term perspective to understanding what change has been enacted. There is a still a tendency, especially in popular narratives, to romanticise the onward march of progress in the postwar decades: to tell tales of longer lifespans, liberalising legislation, and liberation, while glossing over the injustices that called laws and activist movements into being and the inequalities that remain. Across this volume, authors explore how diverse groups – adolescents, patients, housewives, mothers, LGBTQ+ people, feminists, disability activists – negotiated the restrictions on their lives and reshaped understandings of their bodies and selves. These chapters do not ignore the pervasive power of state bureaucracies, social hierarchies, and stigmatising beliefs but they always pick out the agentic capacities of individuals and groups.

The concept of 'everyday health' helps us to consider agency, power, and resistance in more open-ended ways. Placing day-to-day experience at the centre of our understanding forces us to move towards fluidity and emphasis on the multiple networks people operate within during their everyday lives, and away from top-down models that petrify their more passive status at particular moments, but without denying the existence or importance of those moments. In this volume, Hannah Froom tells how a young girl without tampons feared going swimming at school but wore multiple pairs of underwear under her costume and went anyway; her choices were limited, but she took what action she could. Grace Redhead details the ignorance and racist assumptions that Black women faced in negotiating sickle cell anaemia, but also how they worked to support others in patient groups and became doctors. Beckie Rutherford describes how a disabled woman excluded from an inaccessible feminist disco wrote a play about the experience and joined a radical group that set up its own socials. Other chapters offer similar examples of agentic action within externally imposed boundaries – this tells us something about how people make 'everyday health' and helps us to consider anew what constitutes power and resistance, both in and beyond activism. Crucially, emphasising embodied experiences also maintains the focus on subjectivities rather than structures, and agency rather than powerlessness. As Kathleen Canning argues, understanding the body as a complex site of inscription, subjectivity, and resistance offers an intricate way of retheorising agency.[32]

Introduction: 'Everyday health'

Structures do matter, but they are not everything. Where activism around 'everyday health' is inspired by the desire to resist and rework the top-down operation of power, it can shed new light on the relationship between state and citizens. We might think here of anti-vaccination and anti-fluoride movements that resist state intervention because of fears about the unknown and potentially negative effects of measures to improve health, and in doing so lay bare the extent and limitations of state power, and the capacities of private citizens to withstand its reach.[33] Because activism around bodies and health often arises out of the 'everyday', from experience rather than on abstract grounds, it can also challenge more traditional ideas of what activism *is*. In Fleur MacInnes' chapter in this volume, we see how friendship and mutual aid were powerful forces enabling trans people to connect and form communities. In some circumstances, becoming visible to yourself and others is not only an important precursor to activism, but an essential part of what it means.

This 'everyday' basis for action is found across multiple activist movements, each containing contests for power within the movement, as well as fighting more established structures outside. The Women's Liberation Movement (WLM) slogan 'the personal is political' formed the basis for Women's Health Movement (WHM) activism that sought not only to validate women's bodily experiences but to demonstrate the inseparability of subjective experience from its social and political context. At the same time, campaigns against misuse of the injectable contraceptive Depo-Provera by Black feminists complicated the notions of 'choice' promoted by white feminist health campaigners.[34] Meanwhile, in activism around specific health crises, including AIDS Coalition To Unleash Power (ACT UP), Fat Liberation, and sickle cell campaign groups, 'experientially-inspired' activists have been forced to seek coalitions with medical experts – representatives of the wider system they fought against.[35] Activism can incorporate negotiation as fightback. Looking through the lens of 'everyday health' shows how people used their embodied health experiences to resist, inform, and reformulate dominant modes of understanding, and how they have forged new discourses, spaces, and communities on the basis of these shared experiences.

Thinking about and through the 'everyday' enables the location of different sites and/or nodes of agency, power, and resistance and

10   *'Everyday health', embodiment and selfhood*

different historical actors. Not all acts of agency, power, and resistance can be described as 'activism'. A more multifaceted approach incorporates acts as simple as buying or boycotting consumer products or making complaints.[36] It brings in those who, like the readers of *Chatelaine* discussed by Whitney Wood, wrote to magazines for guidance.[37] It makes visible people who found out about 'everyday health' from television chat shows like those Fabiola Creed analyses. It includes those who, like the disabled women and their families who contested assessments of their capacity for work inside the home cited in Gareth Millward's chapter, advocated for themselves and family members in day-to-day interactions with medical and other authorities. It embraces acts of individual rather than collective resistance such as the development of self-care strategies that circumvent medical authority; a strategy Carol Tulloch deployed when, stuck at home in lockdown, she fell back on her knowledge as an academic and the resources of her wardrobe to create new styles and to renew herself.[38] This approach contributes to a bottom-up history in which individuals and groups draw on the resources available to them to understand and to act, in circumstances of and not of their own choosing – in this way enacting agency, power, and/or resistance.

Visibility, invisibility, and hypervisibility

'Study the historian before you begin to study the facts', urged E.H. Carr in *What is History?* (1961), a text that is still a standard feature of undergraduate historiography modules.[39] Carr argued that every decision about what aspect of the past to research involves judgements about what is or is not important. History is perspectival. These research decisions are made by humans who exist in particular positions in time and space. To understand the history in front of you, study the historian before you begin to study the facts. And so Carr set in motion a torrent of critical reviews and historiographical essays in which undergraduate students, struggling to grasp a complex philosophical position that undermines pretty much everything in their historical training to date, tried to study the historian: 'Sheila Rowbotham writes women's history. She is biased because she is a woman.' This is progress of a kind. It shows that women's history

Introduction: 'Everyday health' 11

is on the curriculum now. E.H. Carr only ever referred to the historian as 'he'.

There are different kinds of invisibility. We are used to thinking about marginalised groups 'hidden from history' and research that is framed as a recovery mission – making the invisible visible to redress historical imbalances of power. We are perhaps less used to thinking about the invisibility of power, or at least not in those terms. But invisibility is the privileged status of the male historian never described as 'biased' because he is a man who writes about men – after all, who else should be a historian or the proper subject of history?[40] It is the advantage of the male bodies assumed as the norm in most scientific and medical research – after all, why would the effects of the menstrual cycle on athletic performance matter to sports science?[41] It is the claim to life of the white female reproductive bodies that exist as the norm for obstetrics and gynaecology – after all, what is there to gain from investigating why Black women are four times more likely to die in pregnancy or childbirth than white women?[42] It is the extra money in the bank account of the able-bodied student not charged extra for 'accessible' accommodation – after all, is it really a basic right to be able to move around easily in your own home?[43] As anyone catcalled, harassed, abused, or manhandled on the street because of misogyny, homophobia, racism, or ableism could tell you, in some places, some bodies are invisible, and that invisibility is a mark of power, not its absence.

The reverse of invisibility is not always visibility, but hypervisibility. In the recovery model of history, to come to notice is to be made visible – to be seen, heard, and validated; to claim power. In the example of street harassment, to come to notice is to be made hypervisible – to be objectified, silenced, and delegitimised; to be forcibly reminded of your lack of power. The hypervisibility of some people could not exist without the invisibility of others. In her history of infertility, Naomi Pfeffer cites the case of a childless woman who, over a two-year period in the late 1940s, underwent two dilation and curettage operations, a tubal insufflation, a salpingogram, an endometrial biopsy, and a host of injections, courses of tablets, and douches, before her husband's semen was tested and found to contain no spermatozoa.[44] Within the patriarchal medical culture that positioned women as reproductive vessels, this man's body was invisible while his wife's body became hypervisible, the object of

12   *'Everyday health', embodiment and selfhood*

incisions, scrapings, piercings, distension, and ingestion. Those who hold power can also hold the dual status of invisible/visible; the rule that determines the exception, the person who can speak and know they will be heard. Those who do not hold power more often occupy the contradictory position of invisible/hypervisible; ignored until their existence is questioned, treated as though claiming unjustified privilege for daring to come to notice. For the powerless, the pendulum does not swing from invisibility to visibility without a barrage of outraged questions about why there isn't an International Men's Day or White History Month or Straight Pride.[45]

The concept of 'everyday health' simultaneously sidesteps and confronts this bind. When we place day-to-day experience at the centre of our histories, our immediate question is what everyday life looks like *for that person*. At the conceptual level, this approach is de facto inclusive and intersectional. It also makes us better able to avoid assumptions about what constitutes the 'everyday'. At the same time, thinking through the 'everyday' pitches us into questions about allied categories – the mundane, ordinary, normal, and natural – and reveals their status as constructions rather than descriptions. This is one reason why 'everyday health' holds radical potential. In this volume, reading Ben Mechen's analysis of *The Joy of Sex* next to Karissa Patton's examination of the work of feminist volunteers at the Calgary Birth Control Association (CBCA) underlines the contingency of classifications of the 'everyday' and their relation to power. The sexologist Alex Comfort saw liberation as stripping sex back to the 'natural', while CBCA workers understood the legal and political structures that shaped sex, and the degree of foreplanning and aftercare necessary for women to have sex safely. Comfort's (hetero)sexual man exists on the same spectrum as Carr's male historian – the norm, unless you exist outside the boundaries of his discourse.

This interrogation of the 'everyday' that the concept of 'everyday health' invites therefore also exposes who or what is visible, invisible, or hypervisible. We might pause here on 'youth' and 'older age', categories invoked across many chapters in this volume. From the 1950s onwards, social scientists and then cultural studies scholars demonstrated keen attention to youth and, to a lesser extent, older age.[46] In contrast, historians mostly neglected 'youth' and 'older age' until quite recently.[47] Likewise, although age is an integral aspect of lived experience, and should be central to genuinely intersectional analysis, such approaches rarely foreground it.[48] Asking why 'youth' and 'older age' are not visible in historical scholarship reveals aspects of their cultural invisibility/hypervisibility that are tied to power relations. There is a sharp disparity between the worship of youth and the invisibility of older people in mass culture, but neither status carries power.[49] Rather, as Caroline Rusterholz and Rosie Gahnstrom, Lucy Robinson, and Rachel Thomson show in their contributions to this volume, the media positioning of young people (and especially young girls and women) as at-risk goes hand in hand with the assumption that young people are spoken *for* and *about* – in other words, they should be seen and not heard. In this case, putting the perspectives of young people at the centre of our histories as demanded by the lens of 'everyday health' complicates tendencies to look at experiences of youth through adult eyes.[50] Meanwhile, in a nice counterbalancing gesture, Kate Mahoney shows that bringing intergenerational dynamics into play reveals aspects of the perspectives of younger/older people that might be missed through exclusive focus on either life stage.

The reparative work of 'everyday health' is to try to bring those who are invisible/hypervisible to ordinary visibility – to write our/their histories in ways that represent but do not objectify, sensationalise, or deny the conditions of oppression. This is no easy task, as Daisy Payling discusses in her chapter, on creating and adapting a public engagement activity for young/adult and queer/non-queer audiences. These acts might become easier as structures open up/are broken down, as the 'we' who speaks in academic texts more often shares ground with the 'them' who are written about, and as the business of writing from and about experience, embodiment, and the self attains more prestige. We are some way off this state of affairs. We have been able to include histories of Black, disabled, and trans 'everyday health' in this volume, but this is good fortune. In the UK the Black health and medical humanities is still an emergent area.[51] The histories of disabled and trans people have been viewed through pathologising medical lenses for so long that the shift to 'everyday health' is especially fraught.[52] Black, disabled, trans, and non-binary scholars are underrepresented in the historical profession,

14   *'Everyday health', embodiment and selfhood*

and the formal structures of the Research Exercise Framework make contributing to edited collections a risky business for those in insecure positions.[53]

The distinction between invisibility/visibility and invisibility/hypervisibility comes into play too. The volume includes two male authors but not a single chapter deliberately centred on male experience. It is difficult to avoid the conclusion that male historians are not researching 'everyday health' partly because Man as abstract category still holds the status of unquestioned norm and rational non-bodied subject – with all the implications that holds for the abstract category of Woman and the lived experience of women. There is a lot of work to do.

The local, national, and global

An own-brand packet of paracetamol tablets from the UK chemist Boots currently costs less than one quarter of some brand rivals. It is one of the most mundane and affordable items in the home medicine kit. The tablets are manufactured in Barnsley, South Yorkshire and distributed by The Boots Company PLC, based in Nottingham.[54] The tablets, constituted from pregelatinised maize starch, sodium metabisulfite (E223), and magnesium stearate, are much the same as those marketed elsewhere in the world under the brand names Tylenol (USA), Calonal (Japan), Captin (Germany), or Napa (Bangladesh).[55] The synthesis of paracetamol was first achieved by the North American chemist Harmon Northrup Morse, first tried on humans by the German clinical pharmacologist Joseph von Mering, and 'rediscovered' as the result of a paper by the Jewish-English emigré Bernard Brodie and his colleague Julius Axelrod, the New York-born son of Jewish immigrants from Poland.[56] Paracetamol is an international phenomenon. So too, it turns out, is Boots; 'the nation's chemist' appointed its first agent to India in 1919, expanded its international networks in subsequent decades, and by the 1960s was 'an international player of worldwide significance'.[57] It is currently owned by the North American pharmaceutical giant Walgreens and trades across six countries and two continents.[58]

The simple act of reaching for a tablet when we have a headache enmeshes us in a global network.[59] We live in localities and hold

Introduction: 'Everyday health' 15

national passports but our lives, and therefore our experiences of 'everyday health', are global as well as local and national. This is not just because we live in the age of the internet and instant connectivity. This introduction earlier outlined major political, economic, social, and cultural shifts since 1950; these developments occurred across many parts of the globe in the same period, if to different extents and on different timelines. The rise of welfare states, reshaping of citizenship, transformation in life patterns, revolution in sexual and family life, proliferation of psychological discourses, and access to life-changing technologies – these transformations are apparent in whole or substantial part across the western world. Their effects on experiences of 'everyday health' simultaneously transcended national boundaries and were refracted through local healthcare systems, organisations, structures, and traditions.[60] This means that while the majority of case studies in this volume focus on the UK, they will also be of use to future scholars of 'everyday health' as they seek to find suitable sources, develop research methods, establish patterns, and separate out local from global effects.

We include chapters that do not centre on the UK – Karissa Patton on the Calgary Birth Control Association, Evangelia Chordaki on the Greek women's movement, and Whitney Wood on Canadian responses to 'natural birth' – in part because these case studies provide opportunities to trace transnational exchange of ideas and practices related to 'everyday health' and in this way also reframe the British history chapters within an international context. Chordaki and Patton explore local and national manifestations of the global feminist self-help health movement. The other authors who examine activist movements, MacInnes and Rutherford, explore local case studies that branched out to the edges of the nation and beyond. The analytical frames of all four chapters draw on scholarship from across the globe, reflecting the soft internationalism of radical politics in these decades. Likewise, Wood shows the role of mass-market magazines as vehicles for the dissemination within and across borders of ideas about 'everyday health'. Chapters by Froom, Rusterholz, Payling, and Gahnstrom, Robinson, and Thomson also draw on mass-market magazines and show the same processes at work in the UK, underlining a central feature of mass media wherever it is found. Moreover, the conscious effort to avoid lazy assumptions about what is global and what is local makes us think differently

16   *'Everyday health', embodiment and selfhood*

about other mediums of communication: social media platforms like Instagram, as Louise Morgan discusses in relation to clean eating, operate across the globe, but most accounts do not achieve worldwide followings, and the influencers she considers are not household names outside the UK.

This 'internationalised' approach relates to our vision of the history of 'everyday health' as a political project. In recent years, British history was first subjected to Michael Gove's attempts to narrow it back to an 'island story' and then co-opted into the culture wars concocted by right-wing agitators and enthusiastically endorsed by Conservative politicians.[61] Those of us whose identities are global not local, who see ourselves as connected to diasporic peoples, LGBTQ+ siblings, or workers of the world, over and above our national identities, want to understand how those histories link up to the times and places in which we stand now; those of us who see history as perspectival want more perspectives, not fewer; those of us who care about History and its future are saddened and angry at this continuous attack on what it is and can be. There are more histories of 'everyday health' in the UK than elsewhere in the world partly because for decades the Wellcome Trust has funded the health and medical humanities here. The predominance of these histories in this volume reflects that research strength. But we also want this volume to acknowledge the place of the UK in the wider world and to acknowledge the powerful impulses towards transnationalism within the wider historical discipline over the twenty-first century's opening two decades.[62]

The pursuit of this vision is justified by the extensive and unforced connections across borders that can be traced in every chapter in this volume. As well as those already mentioned, we find a British physician writing a work on sex that drew on sexological research from North America and elsewhere and achieved bestseller status in many parts of the globe (Mechen); UK television personalities adapting the American talk show model for their national audience (Creed); European Economic Community rulings causing problems for the Conservative government's position on disability benefits in the late 1970s and 1980s (Millward); Black British women drawing on family diasporic histories to make sense of and explain their lives (Redhead and Tulloch); and oral historians writing from the self,

Introduction: 'Everyday health' 17

but drawing on scholarship from a subfield unusually international in scope because it speaks to method more than content (Mahoney and Loughran). Understanding 'everyday health' means working out its meanings at the local level, but to grasp the concept in its fullest dimensions, we also need to look to the network of relationships between the local, national, and global.

Conclusion

In Deborah Levy's *Hot Milk* (2016) the narrator, an anthropologist by training, takes her mother to a Spanish clinic to seek treatment for her psychosomatic paralysis. She describes watching the nurse take her mother's case history:

> My mother is giving a history of her present illness. Where does that history start? It moves around in time and merges into past history, childhood illness and all the rest of it. This is not chronological time. Julieta will have to later transcribe Rose's words and author her case history. I have been trained to do something similar, except I am not a physiotherapist, I am an ethnographer. Julieta will at some stage have to describe the complaint that brought the patient to her clinic. Symptoms and their presentation. It is not one complaint. It is not even six. I overheard twenty complaints but there were more. The past the present and the future are simultaneously present in all these complaints.[63]

The entanglements of 'everyday health' similarly move between body and mind, self and other, past and present. There is a lot of history to chart.

This volume spans decades and continents, but it is only a starting point in explorations of 'everyday health'. It draws together exciting new research on this underexplored area but is also intended as a spur to future studies. Many histories of 'everyday health' remain to be written. This volume reflects the current state of scholarship, which in turn reflects historic imbalances of power and the complex positioning of different groups. Future histories of 'everyday health' will have to explicitly address the effects of globalisation, and work out how to combine historical specificity with awareness of the extent of transnational exchange. The history of 'everyday health'

18   *'Everyday health', embodiment and selfhood*

is barely out of the starting blocks, and there is much to look forward to from here.

Where future scholars might most directly benefit from this volume is in the conceptual and methodological approaches it puts forward for researching and writing about 'everyday health'. The history of 'everyday health' starts by centring experience. There are many ways we might try to understand that experience. We can examine the external influences on it or we can try to capture subjectivity through direct testimonies. Because 'everyday health' is an expansive concept, it generates methodological eclecticism. In this volume, scholars draw on state records, social surveys, newspapers and magazines, television shows, personal, activist, and voluntary sector archives, oral histories, and the resources of the self. They employ diverse theoretical and conceptual frameworks, including queer theory, feminism, autoethnography, phenomenology, and science and technology studies. These different approaches hang together, like glass beads of different colours and shapes on a necklace string, through authors' commitment to locating and representing ground-up histories of health, subjectivity, and embodiment. As an endeavour, the history of 'everyday health' is therefore creative and experimental.

The creativity is apparent above all in these scholars' ways of recapturing voices that would otherwise be lost. It is not easy to locate direct testimony about intimate aspects of selfhood, and even when this can be found (or created) it is not a straightforward guide to what people thought or felt at the time.[64] We are all unreliable narrators. We write for audiences, we speak to our interlocutors as much as for ourselves, we forget because we will or we must, we rearrange our thoughts and feelings so that we can live with them. But how much more difficult when there is no direct testimony! The contributors to this volume seek out the voices of past people in tribunal records, newspaper reports, and letters to newsletters and magazines. These voices are heavily mediated, but an echo is better than a silence. Thinking about 'everyday health' raises questions about who is represented, who has the power to speak, and who is listened to – but also how we, as historians, can access and hear these voices.

This volume has started this work, and its chapters demonstrate what can happen when we place 'everyday health' at the centre of

Introduction: 'Everyday health'   19

our histories. Benefits include complicating understandings of power and resistance; deepening and extending notions of identity and intersectionality; and encouraging and celebrating methodological diversity. As we centre 'everyday health', however, we must be alive to the need to continually incorporate more and diverse experiences, and to the shifting nature of the 'everyday' itself. What we think is 'everyday' in the present will inevitably shape the questions about 'everyday health' that we ask of the past. We need to find the right starting points, the ones that will not blind us to the messiness of the histories that we might encounter, their many possible ways of ripening, and the multitudes that coexist within even one subjectivity, one past, one potential future.

Notes

1 'How Bodyform took the "toxic shame" out of periods', *Marketing Week*, 18 October 2018: www.marketingweek.com/how-bodyform-took-the-toxic-shame-out-of-periods/ (accessed 22 June 2023).

2 Daisy Payling, 'Selling shame: feminine hygiene advertising and the boundaries of permissiveness in 1970s Britain', *Gender & History*, 35:3 (October 2023); Claire Rayner, 'Legal, decent, honest, and banned from TV', *Independent*, 11 January 1993: www.independent.co.uk/life-style/legal-decent-honest-and-banned-from-tv-claire-rayner-is-angry-about-the-decision-to-take-her-advert-for-sanitary-towels-off-our-screens–1477860.html (accessed 22 June 2023); Claire Cozens, '"Disgusting" Lil-lets ad offends viewers', *Guardian*, 23 May 2003: www.theguardian.com/media/2003/may/23/advertising (accessed 22 June 2023); Hannah Froom, 'Menstruation, Subjectivity and Constructions of Girlhood in Britain, 1960–1980' (PhD thesis, University of Essex, 2022).

3 Ela Przyblo and Breanne Fahs, 'Empowered bleeders and cranky menstruators: menstrual positivity and the "liberated" era of new menstrual product advertisements', in Chris Bobel, Inga T. Winkler, Breanne Fahs, Katie Ann Hasson, Elizabeth Arveda Kissling, and Tomi Ann-Roberts (eds), *The Palgrave Handbook of Critical Menstruation Studies* (Basingstoke: Palgrave Macmillan, 2020); Camilla Mørk Røstvik, *Cash Flow: The Businesses of Menstruation* (London: UCL Press, 2022), especially pp. 1–34, 177–200.

4 Tricia (a pseudonym) was interviewed for the project 'Body, Self, and Family: Women's Psychological, Emotional, and Bodily Health in Britain,

20   *'Everyday health', embodiment and selfhood*

c. 1960–1990'. These interviews will be archived at the British Library in 2024–25.

5 Laura Carter, *Histories of Everyday Life: The Making of Popular Social History in Britain, 1918–1979* (Oxford: Oxford University Press, 2021); Ben Highmore (ed.), *The Everyday Life Reader* (London and New York: Routledge, 2002); Matthew Hilton, '"Politics is ordinary": non-governmental organisations and political participation in contemporary Britain', *Twentieth Century British History*, 22 (2011); Claire Langhamer, '"Who the hell are ordinary people?" Ordinariness as a category of historical analysis', *Transactions of the Royal Historical Society*, 28 (December 2018); Jennifer Crane, *Child Protection in England, 1960–2000: Expertise, Experience, and Emotion* (Basingstoke: Palgrave Macmillan, 2019).

6 Paul Addison, *No Turning Back: The Peacetime Revolutions of Post-War Britain* (Oxford: Oxford University Press, 2010).

7 Matthew Grant, 'Historicising citizenship in post-war Britain', *Historical Journal*, 59:4 (2016); Teri Chettiar, *The Intimate State: How Emotional Life Became Political in Welfare-State Britain* (Oxford: Oxford University Press, 2023).

8 Peter Stearns, *Consumerism in World History: The Global Transformation of Desire*, 2nd edn (London and New York: Routledge, 2006); Gillian Swanson, *Drunk with the Glitter: Space, Consumption and Sexual Instability in Modern Urban Culture* (London and New York: Routledge, 2007).

9 Celia Hughes, *Young Lives on the Left: Sixties Activism and the Liberation of the Self* (Manchester: Manchester University Press, 2015); Lucy Robinson, *Gay Men and the Left in Post-War Britain: How the Personal Got Political* (Manchester: Manchester University Press, 2007); Daisy Payling, *Socialist Republic: Remaking the British Left in 1980s Sheffield* (Manchester: Manchester University Press, 2023).

10 Alex Mold, Peder Clark, Gareth Millward, and Daisy Payling, *Placing the Public in Public Health in Post-War Britain, 1948–2012* (Basingstoke: Palgrave Macmillan, 2019).

11 Nikolas Rose, *Governing the Soul: The Shaping of the Private Self* (London and New York: Routledge, 1989); Robert Crawford, 'Healthism and the medicalization of everyday life', *International Journal of Health Services*, 10:3 (1980).

12 Kathy Davis, *The Making of Our Bodies, Ourselves: How Feminism Travels Across Borders* (Durham, NC: Duke University Press, 2007); Kate Mahoney, *Feminist Mental Health Activism in England, c. 1968–1995* (Manchester: Manchester University Press, 2023); Tommy Dickinson, *'Curing Queers': Mental Nurses and Their Patients, 1935–74*

Introduction: 'Everyday health' 21

(Manchester: Manchester University Press, 2015), pp. 200–30; Suman Fernando, *Institutional Racism in Psychiatry and Clinical Psychology: Race Matters in Mental Health* (Basingstoke: Palgrave Macmillan, 2017).

13 Susan Oman, *Understanding Well-being Data: Improving Social and Cultural Policy, Practice and Research* (Basingstoke: Palgrave Macmillan, 2021), pp. 35–66; Jina B. Kim and Sami Schalk, 'Reclaiming the radical politics of self-care: a crip-of-color critique', *South Atlantic Quarterly*, 120:2 (2021).

14 Tracey Loughran, Kate Mahoney, and Daisy Payling, 'Women's voices, emotion and empathy: engaging different publics with "everyday" health histories', *Medical Humanities*, 48:4 (2022), 394.

15 On intersectionality, see Kimberlé Crenshaw, 'Mapping the margins: intersectionality, identity politics, and violence against women of color', *Stanford Law Review*, 43:6 (July 1991); Anna Carastathis, *Intersectionality: Origins, Contestations, Horizons* (Lincoln, NE: University of Nebraska Press, 2016); Ange-Marie Hancock, *Intersectionality: An Intellectual History* (Oxford: Oxford University Press, 2016).

16 For an overview of these historiographical trends, see Joan Scott, 'The evidence of experience', *Critical Inquiry*, 17 (1991); Kathleen Canning, 'The body as method? Reflections on the place of the body in gender history', *Gender & History*, 11:3 (1999); Michael Roper, 'Slipping out of view: subjectivity and emotion in gender history', *History Workshop Journal*, 59:1 (2005); Geoff Eley, *A Crooked Line: From Cultural History to the History of Society* (Ann Arbor, MI: University of Michigan Press, 2005), pp. 133–48, 158–61, 171–2.

17 Victoria Bates, 'Healthcare, health and wellbeing', in Francesca Carnevali, Nicole Robertson, John Singleton, and Avram Taylor (eds), *20th Century Britain: Economic, Cultural and Social Change*, 3rd edn (London and New York: Routledge, 2023); Mary Shaw, Daniel Dorling, David Gordon, and George Davey Smith, *The Widening Gap: Health Inequalities and Policy in Britain* (Bristol: Policy Press, 1999); Stephen Jivraj and Ludi Simpson (eds), *Ethnic Identity and Inequalities in Britain: The Dynamics of Diversity* (Bristol: Policy Press, 2015).

18 Mathew Thomson, *Psychological Subjects: Identity, Culture and Health in Twentieth-Century Britain* (Oxford: Oxford University Press, 2006); Mark Jackson (ed.), *Stress in Post-War Britain, 1945–85* (London and New York: Routledge, 2016); Jill Kirby, *Feeling the Strain: A Cultural History of Stress in Twentieth-Century Britain* (Manchester: Manchester University Press, 2019).

19 Kathleen Paul, *Whitewashing Britain: Race and Citizenship in the Postwar Era* (Ithaca, NY: Cornell University Press, 2081); Kennetta Hammond Perry, *London is the Place for Me: Black Britons, Citizenship, and the*

22   *'Everyday health', embodiment and selfhood*

Politics of Race (Oxford: Oxford University Press, 2018); Roberta Bivins, *Contagious Communities: Medicine, Migration, and the NHS in Post-War Britain* (Oxford: Oxford University Press, 2015), Part III.

20 Rob Baggott, Judith Allsop, and Kathryn Jones, *Speaking for Patients and Carers: Health Consumer Groups and the Policy Process* (Basingstoke: Palgrave Macmillan, 2005); Christine Hogg, *Citizens, Consumers and the NHS: Capturing Voices* (Basingstoke: Palgrave Macmillan, 2009).

21 Adrian Horn, *Juke Box Britain: Americanisation and Youth Culture, 1945–60* (Manchester: Manchester University Press, 2010); Penny Tinkler, '"Are you really living?" If not, "get with it!" The teenage self and lifestyle in young women's magazines, Britain 1957–70', *Cultural and Social History*, 11:4 (2015).

22 Pat Thane, 'Old age', in Roger Cooter and John V. Pickstone (eds), *Companion of Medicine in the Twentieth Century* (London and New York: Routledge, 2002); C.C. Harris, 'Social ageing in the Macmillan era', *Continuity and Change*, 2:3 (1987).

23 B. Jane Elliott, 'Demographic trends in domestic life, 1945–1987', in David Clark (ed.), *Marriage, Domestic Life and Social Change: Writings for Jacqueline Burgoyne (1944–88)* (London and New York: Routledge, 1991); Pat Thane, 'Population politics in post-war British culture', in Becky Conekin, Frank Mort, and Chris Waters (eds), *Moments of Modernity: Reconstructing Britain, 1945–1964* (London: Rivers Oram Press, 1999); Jeffrey Weeks, *Sex, Politics, and Society: The Regulation of Sexuality since 1800*, 3rd edn (Harlow, Essex: Pearson, 2012), pp. 321–426.

24 Hera Cook, 'The English sexual revolution: technology and social change', *History Workshop Journal*, 59 (Spring 2005); David Geiringer, *The Pope and the Pill: Sex, Catholicism and Women in Post-War England* (Manchester: Manchester University Press, 2019).

25 Ann Oakley, *Housewife* (Harmondsworth: Penguin, 1974); Ina Zweiniger-Bargielowska, 'Housewifery', in Ina Zweiniger-Bargielowska (ed.), *Women in Twentieth-Century Britain* (Harlow, Essex: Pearson Education, 2001).

26 Oakley, *Housewife*; Zweiniger-Bargielowska, 'Housewifery'; Tracey Loughran, '"The most helpful friends in the world": letters pages, expertise and emotion in British women's magazines, c. 1960–1980', in Laurel Forster and Joanne Hollows (eds), *Women's Periodicals and Print Culture in Britain, 1940s–2000s: The Postwar and Contemporary Period* (Edinburgh: University of Edinburgh, 2020); Kelly Loughlin, 'The history of health and medicine in contemporary Britain: reflections on the role of audio-visual sources', *Social History of Medicine*, 13:1 (2000); Fabiola Creed, 'From "immoral" users to "sunbed addicts": the

media–medical pathologising of working-class consumers and young women in late twentieth-century England', *Social History of Medicine*, 35:3 (2022); Katherine Dow, 'Looking into the test tube: the birth of IVF on British television', *Medical History*, 63 (2019); European Centre for Disease Prevention and Control, Institute for Social Marketing (Great Britain), Health Promotion Research Centre, and Clinica Universidad de Navarra, *A Literature Review on Health Information-Seeking Behavior on the Web: A Health Consumer and Health Professional Perspective: Insights into Health Communication* (Stockholm: European Centre for Disease Prevention and Control, 2011).

27 Mold et al., *Placing the Public*, pp. 33–65.

28 Hannah Gavron, *The Captive Wife: Conflicts of Housebound Mothers* (Harmondsworth: Penguin, 1968), pp. 36, 45.

29 Helen McCarthy, 'Social science and married women's employment in post-war Britain', *Past & Present*, 233:1 (November 2016), 270.

30 Jeremy Gavron, *A Woman on the Edge of Time: A Son's Search for His Mother* (London: Scribe Publications, 2015), pp. 83, 241.

31 Gavron, *A Woman on the Edge of Time*, p. 146.

32 Canning, 'The body as method?', 503–5; Canning, 'Feminist history after the linguistic turn: historicizing discourse and experience', *Signs*, 19:2 (1994), 397.

33 Amy Whipple, '"Into every home, into every body": organicism and anti-statism in the British anti-fluoridation movement, 1952–1960', *Twentieth Century British History*, 21:3 (2010); Gareth Millward, '"A matter of commonsense": the Coventry poliomyelitis epidemic 1957 and the British public', *Contemporary British History*, 31:3 (2017).

34 Beverley Bryan, Stella Dadzie, and Suzanne Scafe, *Heart of the Race: Black Women's Lives in Britain*, reissue (London: Verso, 2018), pp. 105–6; Caitlin Lambert, '"The objectionable injectable": recovering the lost history of the WLM through the Campaign Against Depo-Provera', *Women's History Review*, 29:3 (2020).

35 Deborah B. Gould, *Moving Politics: Emotion and ACT UP's Fight Against AIDS* (Chicago, IL: University of Chicago Press, 2009), pp. 292–9; Charlotte Cooper, *Fat Activism: A Radical Social Movement* (Bristol: HammerOn Press, 2016), pp. 23–4; Grace Redhead, '"A British problem affecting British people": sickle cell anaemia, medical activism and race in the National Health Service, 1975–1993', *Twentieth Century British History*, 32:2 (2021).

36 Jane Hand, 'Marketing health education: advertising margarine and visualising health in Britain from 1964–c. 2000', *Contemporary British History*, 31:4 (2017); Mobeen Hussain, 'Combining global expertise with local knowledge in colonial India: selling ideals of beauty and

health in commodity advertising (c. 1900–1949)', *South Asia*, 44:5 (2021); Daisy Payling, '"The people who write to us are the people who don't like us": class, gender, and citizenship in the Survey of Sickness, 1943–1952', *Journal of British Studies*, 59:2 (2020).

37 Laura Kelly, '"Please help me, I am so miserable!": sexual health, emotions and counselling in teen and young adult problem pages in late 1980s Ireland', *Medical Humanities*, 49:2 (2023).

38 Ayesha Nathoo, 'Initiating therapeutic relaxation in Britain: a twentieth-century strategy for health and wellbeing', *Palgrave Communications*, 2:1 (2016).

39 E.H. Carr, *What is History?* (London: Macmillan, 1961), p. 23.

40 We now have histories of masculinity, but there is no subfield of 'men's history'. See Melinda S. Zook, 'Integrating men's history into women's history: a proposition', *The History Teacher*, 35:3 (2002).

41 Jacky Forsyth and Claire-Marie Roberts (eds), *The Exercising Female: Science and Its Application* (London: Routledge, 2018); Lauren Fleshman, *Good for a Girl: My Life Running in a Man's World* (London: Virago, 2023).

42 Hannah Summers, 'Black women in the UK four times more likely to die in pregnancy or childbirth', *Guardian*, 15 January 2021: www.theguardian.com/global-development/2021/jan/15/black-women-in-the-uk-four-times-more-likely-to-die-in-pregnancy-or-childbirth (accessed 22 June 2023); Annabel Sowemimo, *Divided: Racism, Medicine and Why We Need to Decolonise Healthcare* (London: Wellcome Collection, 2023); Candice Brathwaite, *I Am Not Your Baby Mother: What It's Like to be a Black British Mother* (London: Quercus, 2020).

43 UCL Disabled Students' Network, *Disability Discrimination Faced by UCL Students and Recommended Measures* (January 2020): https://studentsunionucl.org/sites/default/files/u318399/documents/disabled_students_network_report.pdf (accessed 2 June 2023); Stephanie Jenkins, 'Constructing ableism', *Genealogy*, 5:3 (2021).

44 Naomi Pfeffer, *The Stork and the Syringe: A Political History of Reproductive Medicine* (Cambridge: Polity Press, 1993), p. 61.

45 International Men's Day does exist and it is held on 19 November: https://internationalmensday.com/ (accessed 22 June 2023). Sadly, Straight Pride also exists: Barbara Ellen, 'It's time gay people stepped aside … hetero whiners have rights too', *Guardian*, 8 June 2019: www.theguardian.com/commentisfree/2019/jun/08/time-gay-people-stepped-aside-hetero-whiners-have-rights-too (accessed 22 June 2023). For a thoughtful exploration of the potential value of a White History Month to reveal who instituted slavery as well as who abolished it, see Sabrina Stevens, 'The case for White History Month', *The Progressive*, 80:4 (2016).

46 On youth, see Mark Abrams, *The Teenage Consumer* (London: London Press Exchange, 1959); T.R. Fyvel, *The Insecure Offenders: Rebellious Youth in the Welfare State* (Harmondsworth: Penguin, 1963); Stanley Cohen, *Folk Devils and Moral Panics: The Creation of the Mods and Rockers* (London: MacGibbon and Kee, 1972); Stuart Hall and Tony Jefferson (eds), *Resistance Through Rituals: Youth Subcultures in Post-war Britain* (London: Hutchinson, 1976); Angela McRobbie, *Feminism and Youth Culture: From Jackie to Just Seventeen* (Basingstoke: Macmillan, 1991). On older age, see Peter Willmott and Michael Young, *Family and Kinship in East London* (Harmondsworth: Penguin, 1962) [originally published 1957]; Peter Townsend, *The Family Life of Old People: An Inquiry in East London* (London: Routledge and Kegan Paul, 1957). Older people who lived outside East London were apparently not of much interest to sociologists.

47 For more recent historical scholarship, see Sîan Pooley and Jonathan Taylor, *Children's Experiences of Welfare in Modern Britain* (London: Institute of Historical Research, 2021); Felix Fuhg, *London's Working-Class Youth and the Making of Post-Victorian Britain, 1958–1971* (Basingstoke: Palgrave Macmillan, 2021); Laura Tisdall, '"What a difference it was to be a woman and not a teenager": adolescent girls' conceptions of adulthood in 1960s and 1970s Britain', *Gender & History*, 34:2 (2022); Peter Laslett, *A Fresh Map of Life: The Emergence of the Third Age*, 2nd edn (Basingstoke: Macmillan, 1996); Pat Thane, *Old Age in English History: Past Experiences Present Issues* (Oxford: Oxford University Press, 2000); Jane Traies, *The Lives of Older Lesbians: Sexuality, Identity and the Life Course* (London: Palgrave Macmillan, 2016); Charlotte Greenhalgh, *Aging in Twentieth-Century Britain* (Oakland, CA: University of California Press, 2018).

48 Jeanne Boyston, 'Gender as a question of historical analysis', *Gender & History*, 20:3 (2008), 565; Diditi Mitra and Joyce Weil (eds), *Race and the Lifecourse: Readings from the Intersection of Race, Ethnicity, and Age* (New York: Palgrave Macmillan, 2014); Has Georg Eilenberger, Annemie Halsema, and Jenny Slatman, 'Age difference in the clinical encounter: intersectionality and phenomenology', *American Journal of Bioethics*, 19:2 (2019).

49 Sue Westwood, '"It's the not being seen that is the most tiresome": older women, invisibility and social (in)justice', *Journal of Women & Aging*, first published online 25 April 2023: https://doi.org/10.108 0/08952841.2023.2197658; Rob Jay Fredericksen, 'Just kill me when I'm 50: impact of gay American culture on young gay men's perceptions of aging', *Anthropology & Aging*, 31:1 (2010).

50 Spyros Spyrou, 'The limits of children's voices', *Childhood*, 18:2 (2011); Katie Wright and Julie MacLeod, 'Public memories and private

26   *'Everyday health', embodiment and selfhood*

meanings', *Oral History*, 32 (2012); Neil Sutherland, 'When you listen to the winds of childhood, how much can you believe?', *Curriculum Inquiry*, 22:3 (1992); Jay Mechling, 'Oral evidence and the history of American children's lives', *Journal of American History*, 74:2 (1987); Anna Mae Duane (ed.), *The Children's Table: Childhood Studies and the Humanities* (Athens, GA: University of Georgia, 2013). With thanks to Laura Tisdall for these suggestions.

51 On Black health and medical humanities, see Amber Lascelles, 'Black health and the humanities', *The Polyphony*, 14 December 2020: https://thepolyphony.org/2020/12/14/black-health-and-the-humanities/ (accessed 22 June 2023); Black Health and the Humanities Project: www.blackhealthandhumanities.org/ (accessed 22 June 2023).

52 See chapter 10 by Beckie Rutherford and chapter 6 by Fleur MacInnes in this volume.

53 On inequalities in the UK historical profession, see the four reports issued by the Royal Historical Society since 2015: Royal Historical Society, 'RHS Reports': https://royalhistsoc.org/publications/rhs-reports/ (accessed 22 June 2023).

54 Boots, 'Paracetamol 500mg tablets: patient information leaflet', January 2023: https://www.boots.com/boots-paracetamol-500mg-caplets-16s-10276369 (accessed 22 June 2023).

55 For an extensive list of common brand names by country, see 'List of paracetamol brand names', Wikipedia: https://en.wikipedia.org/wiki/List_of_paracetamol_brand_names (accessed 22 June 2023).

56 'Paracetamol: history', Wikipedia: https://en.wikipedia.org/wiki/Paracetamol (accessed 22 June 2023).

57 Anna Greenwood and Hilary Ingram, 'Sources and resources: "The People's Chemists": The Walgreens Boots Alliance Archive', *Social History of Medicine*, 31:4 (2018), 862–3.

58 Boots UK, 'About Boots UK: Company information: Walgreen Boots Alliance': www.boots-uk.com/about-boots-uk/company-information/walgreens-boots-alliance/global-presence/ (accessed 22 June 2023).

59 Anna Greenwood and Richard Hornsey are currently researching the international history of Boots: 'Chemists to the nation, pharmacy to the world': www.nottingham.ac.uk/vision/vision-pharmacy-to-the-world (accessed 22 June 2023).

60 Compare for example Gareth Millward, *Vaccinating Britain: Mass Vaccination and the Public since the Second World War* (Manchester: Manchester University Press, 2019) and Dóra Vargha, *Polio Across the Iron Curtain: Hungary's Cold War with an Epidemic* (Cambridge: Cambridge University Press, 2021); Alex Mold, *Making the Patient-Consumer: Patient Organisations and Health Consumerism in Britain*

(Manchester: Manchester University Press, 2015) and Alexander Harmann, *The Evolution and Everyday Practice of Collective Patient Involvement in Europe: An Examination of Policy Processes, Motivations, and Implementations in Four Countries* (Utrecht, NL: Springer International, 2018); Pfeffer, *The Stork and the Syringe* and Margaret Marsh and Wanda Ronner, *The Empty Cradle: Infertility in America from Colonial Times to the Present* (Baltimore, MD: Johns Hopkins University Press, 1996).

61 Nicola Sheldon, 'Politicians and history: the national curriculum, national identity and the revival of the national narrative', *History*, 97 (2012); Matthew Watson, 'Michael Gove's war on professional historical expertise: Conservative curriculum reform, extreme Whig history and the place of imperial heroes in modern multicultural Britain', *British Politics*, 15 (2020).

62 Dipesh Chakrabarty, *Provincializing Europe: Postcolonial Thought and Historical Difference* (Princeton, NJ: Princeton University Press, 2007); Akira Iriye, *Global and Transnational History: The Past, Present and Future* (Basingstoke: Palgrave Macmillan, 2013); Kenneth Pomeranz, 'Histories for a less national age', *American Historical Review*, 119:1 (2014); Willibald Steinmartz (ed.), *The Force of Comparison: A New Perspective on Modern European History and the Contemporary World* (Oxford: Berghahn Books, 2019).

63 Deborah Levy, *Hot Milk* (London: Penguin, 2016), p. 62.

64 Penny Summerfield, *Histories of the Self: Personal Narratives and Historical Practice* (London and New York: Routledge, 2018).

Part I

Experiential expertise

Part I: Introduction

Hannah Froom and Tracey Loughran

In 1973, Barbara Ehrenreich and Deirdre English published *Complaints and Disorders: The Sexual Politics of Sickness*, an excoriating analysis of patriarchal culture's pathologisation of women's bodies and its role in their oppression. As feminist activists, Ehrenreich and English echoed Women's Liberation Movement (WLM) demands for women to refuse the 'sexist ideology' that justified 'sexual discrimination' as simply the logical consequence of biological differences and to seize control of their own bodies. But these political beliefs arose out of day-to-day 'encounters with the medical system' that brought them 'face to face with sexism in its most unmistakeably crude and insulting forms'. They wrote from their 'experiences as women, as health care consumers, and as activists in the women's health movement' – an indivisible trinity of motivations.[1] In their emphasis on experience as a form of expertise, Ehrenreich and English represented not only the WLM but a wider shift within western democracies from the mid-twentieth century that saw 'expertise' reframed to accommodate 'ordinary' or experiential expertise as well as, and sometimes at the expense of, professional or technical knowledge, qualifications, and practice.[2] In the wake of the Second World War, haunted by the terrible consequences of mindless submission to fascist leaders, democratic polities sought to inculcate the twin virtues of autonomy and responsibility in their citizens – a move that necessitated engagement with authority rather than unthinking obedience, and that eventually branched into the questioning spirit of 'permissiveness' and the free-for-all of neoliberalism.[3]

32 *Experiential expertise*

The reshaping of expertise occurred in different forms and on different timelines in different places, but the overall effect was the same: to afford new weight to the importance of lived experience in determining the perceived right of individuals and groups to speak on or intervene in relation to particular issues. In this way, the concepts of 'experience' and 'expertise' came to exist in a new relation to each other.[4] Within welfare states, many factors reinforced this relationship. Citizens felt personal and often emotional investments in healthcare systems that symbolised the rights and responsibilities of democratic citizenship.[5] As consumerism expanded and infiltrated every aspect of life in western democracies, these investments translated into patient consumerism, evident in the proliferation from the 1960s of both patient organisations and new classes of experts from whom individuals could seek help on all aspects of physical and psychological health.[6] From the 1970s, multiple liberation movements also started to challenge medical authorities that explained their suffering as a result of biological or psychological inferiority rather than political and social structures; the Black Power Movement, Gay Liberation Movement, Disabled People's Movement, and WLM all relocated the cause of oppression from their own bodies and minds to the unjust, corrupt, and sick societies that denied their full humanity.[7] Among wider populations, by the closing decades of the twentieth century the cumulative effect of these developments was the transition from near-complete deference to medical authority to the belief that doctors should at least listen to people's own opinions on their bodily and psychological health.

As expertise and experience came to exist in a new relation to each other, they also came into a new relation with the practices of everyday life. The intertwining of expertise with experience meant that expertise was now situated in more and more contexts outside formal healthcare systems or relationships – indeed, claims to experiential expertise needed no justification outside an individual's life history. This is one reason why 'everyday health' is inseparable from embodiment and selfhood, and why researching 'everyday health' means shifting from a top-down to a ground-up perspective and searching for evidence of its manifestations in more diffuse locations. Part I explores the creation and deployment of expertise in forms of 'everyday health' related to sexuality, reproduction, and kinship. It considers the relationship between shifting perceptions

Part I: Introduction

of sexuality, rights, and activism; how 'ordinary' individuals, 'experts', and activists articulated these perceptions in spaces from the bestseller to the clinic; and the rise of experiential expertise in challenging dominant medical discourses. It illuminates the interrelationship of local, national, and international efforts as different groups used their embodied health experiences to resist, inform, and reformulate dominant modes of medical and/or cultural understanding, and how they have forged new discourses, spaces, and communities out of these shared experiences.

Ben Mechen (chapter 1) examines the ambivalent positioning of human sexuality between 'permissiveness' and prescriptiveness in biologist and medical doctor Alex Comfort's bestselling *The Joy of Sex* (1972). Offering up a menu of acts and techniques that couples could combine into enticing new sexual recipes, Comfort saw himself as unshackling sexuality from the chains of conventional morality. He presented this easy-to-follow everyday sex advice as liberatory and leading to healthier relations between men and women. But Comfort's vision was shot through with unacknowledged tensions. The sexual repertoire he set out was expansive in its list of acts but set up new norms that anxious readers worried they might not be able to achieve. It did not step outside certain paradigms; Comfort's sexual revolution was heteronormative and ultimately treated women as sexual objects rather than fully equal agents. Finally, while his text told readers that they could trust his assessments of different sexual positions and techniques because he had personally tried them all, ostensibly flagging his experiential expertise, the jacket of *The Joy of Sex* flagged the professional qualifications of 'Alex Comfort, M.B., Ph.D.'. This example shows that diffuse and overlapping sources of expertise informed late twentieth-century discourse on sex, but also reveals the limits of change. As exemplified by Comfort, the public face of 'permissive' expertise was male, white, heterosexist, and no less prone to normative judgements than his medical and sexological predecessors.

At the same time as *The Joy of Sex*'s sexual libertarianism was climbing bestseller lists on different continents, feminist activists were setting up grassroots initiatives in their local communities and making connections with each other across the globe – in these ways challenging the patriarchal culture that Comfort unwittingly echoed. Karissa Patton (chapter 2) uses the case study of the Calgary

34   *Experiential expertise*

Birth Control Association (CBCA) to examine how the ethos of volunteers and the particularities of local healthcare coalesced to shape the implementation of the principles of the global Women's Health Movement (WHM) at a specific site in the 1970s. In focusing on emotional labour and the ethics of care, Patton shows how the overarching aims of the WHM translated into practice through intimate knowledge of local personnel and provision as well as apparently mundane tasks such as keeping administrative records. These small acts were infused with intense care; at this level, the political had to be carried out with a personal touch. Whereas conventional hierarchies position women as 'naturally' more caring than men, gendered emotional labour always and inevitably involves cultivated effort that enables institutions, organisations, and other cultural bodies to function. What we call expertise, and what we fail to recognise as expertise, is determined by wider power structures and replicates the inequalities of the world around us.

Feminists knew and know this to be true. Evangelia Chordaki (chapter 3) examines the Greek birth control movement in the 1970s and 1980s. Chordaki draws on Sara Ahmed's notion of 'sweaty concepts' to show how experiential expertise can reposition marginalised peoples and ways of knowing at the centre, and in doing so challenge existing systems of knowledge and established practices. Chordaki's emphasis on Greek feminists' pushback against/highly strategic engagement with medicine and science lays bare the underpinning principles that also motivated CBCA volunteers; reading these chapters in tandem shows the multiple ways that feminists in apparently very different local and national contexts, but linked by the global WHM, creatively produced and circulated knowledge in a world that denied their right to do so. Chordaki's analysis of texts produced, translated, and circulated by Greek feminists, and women's movement activists' involvement in international networks, reveals the mechanisms of transmission of the principles that animated the WHM, but also the specific ways that these were put into practice and how, in the process, feminists became sources of authority for each other. Meanwhile, her use of 'informal archives', curated and held by participants in these movements, to trace the movement of knowledge across disciplinary and geographical boundaries shows how important it is to actively preserve, publicise, and remake experiential expertise before it is lost forever.

Part I: Introduction   35

For some, this work of active remembering in order to keep experiential expertise safe and available for use in the present and future is urgent for their own health and that of their children. Grace Redhead (chapter 4) shows how Black women diagnosed with Sickle Cell Disease (SCD) or the sickle cell trait ended up 'on the front line of the medicalisation of family and kinship'. Drawing on oral history interviews, Redhead explores women's 'everyday theorising'. Fighting the ignorance and racist assumptions of formal healthcare systems, as well as pervasive silence around SCD in their communities and in British culture, these women's experiential expertise was crucial to protecting their own and their families' health. In doing so, they did not reject the formal knowledge of biomedicine but appropriated and reshaped aspects of it that could be of use in their immediate situations. Some joined patient groups or became healthcare professionals, working at different points in these systems to challenge and remake them. Their 'everyday theorising' took place within their own bodies and families and drew on the conceptual resources of their day-to-day lives, from medical education to British national myths of resilience, but also incorporated West African forms of knowledge and practices. These women's experiential expertise therefore not only moved between different intellectual and cultural domains but was embedded in their individual and familial histories of migration, demonstrating the porous boundaries of knowledge and understanding in the late twentieth-century world.

It is perhaps a truism that all history is local history. Every person, object, organisation, and so on comes from and exists somewhere – whether we choose to focus on the local dimensions of their existence or not. In the post-Second World War era, all history is also transnational history. Every person, object, organisation, and so on exists within webs of connection, stretching oceans and time zones, that shape the nature of their existence – whether they understand the extent of these networks, or we choose to study them, or not.[8] The chapters in this section (and in Part III: Mass media and networks of communication), underline this fact. *The Joy of Sex* was an international bestseller, by a British scientist who moved between England and California, that formed part of a popular sexological trend apparent across Britain, Europe, and North America. The volunteers at the CBCA drew on their hyperlocal knowledge

36 *Experiential expertise*

to put into practice the principles of the global WHM. Greek feminists translated and redeployed texts from France, Denmark, and North America; they took part in international campaigns and conferences; they contributed to the formation of feminist health practices through creation and re-creation at different sites. Black British women made sense of SCD through western biomedicine and West African knowledge; the family stories they told about illness connected Grenada and London. The local and the global are not separate but intertwined states and ways of being, a point we cannot ignore if we want to recapture what 'everyday health' meant and means – especially for those often relegated to the margins in traditional histories of health and medicine.

If understanding 'everyday health' in the modern era requires ways of seeing that are simultaneously local and global, it also compels us to bring in other voices and ways of knowing that challenge traditional hierarchies, and this brings us back to experiential expertise. Person, perspective, position, place – all mingle in experiential expertise.[9] An experience-centred standpoint often originates from those excluded from traditional forms and sites of knowledge and involves challenging the unspoken assumptions of existing political, social, and cultural institutions. Alex Comfort saw himself as in rebellion against conservative sexual politics, but he was a still a professional man, a scientist – and he still implicitly positioned women and non-heterosexual people/acts as outliers or aberrations. In the chapters in this section, it is Black women, feminists, and patients who are compelled to speak *from* the self in order to speak *back*; who must find forms of creative communication in order not only to connect across distance but to be heard from where they stand; who have to actively negotiate with doctors, scientists, male and/or white professionals of all kinds, or make their own spaces from the ground up, simply to receive care; who, because their gender, 'race', and class mean that they will never be seen as 'objective', are forced to query and demolish the ideal of objectivity itself.

Julia Sudbury explains that a 'focus on location', meaning the situated totality of experience, 'insists on the standpoint of its speakers, yet it does not essentialise'. Rather, this approach 'enables examination of the specificities of the partial story without losing sight of the macro structures which locate and illuminate those

Part I: Introduction   37

details' and 'creates the space for critical analysis of subordinated voices without re-centring those voices which have been deposed'.[10] In this sense, experiential expertise seems almost inevitably to lead to demasculinised, decolonised, activist perspectives, even if there is nothing to stop those who speak from positions of power laying claim to experiential expertise. The chapters in this section both probe and skirt many different kinds of experiential expertise, reflecting different hierarchies of people, sites, and knowledges, in the process illuminating a central aspect of constructions of 'everyday health' from the postwar decades to the present day. More than this, they contribute to the active recovery of at-risk histories. As a form of knowledge primarily claimed and perpetuated by those on the margins, experiential expertise is continually vulnerable to attack, relegation, manipulation, decay, and loss. In insisting on the importance of lived experience and the legitimacy of experiential expertise, these chapters also speak back.

Notes

1 Barbara Ehrenreich and Deirdre English, *Complaints and Disorders: The Sexual Politics of Sickness* (Old Westbury, NY: The Feminist Press, 1973), pp. 9–11.

2 Claire Langhamer, '"Who the hell are ordinary people?" Ordinariness as a category of historical analysis', *Transactions of the Royal Historical Society*, 28 (2018).

3 Frank Biess, 'Introduction: histories of the aftermath', in Frank Biess and Robert G. Möller (eds), *Histories of the Aftermath: The Legacies of the Second World War in Europe* (New York, NY: Berghahn Books, 2010); Nikolas Rose, *Governing the Soul: The Shaping of the Private Self* (London and New York: Routledge, 1989); Mathew Thomson, *Psychological Subjects: Identity, Culture and Health in Twentieth-Century Britain* (Oxford: Oxford University Press, 2006), pp. 209–94; Teri Chettiar, *The Intimate State: How Emotional Life Became Political in Welfare-State Britain* (Oxford: Oxford University Press, 2023).

4 Jennifer Crane, *Child Protection in England, 1960–2000: Expertise, Experience, and Emotion* (Basingstoke: Palgrave Macmillan, 2019), pp. 1–26, 161–95.

5 Roberta Bivins, 'Serving the nation, serving the people: echoes of war in the early NHS', *Medical Humanities*, 46:2 (2020); Jack Saunders, 'Emotions, social practices and the changing composition of class, race

and gender in the National Health Services, 1970–1979: "lively discussion ensued"', *History Workshop Journal*, 88 (Autumn 2019); Jennifer Crane, '"Loving" the NHS: social surveys and activist feelings', in Jennifer Crane and Jane Hand (eds), *Posters, Protests, and Prescriptions: Cultural Histories of the National Health Service in Britain* (Manchester: Manchester University Press, 2022).

6 Graham Smith, 'The rise of the "new consumerism" in health and medicine in Britain, c. 1948–1989', in Jennifer Burr and Paula Nicholson (eds), *Researching Health Care Consumers* (Basingstoke: Palgrave Macmillan, 2005); Alex Mold, *Making the Patient-Consumer: Patient Organisations and Health Consumerism in Britain* (Manchester: Manchester University Press, 2015), pp. 1–17.

7 Natalie Thomlinson, *Race, Ethnicity and the Women's Movement in England, 1968–1993* (Basingstoke: Palgrave Macmillan, 2016); Sarah Browne, *The Women's Liberation Movement in Scotland* (Manchester: Manchester University Press, 2017); George Stevenson, *The Women's Liberation Movement and the Politics of Class in Britain* (London and New York: Bloomsbury Academic, 2019); Kate Mahoney, *Feminist Mental Health Activism in England, c. 1968–1995* (Manchester: Manchester University Press, 2023); R.E.R. Bunce and Paul Field, 'Obi B. Egbuna, C.L.R. James and the birth of Black Power in Britain: Black radicalism in Britain 1967–72', *Twentieth Century British History*, 22:3 (2011); Lucy Robinson, *Gay Men and the Left in Post-War Britain: How the Personal Got Political* (Manchester: Manchester University Press, 2007); Beckie Rutherford, 'Disabled Women Organising: Rethinking Agency within British Liberation Movements, 1976–2000' (PhD thesis, University of Warwick, 2023).

8 Ann Curthoys and Marilyn Lake (eds), *Connected Worlds: History in Transnational Perspective* (Canberra: ANU Press, 2005); Stefan Berger, *History and Identity: How Historical Theory Shapes Historical Practice* (Cambridge: Cambridge University Press, 2022), pp. 261–83.

9 E.M. Castro, T. Van Regenmortel, W. Sermeus, and K. Vanhaecht, 'Patients' expertiential knowledge and expertise in health care: a hybrid concept analysis', *Social Theory & Health*, 17 (2018); Harry Collins and Robert Evans, 'Studies of expertise and experience: a sociological perspective on expertise', in Paul Ward, Jan Maarten Schraagen, Julie Gore, and Emilie M. Roth (eds), *The Oxford Handbook of Expertise* (Oxford: Oxford University Press, 2018).

10 Julia Sudbury, *'Other Kinds of Dreams': Black Women's Organising and the Politics of Transformation* (London: Routledge, 1998), p. 32.

1

Alex Comfort's *The Joy of Sex* and the tensions of liberal sexpertise

Ben Mechen

Introduction

In 1972, the British biologist, physician, and writer Alex Comfort published *The Joy of Sex*, a 256-page 'gourmet guide to love making'. Combining plain speaking with zoological and psychological theories of sexuality, Comfort promised his readers 'a sophisticated and unanxious account' of the 'full repertoire of human sexuality'.[1] *Joy* was dismissive of unnecessary 'hangups', admonished lovers who wore deodorant ('banned absolutely'), and was memorably illustrated with watercolour portraits of a hippyish young couple in the throes of passion – the woman in a floral shift, the man long haired and bearded, his heavy boots at the end of the bed. Its 153 entries mixed instruction on the 'missionary position' and 'mouth music' (oral sex) with obscurities like the '*croupade*' and the '*flanquette*' and cures for common sexual problems. *Joy* became a global bestseller and an instant icon of the counterculture, the 'sexual revolution', and, more broadly, the 1970s, used in museum exhibits and films alike as shorthand for the sexual values of the decade.[2]

Joy made Comfort a star. Over the previous two decades, sex research had been transformed first by Alfred Kinsey and then by William Masters and Barbara Johnson.[3] Comfort placed himself in this lineage while also shifting emphasis from observation of sexual behaviour to instruction. Within months of publication, *Joy* had topped the bestseller lists of *The Times* and the *New York Times*, and in 2012 it was estimated to have sold around ten million copies worldwide.[4] But, despite its (probable) status as the bestselling sex

40 *Experiential expertise*

manual of all time, historians have paid little attention to *Joy*. It is often mentioned, but rarely explored in detail.[5]

This chapter revisits *Joy*'s powerful new libertarian vision of the heterosexual 'sex life'. It was a text attuned to the rising tide of 'permissiveness' in British culture and society that in turn also shaped sexual expression. It emphasised the importance of sexual freedom and pleasure, and domesticated formerly radical ideas about sexual morality and practice, including new sexual positions, 'foursomes and moresomes', and the erotics of everything from earlobes to rubber.[6] Unlike the Kinsey reports, or Britain's own 'little Kinsey' (1949) survey, *Joy* did not claim to hold a mirror to society's sexual habits or fantasies.[7] Instead, it looked to validate and celebrate them, as well as suggest new ones to pick up or imagine. *Joy* hymned the healthiness of everyday sexual exuberance and reassured readers that sex had 'no rules'.[8]

Yet this celebration of sexual freedom and growth hid irresolvable tensions. Most fundamentally, *Joy*'s message of sexual freedom was incompatible with its medium: a work of instruction, written by a well-known and highly credentialed expert. Although Comfort insisted that his text was 'a menu not a rulebook', like its sex manual predecessors *Joy* was a work that defined and set boundaries. Its turn to technique, pleasure, and the sexual lifestyle recalibrated rather than refused the categories of the sexually 'normal' and 'abnormal'.[9] Comfort promoted highly restrictive understandings of the roles of men and women within relationships that were (almost) always assumed to be heterosexual. He counselled that sex must be mutually pleasurable, but nearly everywhere in *Joy* the burdens of sexual labour fell more heavily on women than men, with women seen as best able to reorient domesticity around the endless pursuit of more and better orgasms.

By tracing Comfort's self-construction as a new kind of liberated 'sexpert' with vast personal experience of 'good' sex and a suspicion of conventional morality, we can see how he was able to assume authority over readers while simultaneously decrying the 'anxiety makers' who had previously pronounced on sex. An analysis of Comfort's joys of sex, and the substantial programme of work and self-improvement for men and (especially) women who wanted to get 'with it' in the bedroom reveals further contradictions. These tensions within *Joy*'s liberalism and its version of heterosexuality

Alex Comfort's The Joy of Sex

illuminate the 'attenuated, uneven and partial' nature of postwar sexual liberalisation.[10] Comfort's bestselling vision of 'everyday sex' helped to frame the terms of public debate about sex in 1970s Britain, as well as the terms on which many people encountered questions of sexual technique, attitude, and wellbeing in their private lives.[11] Revisiting *Joy* therefore elucidates how heterosexuality was reconceived during Britain's 'sexual revolution', and how liberalisation was consistently marked by both the setting-up of new anxieties around healthiness and happiness and the endurance of older configurations of gender, class, and sexuality. Contemporaries were encouraged to ask, 'am I free enough?' As historians, we should ask, 'who was this freedom really for?'

Comfort as sexpert

Joy took Comfort only two weeks to write. He had agreed to write a book on 'real sex' at the suggestion of James Mitchell, co-owner of the London publisher Mitchell Beazley.[12] The first draft, a home-made 'blue duplicated octavo volume', was called 'Our ABC' and attributed to 'John and Jane Thomas', pseudonyms for Comfort and his partner Jane Henderson.[13] In keeping with his academic training in the natural sciences, Comfort had kept notes on his and Jane's sex life, and what others might glean from it, for several years. *Joy* extrapolated from these notes.[14] While Comfort framed the book in its preface as the work of a couple, with him as their editor, only his name appeared on the cover.[15] If the book was based on shared experiences, then the words (and the copyright) were his alone.[16] With Jane not taking part in any of the publicity work for *Joy*, the fame would be his too.

Though *Joy* was written in England by an English author, Comfort's intellectual inspiration and intended readership were found in 'modern California', a place he had visited regularly since the late 1960s.[17] California, and especially its countercultural sexual scene, exercised a terrific hold over Comfort's imagination. He saw it as a place 'at grips with the cardinal problems of our time', awash with fresh ideas rather than deadened by tradition.[18] In *Joy*, Comfort wanted to push the countercultural values of sexual experimentation and frankness into the cultural mainstream. He did not think this kind

42 *Experiential expertise*

of diffusion possible in England, at least not yet. If the United States was a country 'where they seem to go in for that sort of thing, or rather books on that sort of thing, more than we do', the '"Anglo-Saxon"' culture, as he put in *Joy*, was one of 'intense taboos' and 'cultural reservation[s]', altogether a 'bad hand for really full and personal sex'.[19] In late 1972 *Joy* was published in the United States, where it quickly hit the *New York Times* 'top ten best seller' list, remaining there for seventy-two weeks.[20] Comfort was initially wary of publishing a version in London, believing that the book would most likely 'be banned, since the law in England [is] a Mickey Mouse operation unworthy of the intelligence of its public'.[21] A British edition, if there was to be one at all, would have to wait.

This wariness was uncharacteristic. For some time, Comfort had cultivated a reputation as a social and cultural iconoclast, becoming one of Britain's foremost exponents of 'the new morality'.[22] In 1963 he had published *Sex in Society*, a work of popular sociology and anthropology later reissued as a Pelican Original. It called for a demystified and rational approach to sex and the formal and informal deregulation of private sexual behaviour.[23] In July of that year, on the television programme *This Nation Tomorrow*, he confirmed his reputation as a champion of the 'permissive society' by claiming that 'a chivalrous boy' was 'one who takes contraceptives with him when he goes to meet his girlfriend' – a comment that prompted the conservative campaigner Mary Whitehouse to write her first letter of complaint to the BBC.[24] After translating into English a medieval Indian sex manual, the *Koka Shastra*, Comfort further caught the anti-authoritarian mood by writing *The Anxiety Makers*, a popular critique of the medical profession's role in enforcing conventional sexual morality.[25] As the 1960s drew to a close, the *Guardian* named him one of their 'Priests and Prophets of Permissiveness', alongside Benjamin Spock, Peter Cook, Lenny Bruce, Allen Ginsberg, and the Beatles.[26]

Despite his initial reticence, Comfort quickly came round to the idea of a British publication of *Joy* and channelled his energies into laying the necessary groundwork. He wanted to 'get into the UK press as much advance discussion [of *Joy*] as possible', including 'publicity in *The Times*' and 'articles in professional journals'. In addition, he thought that by passing the book to sexual therapists and marriage counsellors it would be possible to establish *Joy* as 'a

Alex Comfort's The Joy of Sex   43

fact of medicopsychological life' before its critics had a chance to go on the attack. This plan seems to have worked: when the British edition of *Joy* was published in March 1974, it received favourable reviews in several journals, the *Sunday Times* ran a lengthy piece on it by star journalists Jill Tweedie and Alan Brien ('a couple for whom sex is already a Joy'), and its sales were enormous.[27] The hardback version debuted on the *Sunday Times* non-fiction bestseller list within two weeks of publication, while the 1975 paperback edition remained in the top ten bestselling paperbacks until the end of the year, and sold a further 360,000 copies during 1976.[28] Nevertheless, Comfort's anxieties about the reception of *Joy* in Britain demonstrate the extent to which even the architects of the 'sexual revolution' believed it to remain insecure and unfinished in the early 1970s.

Critics differed as to the book's merits but agreed on its originality. Of course, not everything about *Joy* was new. Comfort's emphasis on sexual pleasure, mutuality, and honesty had clear precedents within the history of popular sex advice. As early as 1918 Marie Stopes' *Married Love* had taught readers the importance to a happy union of the female orgasm, while in the mid-1920s Stella Browne's translation of Theodoor van de Velde's *Ideal Marriage* guided British men and women through diverse sexual positions and counselled the use of foreplay like oral sex.[29] *Joy* therefore joined a long tradition of sexual radicalism refracted through the medium of practical advice and instruction. But, unlike these earlier sex manuals, *Joy* refused to dress up its descriptions of sex in language others might deem medically and morally proper, and instead embraced plain words and slang. *Joy* also did not justify its publication within the terms of religious, reproductive, or conjugal ethics. It was a radical departure from the kinds of sex manual that Jill Tweedie satirised in a 1969 *Guardian* article: it had no 'preface by a member of the clergy', no 'obscure Latin words', no references to the Ancient Greeks or the 'esoteric' practices of African tribes, and few attempts at a 'patina' of respectability.[30] In the words of reviewers, *Joy* was 'one of the least inhibited books on sex ever written', notable for its 'lack of solemnity', 'flashes [...] of humour', and rejection of 'pretentious pompousness', as well as its tone of 'well-judged' 'flippancy'.[31]

In the changing cultural climate of the early 1970s, *Joy*'s sexual frankness meant that many saw it as a book for the times. In March

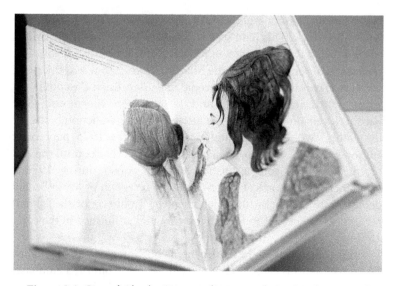

Figure 1.1 One of Charles Raymond's watercolours for the original edition of *The Joy of Sex*. Courtesy of Nils Jorgensen/Shutterstock. All rights reserved and permission to use the figure must be obtained from the copyright holder.

1974, coinciding with the publication of the British edition of *Joy*, *Cosmopolitan* (a women's magazine that also traded on a reputation for sexual openness) included a lengthy excerpt and illustration from *Joy*.[32] This watercolour painting by Charles Raymond, showing the *Joy* couple in a warm embrace, was less explicit than most of *Joy*'s Raymond paintings or black-and-white sketches by Chris Foss. Nevertheless, this use in *Cosmopolitan* demonstrates the centrality of visual design to *Joy*'s success. A large, hardbound book, *Joy* did not look like a typical sex manual. Avoiding both the bright psychedelia of the counterculture and the self-conscious plainness of other predecessors, it embraced white space (as 'dazzling as Easter lilies', thought one reviewer) and blocks of clean black text, interspersed with illustrations: 'lyrical, gentle, *clean* paintings of a modern couple making love'.[33]

The couple were attractive, but not conventionally beautiful, and they were shown as an 'ordinary' couple having 'real' sex.[34] The effect was, wrote Peter Lewis in the *Daily Mail*, 'unusually artistic',

Alex Comfort's The Joy of Sex

the watercolours rendering tasteful what in photographs would have 'crossed the borderline of pornography'.[35] Jill Tweedie praised *Joy*'s use of an ordinary-looking couple, 'innocuous persons neither dauntingly gorgeous nor overly endowed', who suggested *Joy*'s vision of sexuality was available to all.[36] Unlike older sex manuals, *Joy* was not meant to be bought secretly, then hidden away at the back of a drawer or between the covers of a more respectable book; rather, Comfort saw it as a tome for the 'coffee table', with a visual language that was 'tender' rather than 'kinky' or 'sentimental'.[37] 'Clean and fresh-looking' in appearance and full of tasty (and 'tasteful') morsels of advice, it was, suggested the *Liverpool Daily Post*, quite simply the 'Cadbury's Milk Tray' of sex manuals.[38]

Not everybody agreed. Some commentators hostile to *Joy*'s intentions singled out the artwork for criticism; an anonymous reviewer in the *Observer* thought it 'sub-pornographic', even 'sick-making'.[39] The writer Auberon Waugh suggested that *Joy*'s illustrations were 'without exception hideous, embarrassing and dull', offensive not because of their sexual content but rather on account of their cringeworthy hipness; there was a 'stupidity to the faces', and the models looked like 'the sort of people one knows slightly and rather dislikes', certainly not the sort 'one wishes to see showing off their sexual prowess'.[40] Other commentators were more concerned with *Joy*'s overarching message. Peter Lewis suggested that *Joy* might cause more anxieties than it laid to rest, its gourmet menu potentially producing 'an inferiority complex' in couples who had been quite happy 'with plain home cooking'.[41] *Joy*'s most vehement critic was *The Spectator*'s David Holbrook, who viewed *Joy*'s interest in bondage, discipline, and other unorthodox sexual practices as dangerous. He described Comfort as one of the 'New Gangsters of Liberation' making a 'private fortune' by 'ruthlessly bulldozing us into the '"new freedom"', 'buggery' and all.[42]

This story of *Joy*'s writing, publication, popular success, and mixed critical reception, provides insights into the changing status of experts in postwar Britain, including their perceived role as observers and architects of the 'ordinary'. Matthew Hilton has identified the expert as a 'growing authority' in postwar Britain, with 'professional quasi-outsiders' such as physical and social scientists, economists, civil servants, and those employed within the expanding NGO (non-governmental organisation) sector associated

46   *Experiential expertise*

with 'the rise of the technocratic state', although often situated at one remove from it.[43] To an extent, Comfort seems to fit within this narrative, but the success of *Joy* also refocuses attention on how experts mobilised popular culture as a venue for their ideas. Though sex has always had its professional experts, especially doctors, psychoanalysts, and sexologists, the rise from the 1950s of the media-friendly, million-selling *public* expert on sex embodied by a figure like Comfort (but also, as Adrian Bingham has noted, the newspaper agony aunt) was a qualitatively different phenomenon, as was the decidedly liberal bent of Comfort's advice.[44] *Joy* therefore signals that professional sexual expertise aligns with the transformations described by Hilton, and that expertise was central to sexual liberalisation in Britain in the 1960s and 1970s.

But the story of Comfort and *Joy* also complicates and even challenges these narratives about the rise of experts and 'sexperts', as Comfort actually claimed authority by attacking expertise and defining himself as a kind of *anti*-expert. Since the early 1960s, he had courted outrage by pillorying traditional sexual authorities. True to this pattern, Comfort framed *Joy* as a work of 'humane and experienced sense' aimed at counteracting the 'admonitory, weird, religious, naïve, conventional or just plain ignorant' books written by others.[45] He told one interviewer that, 'We have all suffered terribly from the non-playing coaches' of medicine, religion, and psychiatry. Comfort believed that over the years, doctors in particular had proved as useful as 'chocolate teapots' when it came to giving sensible sexual advice.[46] *Joy* tried to undo these evil effects by capturing the experiences of a regular couple who enjoyed sex, albeit overlaid with the editorialising of the scientist (and doctor!) who was that couple's male half.[47]

In this self-conscious project, *Joy* caught the anti-authoritarian mood of the 1960s and 1970s. At the same time, Comfort's peculiar relationship to expert knowledge – as both its keen detractor and a contributor to *new* bodies of expert knowledge – reveals him as a classic case of what Stefan Collini has called the English intellectual's 'paradox of denial'.[48] Collini argues that English intellectual culture's suspicion of the dangerously French idea of 'intellectualism' has resulted in English cultural authorities habitually denying their own status. *Joy* traded constantly on both Comfort's authority to hand out advice and his claim that self-proclaimed authorities on sex

Alex Comfort's The Joy of Sex 47

should rarely be taken seriously. Only the doctor–scientist's personal 'experience' could square this circle.

Cordon bleu sex

Joy was not, wrote one reviewer, 'a book for beginners'.[49] In his introduction on 'Advanced Lovemaking', Comfort opined that there were already 'enough books about the basics' and that readers of the 1970s needed something completely different. Books like Masters and Johnson's *Human Sexual Response* (1966) still had their uses, not least for people only just beginning to 'get rid of worries over the normality, possibility, and variety of sexual experience', but *Joy* aimed to go further by breaking down the last vestiges of anxiety among readers, expanding the realm of the permissible and the pleasurable, and making this pursuit the work of a lifetime.[50]

Comfort's description of *Joy* as a 'gourmet guide to lovemaking' succinctly demonstrates his redefinition of the sex manual. Its predecessors had been positioned as texts to help readers make their first, tentative steps out of sexual ignorance, perhaps in the early days of marriage.[51] *Joy*, on the other hand, started 'at the point where people know how to prepare and enjoy food' but 'want to go on from there'.[52] Accordingly, where sex manual advice had often been vague in detailing the 'hows' of sex, or limited in the techniques covered, *Joy* was meticulous and candid in its descriptions, and generous in its definition of healthy and permissible ways of having sex: it included oral sex, anal sex, group sex, and multiple sexual positions, all absent or downplayed in previous texts.

For Comfort, the possibility of 'gourmet sex' had to be temporally positioned. Beyond even the work of pioneering sexologists, he felt it was the availability of reliable contraception that had altered the sexual landscape, by conclusively separating sex and reproduction. *Joy* claimed the oral contraceptive pill as 'the discovery which more than any other makes carefree sex possible', the 'security' against conception it offered allowing women for the first time to 'discover the play-function of sex'.[53] Hera Cook has argued that before widespread access to reliable contraception, the ever-present danger of pregnancy made women (and men) more risk averse. Their sexual mores and behaviour were shaped by the desire to avoid unplanned

48   *Experiential expertise*

pregnancies, resulting in strategies such as abstinence that reduced women's exposure to sex.[54] *Joy* instead elaborated a putatively *post*-reproductive sexuality, in which mores and behaviour could be relaxed to suit an era in which sexual abundance rather than abstinence was newly possible (though perhaps not as easily as Comfort assumed; only in 1974 was the oral contraceptive pill made available to unmarried women free of charge on the National Health Service). *Joy* framed this shift as the 'difference between sex as the last generation came to accept it and sex as it can be': removing pregnancy from the equation could open up possibilities for sex as experiment and self-expression.[55]

Joy also implicitly positioned its approach to sex within a class-based cultural hierarchy. By the 1970s, the cookbook was a form highly symbolic of middle-class domesticity. In *Joy*'s world, sex was a culinary art with 'Starters', 'Main Courses', 'Sauces and Pickles', and, in a nod to the vogue for French cookery, its *cassolette*, *croupade*, and *cuissade*.[56] It was a musical art too, complete with 'duets', 'solos', and 'concerts', calling for readers to be as talented in the bedroom as Menuhin was on the violin.[57] *Joy* also tried to show sex as a worthy subject of serious artists. Looking to break apart the association between sexual explicitness and the pornographic, *Joy* placed Raymond's delicate watercolours of the '*Joy* couple' alongside selections from medieval and early modern Indian and Japanese erotic art. This situated *Joy* within a long tradition of works that looked to titillate the West by eroticising the East.[58] These purposeful references to the cornerstones of middle-class taste suggested that the appreciation of good sex, like that of food, music, and painting, was a pursuit open to connoisseurship: the cultivation of specialist knowledge and talents, the accumulation of new specimens and experiences, and the ability, above all, to discern between the perfect and the merely good.

This alignment of good sex and good taste was freighted with meaning. The 1970s were, as one historian of the period has labelled it, 'the decade that taste forgot'.[59] *Joy* represented an attempt to rescue sex from the 'permissive populism' of *The Benny Hill Show* (1955–89), the *Carry On* film series (1958–92), and *Confessions of a Window Cleaner* (the highest-grossing film of 1974).[60] Comfort tried to persuade readers that sex was not a joke. *Joy*'s idea of sexual good taste was a version of the 'taste of liberty' or 'luxury' in eating

Alex Comfort's The Joy of Sex   49

habits that Pierre Bourdieu saw as an ongoing marker of middle-class distinction, a 'shift in emphasis' from privileging how filling or cheap a foodstuff is ('the taste of necessity' of the working class) to privileging the 'manner' of its consumption.[61] *Joy*'s elaboration of sexual technique and variety proposed a similar shift, from simply *having* sex to adopting a whole sexual lifestyle in which *how* you did it, and the meanings you invested in it, became everything: as one reviewer noted, *Joy* marked the distance between the 'gourmet' cooking of the sexual sophisticate and 'the Saturday evening bellyful of Guinness and chips' that satisfied the appetites of the sexually humdrum.[62]

In Comfort's view, sexual connoisseurship required both high levels of personal commitment and expert instruction from a book like *Joy*: just as 'it's hard to make mayonnaise by trial and error', 'cordon bleu sex' 'doesn't happen naturally'. He framed earth-shattering sex as a pursuit just as desirable and just as learnable as the middle-class hobbyist's aspiration of 'chef-grade cooking'.[63] Indeed, *The Joy of Sex* looked to do for sex what Irma Rombauer's *The Joy of Cooking* had already done for food: where Rombauer had explained in 'unruffled detail' how to 'tackle a live lobster' or 'fix a chateaubriand', Comfort showed readers 'what to do about [...] premature ejaculation', 'how to manage oral sex', or 'how to treat a partner who is "hip" for discipline'. Through provision of 'practical details', *Joy* promised privileged access to the tastiest fruits of the sexual revolution without having to leave the home or mix in the unfamiliar milieus of hardy sexual experimentalists like Comfort himself.[64] In this sense, Comfort's sexual expertise was alchemical, taking the sexually far-out and making it, through careful use of language, structure, and signification, tasteful.

At £6.50 in its hardback edition, *Joy* was an expensive book – 'overpriced', according to the *Observer*.[65] But the reclassification of good sex as a dimension of good taste, with a price tag to match, was designed to make sexual improvement more appealing to a middle-class readership. It rendered the path to thrilling sex a hospitable and familiar, rather than hostile and strange, terrain. This reconfiguration of the relationship between sex, taste, and respectability led Jill Tweedie to suggest that *Joy* made 'even the rudest Soho-type goings-on seem the sort of activities you might just get away with at a trendy vicar's tea-party'.[66] *Joy*, as was surely

50 *Experiential expertise*

Comfort's intention, and as was surely one of the reasons for its popular success, was a book both strikingly racy and strangely respectable.

The conscious development of sexual good taste required commitment to variety and experimentation: if *Joy* described 'the full repertoire of human sexuality', the idea was less to pick and choose than to learn it all. *Joy* organised its 'goings-on' into three broad types of sexual activity: the 'basic ingredients' ('Starters'), those 'which everyone needs' ('Main Courses'), and those to be saved 'for special occasions' ('Sauces and Pickles').[67] A healthy sexual diet meant balance, perhaps moving within the same encounter between 'regular' coitus, 'handwork' and oral sex, or highly engaged role play and languorous cuddling, whilst allowing room for more unconventional activities like anal or group sex if the mood or opportunity struck. Couples were also to rotate through the full range of sexual positions, adopting 'five, ten or twenty postures at a single session' in an athletic routine that would become almost 'automatic' with practice.[68]

This careful accumulation of experiences and techniques was not an empty 'intellectual classificatory exercise' for Comfort, but an important route to sexual satisfaction and continued interest and excitement.[69] *Joy* tried to reconfigure everyday heterosexual practice by pushing to its centre pleasure rather than 'normality'. The 'matrimonial' or missionary position, though 'uniquely satisfying' and 'the most reliably mutual finishing-point for orgasm' had been privileged for far too long.[70] By comparison, 'Sauces and Pickles', the activities that made sex a thrillingly diverse experience, had been considered unnecessary or unnatural. Comfort tried to remove the anxiety-inducing libel of 'perversion' from even the most eccentric acts. Though these practices should never entirely replace 'full, let-go intercourse', they were necessary addenda: a 'genital kiss' or the exploration of a strange fantasy could be a 'supplement', 'overture', or 'interlude' that brought the whole thing together.[71] Adapting the psychologist Abraham Maslow's idea that there was no such thing as intrinsically perverted acts, only perverted individuals, Comfort argued that if doing x, y, or z made you both happy, that was all that mattered.[72]

Joy's frank discussions of the possibilities of anal eroticism within heterosexual relationships serve as a case in point, representing a

Alex Comfort's The Joy of Sex   51

significant transformation in the dominant discourse of heterosexuality. Whereas its sex manual predecessors had routinely excluded discussion of such practices, *Joy* neutrally framed anal eroticism as 'something which nearly every couple tries once'.[73] Again making mutual pleasure the most important index of sexual value, *Joy* considered both the possible rewards of anal sex ('intenser feelings than the normal route' for women, a 'pleasantly tight' sensation for men), and its ability to cause pain or even physical damage, especially to women. *Joy*'s considerations of '*postillionage*' ('putting a finger in or on your partner's anus just before orgasm'), and the '*feuille de rose*' ('tongue stimulation of the anus [...] in either sex'), also widened the sphere of anal eroticism beyond male penetration of women.[74] Alongside *Joy*'s lengthy explorations of 'bondage' and 'discipline', these ruminations elaborated alternative erotic domains as legitimate forms of heterosexual sexual behaviour.

Sex as good housekeeping

But such inclusions also reveal the paradox at the heart of *Joy*. On the one hand, *Joy* instructed readers to be free, and in places admonished them for not being free enough. On the other, and despite its protestations, it outlined a particular set of sexual acts as the most satisfying, and necessary to a contented and stable sexual relationship. Though Comfort criticised hung-up societies' resort to 'classification' in order to make the sexually transgressive intelligible and subject to regulation, *The Joy of Sex* was itself a work of classification: a codification of what made sex 'joyous'.[75] In this way, *Joy* actually belonged to the long sexological tradition Comfort criticised. In a formal, if not a dispositional, sense, not much separated *Joy*'s methodical, alphabetically organised lists of sexual 'recipes' from Richard von Krafft-Ebing's *Psychopathia Sexualis* (1886), the *magnum opus* of sexological taxonomising. Both were concerned with organising sexual knowledge in new ways, and both developed rules about what sex should (and should not) be like. This tension was not lost on *Joy*'s critics. In his review for fashionable women's magazine *Nova*, Auberon Waugh signalled his suspicion at a book that tried quite so hard to wrest people out of one way of doing things, only to push them into another. Unlike Comfort,

Waugh liked deodorant, disliked 'armpit hair in a woman', and found 'the whole idea of shaved pubic hair disgusting'. He did not believe in absolute standards of right or wrong in sexual taste, but questioned why anyone should pay 'to have someone else's turn-ons thrust at one as if they were best'.[76]

Crucially, *Joy*'s programme for good sex was structured by differential understandings of men and women's sexual talents, roles, and capabilities. The book's expert voice was nearly always that of a sexually demanding man, even though Comfort argued elsewhere that any decent book on sex should be co-authored by a 'really turned-on woman'.[77] *Joy* included a section called 'By her (for him)', but it was only a few pages long.[78] *Joy*'s gendered approach to sexual mutuality surfaced in its discussion of different techniques. In evaluations of positions like the '*negresse*' (note the misogynoir), 'a very deep position [...] apt to pump her full of air' but 'otherwise excellent', Comfort's cool and one-sided tone pointed to his focus on male satisfaction, as did his recommendations of 'intermammary intercourse', 'a good expedient when she is closed to the public', or sex from behind, which offered men 'the sight of a pretty rear view'.[79]

Indeed, the meaning of mutuality was frequently skewed in *Joy*. Comfort paid lip service to the equitable division of pleasures, but framed the woman's role as to produce pleasure, and the man's role as to consume it. *Joy* contained numerous addresses to female readers on how to master sexual techniques, especially the 'solos' they might perform on their lover. These addresses were precise and anatomical, where those directed to men were usually vague and impressionistic. *Joy* assumed women to require more explicit tutoring in the arts of love than their partners. When it came to 'masturbating' a man 'well', for instance, women were informed, with the exactitude of a car manual, that the 'best grip is just below the groove, with the skin back as far as it will go, and using two hands, one pressing near the root, holding the penis steady, or fondling the scrotum, the other making a thumb-and-first finger ring or a whole hand grip'.[80] Instructions like these afforded little room for misunderstanding but also little room for error: they levelled the kind of heavy demands at women that made anyone 'who does not whip up and over her lover like a tornado scented with musk', according to the *Nova* columnist Irma Kurtz, a suitable case for treatment.[81]

Alex Comfort's The Joy of Sex   53

Beyond the acquisition of new techniques, Comfort also expected of women new states of mind, including an 'intuitive empathy' with a penis and a 'real enjoyment' of its presence. Such injunctions reveal Comfort's residual belief in women's basic 'frigidity'. Only by a dual technical and mental transformation could a woman's lovemaking become truly 'advanced' so that she would become a 'superlative' rather than merely proficient partner.[82] In Comfort's imagined post-reproductive world in which the burdens of pregnancy had been removed from women, the burdens of perfecting 'cordon bleu sex' took up their place.

Comfort further implied that their transformation into sexually superlative beings would allow female readers to resume their natural place as the keepers of a contented home. *Joy*'s re-idealisation and eroticisation of the domestic demanded a redefinition of women's role as 'the angel in the house', where women's exemplary virtues would no longer be sexual naivety or purity, but their ability to practise the 'divine gift of lechery' (a phrase Comfort attributed to the eighteenth-century libertine John Wilkes). This new lechery meant willingness to become an 'initiator' – 'starting the plays', using their 'stimulatory equipment' freely and ably, and 'giving' things 'ahead of being asked' – and the ability to 'meet her partner's needs as fully as a professional'.[83] *Joy* therefore elaborated experimental, virtuosic sex as a domestic possibility rather than something to be sought by men outside the home, in which women's management of good sex became part of the definition of good housekeeping.

Conclusion

Joy directed readers to regularly *practise*, rather than simply *have*, sex. At first glance this looked like reassurance: 'The right frequency for sex is as often as you both enjoy it'; 'Don't enforce a timetable.' On closer inspection, however, this slid into new norms to measure oneself against: 'Two or three times a week is a common rate'; 'Some people do stick to a pretty regular schedule.'[84] By framing sex as a permanent training programme with *Joy* its handbook, and by raising both variety and technical proficiency to hitherto unprec-edented levels of importance, *Joy* demanded from its readers a permanent state of watchfulness, of both the self and others. Am I

54 *Experiential expertise*

(or are we) doing it right? Am I (or are we) doing it enough? And is this or that technique more pleasurable?

Joy's version of everyday sex therefore set up new norms that, internalised by readers, could affect perceptions of what a healthy sex life could or should look like. In this way, liberal sexpertise might actually lead to heightened self-consciousness, self-criticism, and disappointment; a newly minted form of everyday unhappiness that caused emotional and psychological dis-ease. Several of *Joy*'s reviewers were alive to this prospect. For them, *Joy* represented a rationalisation, technicalisation, or even disenchantment of sex that was wholly unwelcome. For Peter Lewis, *Joy* made sex look a tick-box exercise in which couples could find happiness by selecting positions from an 'itemised menu'.[85] Jill Tweedie, meanwhile, thought that *Joy*'s attempts to transmit precise technical knowledge to readers proved that Comfort was unaware that 'true art must incorporate a soupçon of artlessness'.[86]

These critiques are reinforced by a letter published in the May 1974 issue of *Cosmopolitan*, two months after its excerpts from *Joy*. 'I know what my problem is,' the reader lamented: 'I know too much.' Experts' endless commentary on sex and sexual technique had left her, like 'most girls of [her] age', feeling 'gauche', as though sex was unnecessarily 'complicated', and wondering what it meant to be 'properly fulfilled'. A combination of Freud, Germaine Greer, and sex manuals had left her an anxious 'product of over-education'.[87] These comments illustrate that the kind of sexual freedom *Joy* preached often brought its own worries, especially for women. Comfort himself recognised that 'liberal enthusiasms', including sexual ones, could 'themselves create as much anxiety as repressive enthusiasms'.[88] 'The human capacity for punishment', he thought, was 'endless'.[89] But, in its notion of healthy, happy sex as 'cordon bleu sex', *Joy* itself set a high bar, perhaps an impossibly high one: every couple would fall short, some (or most) of the time. How many 'Menuhins', after all, could there ever really be?

Notes

1 Alex Comfort, *The Joy of Sex: A Gourmet Guide to Lovemaking* (London: Quartet Books, 1974), p. 6.

Alex Comfort's The Joy of Sex 55

2 'The Institute of Sexology', exhibition, Wellcome Collection, London, 20 November 2014–20 September 2015: https://wellcomecollection.org/exhibitions/W31ooSkAACIAP4So (accessed 3 October 2023); *Sex Tape* (dir. Jake Kasdan, 2014).

3 Alfred Kinsey et al., *Sexual Behavior in the Human Male* (London: Saunders, 1948); Alfred Kinsey et al., *Sexual Behavior in the Human Female* (London: Saunders, 1953); William Masters and Virginia Johnson, *Human Sexual Response* (London: Churchill, 1966).

4 Cordelia Hebblethwaite, 'How *The Joy of Sex* was illustrated', *BBC News Magazine* (26 October 2011): http://www.bbc.co.uk/news/magazine-15309357 (accessed 3 October 2023).

5 This applies to histories of sexuality and general histories of Britain. See Hera Cook, *The Long Sexual Revolution: English Women, Sex, and Contraception, 1800–1975* (Oxford: Oxford University Press, 2004), p. 244; Roy Porter and Lesley Hall, *The Facts of Life: The Creation of Sexual Knowledge in Britain, 1650–1950* (New Haven, CT: Yale University Press, 1995), p. 274; Dominic Sandbrook, *State of Emergency: The Way We Were: Britain, 1970–1974* (London: Allen Lane, 2010), p. 428; Francis Wheen, *Strange Days Indeed: The Golden Age of Paranoia* (London: Fourth Estate, 2009), p. 135; Paul Addison, *No Turning Back: The Peacetime Revolutions of Post-war Britain* (Oxford: Oxford University Press, 2010), p. 347.

6 Comfort, *The Joy of Sex*, pp. 168, 106, 132, 211, 201, 153, 163.

7 Adrian Bingham, 'The "K-Bomb": social surveys, the popular press, and British sexual culture in the 1940s and 1950s', *Journal of British Studies*, 50:1 (2011).

8 On *Joy*'s mission of 'reassurance', see University College London (hereafter UCL) Special Collections, Comfort Papers, Box 41, Correspondence A, 1971–73, Alex Comfort to William Miller, 9 February 1972. On sex without rules, see Comfort, *The Joy of Sex*, p. 9.

9 Comfort, *The Joy of Sex*, p. 8. For understandings of sexual 'normality' in the wake of the Kinsey reports, see Peter Cryle and Elizabeth Stephens, *Normality: A Critical Genealogy* (Chicago, IL: University of Chicago Press, 2017), pp. 333–51.

10 Matt Cook, 'Sexual revolution(s) in Britain', in Gert Hekma and Alain Giami (eds), *Sexual Revolutions* (Basingstoke: Palgrave Macmillan, 2014), p. 122.

11 See also Ben Mechen, 'Everyday Sex in 1970s Britain' (PhD thesis, University College London, 2016).

12 Claire Rayner, 'Obituary: Alex Comfort', *Guardian* (28 March 2000): https://www.theguardian.com/news/2000/mar/28/guardianobituaries (accessed 3 October 2023).

13 Kinsey Institute Library, Bloomington, IN, Alex Comfort Collection, Series II, Part C, Correspondence, Folder 7, Alex Comfort to the Library of the Kinsey Institute, 16 July 1976.

14 UCL Special Collections, Comfort Papers, Box 6, Cuttings Book, Jean Sharley Taylor, 'Sex manual sans plain brown wrapper', *Los Angeles Times*, 'View' supplement, 5 November 1972.

15 Comfort, *The Joy of Sex*, p. 7.

16 Stylistic comparison between *Joy* and Comfort's other writings strongly indicates that Comfort was the book's primary author, as do suggestions in Comfort's private correspondence.

17 Kinsey Institute Library, Alex Comfort Collection, Series II, Part D, Manuscripts, Folder 2, Alex Comfort to William Miller, 17 November 1972.

18 UCL Special Collections, Comfort Papers, Box 6, Cuttings Book, Comfort to *Los Angeles Times*, published as 'Taking Comfort in California's variety', 15 July 1973.

19 Comfort quoted in Derrick Hill, 'Take Comfort: it's just what the doctor ordered', *Liverpool Daily Post*, 23 March 1974, p. 5; Comfort, *The Joy of Sex*, p. 10.

20 Hawes Publications, 'Adult New York Times adult hardcover best seller listings': http://www.hawes.com/pastlist.htm (accessed 3 October 2023).

21 Kinsey Institute Library, Alex Comfort Collection, Series II, Part D, Manuscripts, Folder 2, Alex Comfort to William Miller, 17 November 1972. For the workings of obscenity law in the 1960s–70s, see Christopher Hilliard, *A Matter of Obscenity: The Politics of Obscenity in Modern England* (Princeton, NJ: Princeton University Press, 2021), pp. 88–187.

22 John A.T. Robinson, *Honest to God* (London: SCM Press, 1963), p. 105.

23 Alex Comfort, *Sex in Society* (London: Duckworth, 1963).

24 Marjorie Proops, 'TV doctor's amazing sex talk', *Daily Mirror*, 15 July 1963, p. 1; Mary Whitehouse, *Whatever Happened to Sex?* (Hove: Wayland, 1977), pp. 16–17; Dennis Barker, 'Obituary: Mary Whitehouse', *Guardian* (24 November 2001): http://www.theguardian.com/media/2001/nov/24/guardianobituaries.obituaries (accessed 3 October 2023).

25 *The Koka Shastra*, trans. Alex Comfort (London: Allen & Unwin, 1964); Alex Comfort, *The Anxiety Makers: Some Curious Preoccupations of the Medical Profession* (London: Nelson, 1967).

26 *The Permissive Society: The Guardian Inquiry* (London: Panther, 1969), pp. 35–9.

27 Kinsey Institute Library, Alex Comfort Collection, Series II, Part D, Manuscripts, Folder 2, Alex Comfort to William Miller, 17 November

Alex Comfort's The Joy of Sex 57

1972; Jill Tweedie and Alan Brien, 'Look! Gourmet sex...whipping up the appetite', *Sunday Times*, 31 March 1974, p. 42.

28 'Best-sellers', *Sunday Times*, 14 April 1974, p. 13; Suzanne Hodgart, 'Paperbacks: success stories', *Sunday Times*, 27 February 1977, p. 25.

29 Cook, *The Long Sexual Revolution*, pp. 187–202.

30 Jill Tweedie, 'The socio-sexual whirl', *Guardian*, 6 October 1969, p. 9.

31 UCL Special Collections, Comfort Papers, Box 6, Cuttings Book: Anthony Storr, 'Bed is the place to play', *Washington Post*, 2 October 1972; Peter Lewis, 'Love is tenderness and Joy and a bestseller', *The Daily Mail*, 28 March 1974, p. 7; Sam Hutt, '*The Joy of Sex*', review, *FP News* (the newspaper of the Family Planning Association), June 1974; John Bancroft, '*The Joy of Sex*', review, *British Journal of Psychiatry*, 1 January 1975, p. 100.

32 Alex Comfort, 'The joy of sex', *Cosmopolitan* (UK), June 1974, pp. 76–7, 138.

33 Taylor, 'Sex manual sans plain brown wrapper'.

34 Comfort, *The Joy of Sex*, p. 4.

35 Lewis, 'Love is tenderness', p. 7.

36 Tweedie and Brien, 'Look! Gourmet sex', p. 42.

37 Comfort in Hill, 'Take Comfort', p. 5.

38 Hill, 'Take Comfort', p. 5.

39 '*The Joy of Sex*', review, *Observer*, 31 March 1974, p. 39.

40 Auberon Waugh, 'Well, if you insist ...', *Nova*, January 1974, p. 64.

41 Lewis, 'Love is tenderness', p. 7.

42 David Holbrook, 'Pornography', *The Spectator*, 6 April 1973, p. 425.

43 Matthew Hilton, 'Politics is ordinary: non-governmental organizations and political participation in contemporary Britain', *Twentieth Century British History*, 22:2 (2011), pp. 232, 253–4.

44 Adrian Bingham, 'Newspaper problem pages and British sexual culture since 1918', *Media History*, 18:1 (2012).

45 Comfort, *The Joy of Sex*, pp. 6–7.

46 Comfort quoted in Taylor, 'Sex manual sans plain brown wrapper'.

47 On sex and 'ordinariness' in this period, see Ben Mechen, '"Instamatic living rooms of sin": pornography, participation and the erotics of ordinariness in the 1970s', *Contemporary British History*, 26:2 (2022).

48 Stefan Collini, *Absent Minds: Intellectuals in Britain* (Oxford: Oxford University Press, 2006), p. 2.

49 P.T. Brown, '*The Joy of Sex*', review, *Marriage Guidance*, 15:7 (January 1975), p. 272.

50 Comfort, *The Joy of Sex*, pp. 8, 153.

51 Cook, *The Long Sexual Revolution*, pp. 197–8.

58   *Experiential expertise*

52 Comfort, *The Joy of Sex*, p. 8.
53 Comfort, *The Joy of Sex*, p. 54.
54 Hera Cook, 'Sexuality and contraception in modern England: doing the history of reproductive sexuality', *Journal of Social History*, 40:4 (2007).
55 Comfort, *The Joy of Sex*, p. 8.
56 Comfort, *The Joy of Sex*, pp. 104–6.
57 Comfort, *The Joy of Sex*, pp. 112, 132, 166, 205.
58 Comfort, *The Joy of Sex*, pp. 17–48, 177–92.
59 Sian Barber, *Censoring the 1970s: The BBFC and the Decade that Taste Forgot* (Newcastle: Cambridge Scholars, 2011).
60 Leon Hunt, *British Low Culture: From Safari Suits to Sexploitation* (London: Routledge, 1988), p. 2.
61 Pierre Bourdieu, *Distinction: A Social Critique of the Judgement of Taste* [1979], trans. Richard Nice (Cambridge, MA: Harvard University Press, 1984), p. 6.
62 UCL Special Collections, Comfort Papers, Box 6, Cuttings Book, Dick Richards, '*The Joy of Sex*', review, *British Journal of Sexual Medicine*, date unknown.
63 Comfort, *The Joy of Sex*, p. 8.
64 Comfort, *The Joy of Sex*, p. 6.
65 '*The Joy of Sex*', *Observer*, p. 39.
66 Tweedie and Brien, 'Look! Gourmet sex', p. 42.
67 Comfort, *The Joy of Sex*, pp. 49, 99, 149.
68 Comfort, *The Joy of Sex*, p. 113.
69 Comfort, *The Joy of Sex*, p. 113.
70 Comfort, *The Joy of Sex*, p. 124
71 Comfort, *The Joy of Sex*, pp. 11–12.
72 Kinsey Institute Library, Alex Comfort Collection, Series III, Part A, Box 2, 'Norms' subject file, clipping from Maslow's contribution to M.F. DeMartino (ed), *Sexual Behavior and Personality Characteristics* (New York: Grove Press, 1966), pp. 103–5.
73 Comfort, *The Joy of Sex*, pp. 129, 150.
74 Comfort, *The Joy of Sex*, pp. 150, 168, 209.
75 UCL Special Collections, Comfort Papers, Box 6, Cuttings Book, Alex Comfort, 'All sorts and conditions', review of Colin MacInnes, *Loving Them Both*, publication unknown, 5 July 1973.
76 Waugh, 'Well, if you insist …', 64.
77 Alex Comfort, 'A girl needs a father', *The Listener*, 26 April 1973, p. 550 (review of Seymour Fisher, *The Female Orgasm*).
78 Comfort, *The Joy of Sex*, p. 97.
79 Comfort, *The Joy of Sex*, pp. 100, 132, 139.

Alex Comfort's The Joy of Sex

80 Comfort, *The Joy of Sex*, p. 116.
81 Irma Kurtz, 'Sex is vastly over-rated and most of us don't dare say so', *Nova*, November 1974, p. 98.
82 Comfort, *The Joy of Sex*, pp. 116–18.
83 Comfort, *The Joy of Sex*, pp. 72, 248.
84 Comfort, *The Joy of Sex*, pp. 66–7.
85 Lewis, 'Love is tenderness', p. 7.
86 Tweedie and Brien, 'Look! Gourmet sex', p. 42.
87 'Too much advice', *Cosmopolitan*, May 1974, p. 188.
88 Alex Comfort, 'Anxiety in adults', *Public Health*, 82:6 (1968), p. 284.
89 UCL Special Collections, Comfort Papers, Box 6, Cuttings Book, Alex Comfort, 'Don't think twice, it's alright', *Washington Post Book World*, 28 January 1973, p. 8.

2

'Two more calls, one in tears ...': emotion, labour, and ethics of care at the Calgary Birth Control Association, 1970–79

Karissa Robyn Patton

Introduction

On 15 December 1972, Calgary Birth Control Association volunteer Jean Phillips recorded the details of her shift in the Association's volunteer logbook.[1] She wrote,

> Two more calls, one in tears, wanting to come in tomorrow.
>
> To one in tears, 'Pull yourself together. Here we accomplish the impossible. Together we will think of something tomorrow.'
>
> She says, 'I feel better already.'[2]

Jean's notes demonstrate the intense emotions of some clients who reached out to the Calgary Birth Control Association (hereafter, CBCA, or the Association) for help with reproductive and sexual health matters. Jean's response to the client also illustrates her familiarity in addressing these emotion-filled interactions. This client was one of many women who contacted local birth control centres in tears upon finding out about an unwanted pregnancy, following a bad experience at a doctor's office, or after being diagnosed with a venereal disease (VD).[3] This interaction is just one example of how 1970s women's health centres, like the CBCA, were unique spaces where women came together to discuss deeply emotional issues and provide or receive emotional support.

Histories of the women's health movement in North America have outlined the development of feminist models of health in the 1970s that sought to bring women's healthcare into their 'own

'*Two more calls, one in tears ...*'   61

hands'.[4] The women's health movement saw the medical establishment as inherently patriarchal, and created centres offering an alternative model of health and service provision based on 'how they themselves wanted to be treated'.[5] Feminists strategically mobilised programmes and services that encouraged women to reclaim control over their own bodies and wellbeing. Educational programmes and literature were created to teach women about reproductive physiology, contraceptive choices, and other common women's health matters.[6] Service-based initiatives offered pregnancy testing, contraception and abortion counselling, and, on some occasions, facilitated abortion travel.[7] The women running these centres also offered consciousness-raising sessions about women's autonomy and liberation.[8] Through these activities women's health centres offered safe spaces for women to reclaim knowledge about their own bodies, reproduction, sexuality, and liberation.

The emotional labour and other labours of care provided within these women's health centres also became an essential part of the 1970s feminist model of health. Recent scholarship applies emotion as a lens of analysis to 'rethink histories of work and labour and of wider social and cultural life', underscores the historical links between women, work, and emotions, and demonstrates how women's everyday labour as caretakers is often under-recognised.[9] Building on this body of work, I analyse the history of the CBCA as part of the broader women's health movement through the lenses of emotion, care, and labour. Placing the history of the 1970s feminist model of health in conversation with feminist philosophies of care adds to the histories of women's health activism, 1970s feminism, women's labour, and health and healthcare.

The case study of the CBCA epitomises how gendered and undervalued labours of care became woven into feminist health models during the 1970s. Sources like Jean's volunteer 'diary', letters of appreciation from clients, and other CBCA administrative files show that CBCA workers embraced gendered notions of care for their own benefit and the benefit of their clients. Labours of care became essential to the success of both the service-based activism and the broader women's liberation goals of the CBCA. The daily labour of emotion management, relationship maintenance, and caretaking became essential to the CBCA's women-centred healthcare. The women at the CBCA grappled with a nuanced understanding

62 *Experiential expertise*

of labours of care. They critiqued the systemic gender binaries that essentialised, devalued, and dismissed these labours of care as women's work within the domestic sphere. But they also recognised the need for and value of labours of care within their communities and intentionally reclaimed these labours in juxtaposition to the misogynistic medical establishment. Ultimately, the women who worked at the Association intricately entwined feminist concepts of care and models of health to push back against patriarchal notions of objectivity and paternalism within mainstream medical spaces.

Caring away the patriarchy: feminist concepts of labours and ethics of care

Feminist explorations of gendered labour have demonstrated how the often-invisible labour of women and other marginalised groups is crucial to the everyday functioning of families, workplaces, and society.[10] In 1982, Arlie Russell Hochschild coined the terms 'emotional labour' to describe the management of emotions as part of a paid position, and 'emotion work' to describe non-paid work to manage emotions in private settings.[11] Hochschild's work provided a significant foundation for research about emotional interactions both within and outside the workplace.[12] Recently, scholars have blurred the lines between paid and unpaid labour, revealing the nuanced intersections of care, work, and gender in both public and private spaces. Eileen Boris and Rachel Salazar Parreñas introduced the concept of intimate labour to describe 'labours, both paid and unpaid, that sustain the day-to-day work that individuals and societies require to survive – and flourish', which encompass intimate needs like 'sexual gratification but also our bodily upkeep, care for loved ones, creating and sustaining social and emotional ties, and health and hygiene maintenance'. This concept highlights the intersections of emotional labour, intimate labour, the mental load, as well as domestic and reproductive work in how women, in particular, perform labours of care and shows that it is often impossible to separate 'home from work, work from labor, and productive from non-productive labor'.[13]

In addition to feminist concepts of emotion, care, and labour, feminist ethics of care and justice inform this analysis. Grace Clement's research on care, autonomy, and justice exposes the limits of masculinised and individualised understandings of care and justice and points to the important, yet undervalued, feminised work of relationship maintenance and interpersonal care. She argues that while much of this labour is gendered as feminine and has been used to justify women's subjugation within the private sphere, the broader cultural context that devalues these forms of labour is problematic, rather than the forms of labour themselves. In her view, 'care and autonomy are not mutually exclusive but are in many ways interdependent'.[14] Clement argues for a feminist ethic of care and justice that values the gendered labour of care for the purpose of justice against systemic patriarchy.

Using feminist concepts of emotional labour, intimate labour, and ethics of care and justice as a framework, this analysis recognises the CBCA as a local example of how emotion, care, and labour intersected in everyday healthcare provision. Concepts of emotional labour and intimate labour provide a framework to highlight the CBCA as a unique site of deep emotions and intimate discussions. The women working at the Association discussed intimate matters of sexual hygiene, sexual gratification, general wellbeing, and relationship maintenance with clients, which generated emotional conversations about contraceptive and abortion decisions, unwanted and wanted pregnancies, medical experiences, and day-to-day relationship joys and woes. Feminist ethics of care and justice provides a lens to understand how these labours of care were eventually politicised. Like Clement, the women running the CBCA both condemned the cultural gender roles used to confine women to the domestic sphere and recognised the value of gendered labours of care.

The Association staff and volunteers eventually emphasised the labours of care they provided to distinguish themselves from the patriarchal medical establishment. Like many women's health centres at the time, the CBCA's initial mandate was to provide immediate and on-the-ground reproductive and sexual healthcare in their communities. As contraceptive and abortion counselling took up more and more of their time, the women running the CBCA quickly realised that health service gaps were not the only issue their clients faced. In

64 *Experiential expertise*

the early 1970s women's health activists rejected medicine's dismissal of characteristics deemed too feminine, like empathy and care, in favour of the apparently more masculine attribute of objectivity.[15] In line with the broader women's health movement, the CBCA increasingly offered critiques of the kind of care clients received in clinics and hospitals as the decade progressed. As their critiques of the medical establishment continued, the women working at the Association developed and politicised their own model of care. They embraced characteristics, like empathy, intimacy, and emotion, that medicine had rejected as unprofessional. How the women at the CBCA provided care to clients did not significantly shift over the decade, but it became increasingly politicised as aligning with women's health critiques of the medical establishment.

The CBCA and women's healthcare in Alberta, Canada

The CBCA was established in the early 1970s and quickly became an important part of reproductive and sexual health services in Alberta, Canada. Originally created as an Abortion Information Centre in 1970 to help local women navigate Canada's new abortion laws (legislated in 1969), its workers rapidly realised that many clients also sought comprehensive information about their bodies, sex, reproduction, and general health.[16] In 1971, as they expanded their services to better fit with local women's needs, the group changed its name to the Calgary Birth Control Association, explaining that they were 'using "control" in its widest sense'.[17] The following year, the group conducted a city-wide survey to investigate what kind of services and education Calgary citizens needed and wanted. They continued to conduct formal feedback initiatives like surveys and questionnaires throughout the decade, as well as to collect informal feedback from volunteer logs, letters of appreciation, and physician information cards. These feedback strategies allowed CBCA workers to centre clients' experiences as they designed services that met on-the-ground needs in their communities.[18]

The CBCA was a particularly important resource, as it filled service gaps within the new provincial healthcare policy. In 1969, Alberta implemented its first provincial healthcare policy.[19] The rollout of this healthcare policy, years in the making, did not include the newly legalised contraception and abortion services. Birth control, abortion, and other reproductive and sexual health services remained in bureaucratic limbo until officially integrated into Alberta Healthcare between 1978 and 1979.[20] In this context, the Association formed an integral part of the healthcare landscape of the province.

By 1971 Calgary was the second-biggest city in Alberta, home to roughly 25 per cent of the province's citizens.[21] Located in a region where rural and urban boundaries blurred, the Association also became a hub for residents of the surrounding smaller cities, towns, and rural communities, including Indigenous women from urban areas and nearby reserves.[22] It served clients as close as the nearby town of Okotoks and the Tsuuit'ina reserve (only a forty- and thirty-minute drive from downtown Calgary, respectively), as well as those as far away as the northern community of Wanham (a ten-hour drive away when the road and weather conditions were good). The CBCA's local and regional programming depended on financial support from the local, provincial, and federal governments throughout the 1970s, and it benefited especially from the combination of Alberta's booming oil economy and a government that invested heavily in infrastructure and public services.[23]

To ensure access to public funds, the CBCA had to tread a careful political line. Like many similar women's health and reproductive rights services, it met with support, ambiguity, and opposition from different sections of the population.[24] This may explain why it is hard to find the words 'feminist' or 'women's liberation' in the CBCA's official and public materials.[25] In order to reach a broad audience, the Association had to frame itself as providing necessary services, but avoid publicly identifying as feminist.[26] But even if the feminist politics of the CBCA and other birth control centres were implicit rather than explicit, these were still radical enterprises. In an oral history interview Terri Forbis, who worked at the family planning centre in Lethbridge, Alberta in the late 1970s, explained the radical nature of on-the-ground service provision: 'it [sex] was just so not talked about, and people were really hungry for [information] [...] But they still had to get it served under the table. That's why the Birth Control and Information Centre was so controversial – it was really putting [sex and reproduction] on the table.'[27] While some of the workers may not have openly identified as feminist, the goals of the CBCA ultimately aligned with broader women's health

66   *Experiential expertise*

goals of liberating women from a patriarchal medical system. The establishment of a birth control centre as an alternative to medical institutions a mere year or two after decriminalisation was ground breaking.

Women's liberation philosophies featured prominently in the CBCA's resources, education materials, and internal organisational files. The women running the Association looked to diverse new and alternative health models as they designed services and education programmes.[28] They often pointed to the World Health Organization's definition of health as 'not simply absence of disease' but 'dependent on environment, nutrition, physical self, contentment, and feeling O.K. with oneself'.[29] They also argued that social and cultural circumstances tying women's self-worth to their husbands' and children's happiness contributed to women's poor health. Their literature and workshops dismantled gender roles, signposted women's independence from men and the state as important parts of reproductive and sexual health education, and emphasised women's ability to legally control their fertility as integral to accessing education and the workforce.[30] Bridging their clients' needs, scientific knowledge on sexuality and reproduction, and women's liberation goals, the CBCA perceived the health of the individual and the community as deeply connected.[31]

For CBCA activists, their clients' experiences revealed the need for not only services but also women's liberation in medical, political, and social spaces. Clients often cited the emotional and practical turmoil of navigating healthcare systems and unsympathetic medical professionals, making tough decisions about unplanned pregnancies, dealing with family conflict and abuse, fighting stigma and shame, and searching for fulfilment outside the confines of motherhood.[32] Women working at the Association knew they could not silo health work from broader women's liberation goals. In a summary of their educational outreach work in 1978 the CBCA education coordinators explained, 'It is apparent that no one working in the field of family planning can avoid becoming concerned with the status of women, and the reverse is equally true.'[33]

CBCA workers therefore often advised clients on issues beyond reproductive and sexual health matters. They heard stories about unpleasant doctors, problems with welfare and healthcare coverage,

'Two more calls, one in tears ...'

colonialist health policies, family and partner abuse, career trouble, sexism at school, relationship issues, and break-ups. They offered support both officially (through referrals to other services, keeping records of safe and blacklisted services, and helping clients access and navigate reproductive healthcare within the medical establishment) and unofficially (through general counselling and support). In doing so, CBCA employees and volunteers offered care unlike Calgary's other medical and educational services. These labours of care became a significant part of the feminist model of health that distinguished the CBCA from the medical establishment.

Caring as a radical act

The 1970s women's health movement challenged the notions of medical and scientific 'objectivity' that underpinned sharply gendered power dynamics within and outside medical spaces.[34] Many feminists argued that existing social and cultural systems were inherently patriarchal and called for the complete restructuring of economic, political, and legal institutions – including medical and scientific establishments.[35] Women's health activists therefore intentionally centred 'feminised' characteristics and labour. They purposely practised a model of healthcare that made space for emotion, experience, and caring as acts of resistance to the traditional, hierarchical doctor–patient relationship. Their conscious performance of emotional labour and labours of care were informed by women's liberation goals and distinguished them from the medical establishment.

The CBCA's archival fonds shows how this model of health functioned, and the labours of care provided within the walls of the Association. Administrative files such as educational programming materials, physician information cards, and letters of appreciation from clients all offer insight into the CBCA's overarching goals. Jean's 'diary' entries from the volunteer logbook, unmatched in detail by any other logbook entries, stand out as providing insights into day-to-day interactions. They reveal how the labours of care undertaken at the CBCA intervened in local medical and social landscapes and power dynamics.

68   *Experiential expertise*

Clients noticed and appreciated these acts of care and recognised the CBCA and the women who ran it as making a difference to their lives. One 1974 letter to the Association's then president, Gunilla Mungan, stated: 'I hope it makes you happy to know you really helped me. I have adjusted to the pill very well [...] Life is generally very happy and this world is a beautiful one with people like you around who care.'[36] Another client sent Jean a card in 1975 and wrote, 'Sorry I couldn't come and thank you personally. My request went through + the operation was Thursday, July 22nd. Everything seems so much brighter now. Thank you for being understanding and helping me. The centre is a very worthwhile cause.'[37] Other letters referred to the CBCA generally as a safe alternative to other social and medical services. In 1977 two clients sent a thank you card to the CBCA. One thanked the Association for not passing judgement: 'you just listen, and as far as I am concerned when a person has another person who will just listen and offer suggestions that person is pretty lucky. I know I sure was. Thanks.' The other signee wrote, 'Thanks for all the help and understanding. I couldn't have made it without you.'[38] These thank you letters and cards speak to the interpersonal care provided at the CBCA, and how much these local alternative health centres mattered in providing on-the-ground care.

The provision of care, not just services, at the CBCA was a labour-intensive and radical act. Attending to clients' personal emotional and social wellbeing, as well as their reproductive and sexual health needs, became inseparable from the CBCA's women's liberation practice and healthcare provision. Understanding the intentionality behind these labours of care is important. Jean's diaries flag that care was central to the CBCA's mission (Figure 2.1). In conversation with two teenagers about unwanted pregnancy, contraception, and abortion, Jean stated, 'we [the CBCA] are here with help, dished out with t.l.c'.[39] This description rhetorically situates the CBCA in opposition to other medical spaces. Jean's emphasis on care suggests that CBCA workers did not perform emotional labour or other labours of care through adherence to gendered notions of caregiving, but to reclaim labours of care previously cast out of biomedical models. The CBCA's model flipped the script about labours of care and emotional labour, turning them into intentional acts to dismantle the medical establishment's systemic

'Two more calls, one in tears ...'

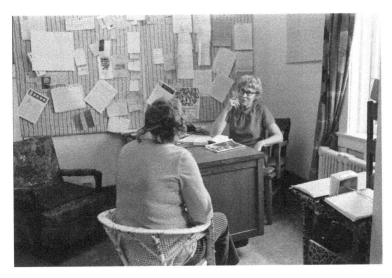

Figure 2.1 'CBCA volunteer, Jean Phillips, gives birth control advice', *Calgary Herald*, 15 January 1973. Courtesy of Glenbow Archives, Archives and Special Collections, University of Calgary. All rights reserved and permission to use the figure must be obtained from the copyright holder.

misogyny. In doing so, the CBCA created a network of care that allowed local reproductive and sexual healthcare to flourish.

Putting the care into healthcare

Throughout the 1970s, clients called, wrote, or visited the CBCA and shared their experiences with local medical professionals and services. Jean's logs outline good and bad encounters with local health professionals. She recorded small details about doctors and nurses encountered when facilitating abortion or contraceptive appointments. In a note about a woman travelling from Calgary to the nearby small city of Drumheller for an abortion, Jean wrote, 'nurse very nice, asked client if she had someone to stay with, etc'.[40] Conversely, one of Jean's notes two days later recorded, 'a girl phoned and said that Dr. [redacted in source] had inserted a

70 *Experiential expertise*

[contraceptive] loop on Wednesday. She said she has never had a child and said she screamed her head off and the nurse had to hold her down.'[41] Jean documented this physician's name and told the woman about a CBCA-approved doctor who would remove the loop and insert an IUD [intrauterine device] under anaesthetic if the pain did not subside soon.[42]

Many volunteers and employees also contributed to a collection of over 130 local medical professionals and services. These 'Physician Information Cards', created in 1972, detailed the services were available at each clinic *and* any bad experiences clients had with specific medical professionals.[43] This detail-oriented labour of record-keeping and relationship management parallels the gendered labour of kinship maintenance outlined in Micaela di Leonardo's foundational scholarship. Leonardo argues that care and emotional and mental management are fundamental to women's kinship work, such as letter and telephone correspondence, organising visits and gifts, establishing and maintaining relationships, and decisions about breaking or strengthening certain relationships, and that these kinds of labour are 'products of conscious strategy [...] sources of women's autonomous power and possible primary sites of emotional fulfilment, and, at times, the vehicles for actual survival and/or political resistance'.[44] The women running the CBCA used similar skills to create and maintain safe networks of care in their local and regional medical communities.

This work was essential to women's wellbeing in the 1970s. After 1969, members of the medical community debated their role as reproductive and sexual health service providers. The CBCA had some medical allies. Local doctor Ruth Simkin, for instance, advocated for the CBCA in the local media, endorsing its provision of integral birth control information and urging 'Calgary doctors to publicly support the work of the birth control association to ensure its continued operation'.[45] However, despite decriminalisation, some physicians believed that contraception and abortion were immoral and refused to offer certain reproductive and sexual health services that did not align with their moral or religious beliefs.[46] The Association flagged one Calgary doctor who was 'not in favour of abortion' after he 'spent ½ hour trying to talk unmarried school girl into having the baby'.[47] Some physicians who did prescribe contraception and abortion referrals regularly shamed unmarried women for being

'Two more calls, one in tears ...'

sexually active outside of marriage. In 1974 the CBCA noted that one physician had scolded a single woman seeking a birth control prescription and told her, 'You shouldn't think of things like that until you're married.'[48]

Other physicians supported provision of abortion and contraception but argued about who should regulate their use. The role of the Therapeutic Abortion Committee (TAC) in particular came to a head in response to feminist calls for 'abortion on demand'.[49] In 1975, the TAC Chairman at one Calgary hospital, Dr K.I. Pearce, directly opposed women's calls for abortion on demand and positioned 'objective' physicians as most capable of making responsible decisions: 'Abortions on demand becomes an unacceptable ethical alternative unless there is a built in careful, informed and personally detached professional examination of the total situation the patient finds herself in and not just the pregnancy alone.'[50] This situation left individual citizens guessing where to turn when in need of contraception, abortion, vasectomy, VD, or pregnancy testing services.

In this context, the CBCA's detailed records of physicians and services provided essential practical information. For example, a 1972 log from Jean stated, 'This client saw a "Dr. M." and [the client] will "call after he has a vasectomy done ... I just asked him to let us know how he liked Dr. M"'.[51] Frequently updated throughout the decade, this directory broke down whether each doctor or clinic would provide abortion referrals, prescribe contraception, insert intrauterine devices, perform voluntary sterilisation surgeries (tubal ligation or vasectomy), and serve the teen population without parental consent (a major factor in providing local teens with contraception or abortion referrals).[52] One entry stated that a local doctor, 'does not require parents' consent for B.C. [birth control]. Will not take referrals for abortion.' Another information card recorded, 'Will take referrals for 18 years and older. Doesn't do IUD. Very pleasant and charming man, sympathetic, but won't be too helpful for young girls or for abortions.'[53]

Like many other women's health services in the 1970s, the CBCA's information cards about clients' experiences with individual physicians were particularly useful. A handwritten note on one card read, 'Aug, 75 – client reported [name redacted] was rude!' Other cards recorded more devastating experiences, like 'he misdiagnosed a woman's

72 *Experiential expertise*

pregnancy. Did not catch error until she was 4 mo. [months along]' and 'one woman mentioned that [name redacted] was a thoroughly repulsive, disgusting man, would only do abortion if she had a tubal [ligation] since she was so irresponsible'.[54] The inclusion of clients' experiences shows that the purpose of the physician information cards was both directive and preventative. The information cards gave the CBCA volunteers and employees the knowledge of where clients could access specific reproductive and sexual healthcare services, but were also critical in building a trusted healthcare network of supportive medical professionals in the region who would treat CBCA clients with the care they deserved.

This record-keeping labour could make a particular difference for low-income clients who dealt with the overlapping burdens of misogyny and classism when seeking reproductive and sexual health services. Canadian Medicare was supposed to equalise access to medical services, and the new provincial healthcare policy covered most of the cost of abortion approved by TACs and general physician appointments, but costs for some prescription appointments, specialised referrals, testing, and anaesthetic were left to individual hospital administrators' and physicians' discretion.[55] For youth, low-income clients, and clients on welfare, it was important to know which clinics and physicians charged fees above Medicare before they went in. The CBCA's physician information cards often recorded the cost of services for individual physicians and clinics, stating, for example, 'charges $50', 'charges $20 for an IUD', or 'does not charge above Medicare'.[56] Jean's notes reveal how important it was to 'bring up the money part' during any healthcare counselling sessions 'so there are no problems when the girl goes for her appointment'.[57] Jean was particularly careful about recording clients' financial situations during her counselling sessions. One note recorded, 'Girl has been out of work for five weeks but can handle money end of it – no help from guy.'[58] Her volunteer log entries also demonstrate how quickly volunteers navigated concerns about cost and access to low-cost reproductive and sexual health services. One entry described:

> Phone call 'I had to go off the pill and I want a loop and my doctor says I will have to pay him $30.00. I am on welfare and can't pay it.'

'Two more calls, one in tears ...'   73

'O.K. phone Family Planning and make an appointment. This is the phone number and these are the times you can see a doctor. Call us if you need us further. Have a good day.'

Doesn't her doctor know about family planning? Or doesn't he care?[59]

For a teen, a single mother, or someone on welfare, the extra cost of a doctor's appointment or procedure was significant. The CBCA's detailed information on costs tried to prevent financial distress for clients.

This approach also helped Indigenous clients navigating the intersecting barriers of misogyny, classism, and colonialist policies. While the Canadian Medical Care Act mandated healthcare across the nation, it made healthcare a provincial power and responsibility. This meant that provinces had to create healthcare policies with their own funding and bureaucratic systems. However, late nineteenth-century treaties made between Indigenous nations and the federal government of Canada stated that the federal government would finance and provide healthcare to Indigenous people. As healthcare programmes were rolled out for non-Indigenous citizens in Alberta in 1969, the federal and provincial governments debated whether Indigenous peoples' healthcare was a federal or provincial responsibility, and resultantly who should pay for these services.[60]

One particularly detailed 1972 entry from Jean (over two pages in length) recorded the bureaucratic hoops an Indigenous client had to jump through because of the political squabbling:

'Sit down and tell me your problem.'

'I have v.d. I've been for a penicillin shot. They gave me some antibiotics too. I told them I was pregnant, and they sent me to the Family Planning Clinic. They wouldn't talk to me there and said to go and see you.' ... 'I am living common-law. We are on welfare and welfare knows me only as Mrs. [name redacted in source]. No, the Indian Affairs wouldn't help [...] We have no money [...] I go to the South Side welfare office.'

All this in answer to my questions. 'Gosh, dear, I just can't send you to a doctor from here, under these circumstances. I'll call your worker and we'll work together.'

Call Social Development, Mr. [name redacted from source], her worker is out for the rest of the day. Talk to his secretary. Yes, welfare pays

74 *Experiential expertise*

her medical expenses, but secretary hasn't run into an abortion case before and just doesn't know.

Make an appointment for Mrs. B. to see Mr. [redacted] Monday morning, December 18, at 9 a.m. (she wouldn't tell me her correct name).

'I have to have another penicillin shot on Monday morning.'

'That's O.K. They open at 8:30. Be there, then head straight for the S.D. office.' [...] Give her the names of Drs. [redacted from source]. They have all handled welfare abortions, waiving their fees over and above. He [welfare worker] can contact them direct or he can work through us, doesn't matter.[61]

'Mrs. B' had been bounced between a local welfare office, the Calgary Family Planning Clinic, and Indian Affairs. She was left with no medical appointments and only the suggestion to visit the CBCA. Jean normally sent low-income and welfare clients to the family planning clinic that provided appointments for VD treatments, contraception prescriptions, and abortion referrals at no cost and directly charged provincial healthcare. But it is likely that Mrs B, as an Indigenous person, was not covered under provincial healthcare. Jean took on the labour to help Mrs B get an abortion referral appointment that no other paid social or health service employee would provide. She even instructed the welfare office secretary through the process of booking abortions that were paid through welfare during the session with Mrs B. It is unclear how much time Jean spent with this client, but her knowledge of the relevant systems demonstrates the impact of the CBCA's sympathetic healthcare network in navigating colonial bureaucracies. This time and care in addressing clients' needs set the CBCA apart from other medical services in Calgary and area.

For these reasons, the Association became locally and regionally known as a safe place to go. Jean herself even became known among local women: 'Phone call from a girl asking for Mrs. Phillips. "Mrs. Phillips, Melanie told me to call you. My sister is pregnant and Melanie said to get in touch with you."'[62] This speaks to the quality of care provided to clients and the success of networks created between clients, the CBCA, and local physicians in 1970s southern Alberta. This strong healthcare network allowed the women working at the CBCA to provide immediate on-the-ground care daily. Their

The care beyond healthcare

Fuelled by broader women's liberation goals, CBCA workers often counselled clients on issues beyond reproductive and sexual health matters. The CBCA's broad definition of health, as well as its calls for social reform, demonstrates its commitment to the physical, emotional, and cultural wellbeing of clients. CBCA volunteers and employees promoted and supported many local and national 'women's' causes and worked with other feminist groups advocating for marriage and property law reform, equal pay, reproductive rights, women's shelters, and rape crisis centres.[63] The women working at the Association knew that ending women's reliance on men as health practitioners was essential to their liberation.

As clients reached out to the CBCA to access local health services, they also sought counsel about family, relationship, and personal issues. During contraceptive and abortion counselling sessions, women discussed their dissatisfaction with their jobs and their aspirations to go to university, confessed to having affairs, and disclosed stories of abuse.[64] CBCA activists developed expertise in helping clients navigate their health and personal quandaries. Jean's 'diary' log entries captured some of these emotionally fraught but common conversations and provide detailed examples of the blurring of health and social wellbeing in CBCA clients' daily lives. Jean noted that when she and Mrs B spoke 'casually' at the end of the VD and abortion counselling session, she heard about Mrs B's relationship woes and financial dependence on her partner:

> 'How did you know you had v.d. Pretty hard for a girl to tell, sometimes.'
>
> 'Bill went down and found out he had it, so they sent for me.'
>
> I wonder – who gave it to who?
>
> 'I want to get married but Bill doesn't want to.' I have to bite my tongue to keep from saying 'so your luck hasn't been all bad.'

76   *Experiential expertise*

'Talk to your worker about some training.'

'I started a course in hairdressing but quit after two months.'

'Life should hold something better than this for you, discuss it with [welfare worker].'

'Yes I will.'[65]

Jean dealt directly with the problem of accessing abortion services while also trying to help this client lead a liberated life, defined by her own career, wants, and needs. Volunteers put women's individual lives and experiences in conversation with social, political, and reproductive contexts to encourage women's liberation. In doing so, they established the centre as space for clients to get reproductive and sexual healthcare beyond clinical care.

Some clients disclosed disturbing stories of abusive family members or partners. Jean recorded one conversation about a pregnant woman and her sister. After Jean helped the client make an abortion referral appointment with a local doctor she asked, 'Well is there anything you would like to tell me.'[66] In response, the client and her sister told Jean about their abusive father:

Non-pregnant girl 'Our dad is a bastard. I had to quit school. He threw me across the room and my spine is wrecked. I just found yesterday I have to have an operation on the top of my spine and they think maybe the lower part too.'

'Why didn't you get the doctor to arrange for you to move out of your home?'

'I moved out on my own and my parents sent the morality squad around and they took me home. You see I am under age.'

'Has he laid his hands on you since?'

'No.'

Pregnant girl 'But he broke my nose last summer. My boyfriend was there and took me to emergency [...] they wanted to send the police around. I begged them not to because I could have moved out, I was working, but life would have been hell for my sister then.' [...]

'O.K. As soon as you start this new job, you must move out. And (to other girl) after your spinal operation, you have to get out of that

'Two more calls, one in tears ...'   77

house.' [...] 'This is my home phone, I want to know how everything went, and if either of you want to talk just give me a call.'

'Oh, we already have your home phone and address. Melanie gave us that in case you weren't here today.'[67]

Clearly this was not the first time Jean had offered her own contact information to young clients. This level of care was labour intensive and emotionally draining, yet Jean and others enthusiastically incorporated it into their volunteer roles because they knew it was necessary in facilitating their clients' overall wellbeing. CBCA workers knew that abandoning the intense labour of caring meant abandoning clients to the medical institutions and systemic patriarchy they sought to disrupt. They were acutely aware that women's health was not confined to healthcare spaces. Rather, they recognised that women's overarching health and wellbeing depended on their liberation in all political and social spaces. The labour, emotion, and care inherent in these counselling sessions provided a necessary and immediate intervention in these clients' situations.

Conclusion

The case study of the CBCA illustrates how the combined lenses of emotion, care, and labour reveal important insights into health history. Examining labours of care, inclusive of emotional and intimate labour, relationship maintenance, and record-keeping, alongside more traditionally discussed forms of labour, like service provision, exposes how healthcare systems functioned on the ground. Jean's logs of daily life within the Association in particular, underscored the deeply emotional conversations, the labour of care performed by volunteers and employees, and the intricate networks of care that CBCA activists created in 1970s southern Alberta. The women running the CBCA recognised work like counselling, relationship maintenance, and record-keeping as essential to navigating the new reproductive and sexual healthcare landscapes and positioned themselves as a distinct alternative to the biomedical establishment. In doing so, they did not separate medical decisions about abortion procedures, VD treatments, or contraceptive choices from their clients' everyday life. They knew that these reproductive and sexual

78 *Experiential expertise*

health matters intersected with clients' home life, relationships, living situations, and jobs. Despite mainstream medical arguments for objective and authoritative medical expertise, the CBCA's dedication to alternative care models exposes the value and legitimacy of gendered labours of care in the functioning of healthcare systems and society in the 1970s.

Notes

1 Glenbow Archives, Calgary, Alberta (hereafter GBA), Calgary Birth Control Association Collection (hereafter CBCA), M-7265-39, 'Diary', volunteer log by Jean Phillips, 1972.
2 GBA, CBCA, M-7265-39, Phillips, 'Diary', 1972.
3 Sandra Morgen, *Into Our Own Hands: The Women's Health Movement in the United States, 1969–1990* (New Brunswick, NJ: Rutgers University Press, 2002); Karissa Patton, 'Con(tra)cepts of Care: Southern Alberta Birth Control Centres and Reproductive Healthcare, 1969–1979' (PhD thesis, University of Saskatchewan, 2021); Beth Palmer, '"Lonely, tragic, but legally necessary pilgrimages": transnational abortion travel in the 1970s', *Canadian Historical Review*, 92:4 (2011).
4 Morgen, *Into Our Own Hands*.
5 Quotation from Laura Kaplan, *The Story of Jane: The Legendary Underground Feminist Abortion Service* (New York: Pantheon Books, 1996), p. x.
6 Wendy Kline, 'The making of *Our Bodies, Ourselves*: rethinking women's health and second-wave feminism', in Stephanie Gilmore and Sara Evans (eds), *Feminist Coalitions: Historical Perspectives on Second Wave Feminism in the United States* (Urbana, IL: University of Illinois Press, 2008), p. 64; Christabelle Sethna, 'The evolution of the *Birth Control Handbook*: from student peer-education manual to feminist self-empowerment text, 1968–1975', *Canadian Bulletin of Medical History*, 23:1 (2006).
7 Wendy Kline, *Bodies of Knowledge: Sexuality, Reproduction, and Women's Health in the Second Wave* (Chicago, IL: University of Chicago Press, 2010), p. 2; Morgen, *Into Our Own Hands*, p. 105; Palmer, '"Lonely, tragic, but legally necessary pilgrimages"'.
8 Hannah Dudley-Shotwell, *Revolutionizing Women's Healthcare: The Feminist Self-Help Movement in America* (New Brunswick, NJ: Rutgers University Press, 2020), pp. 15–16; Loraine Greaves, *Personal and Political: Stories from the Women's Health Movement, 1960–2010* (Toronto, ON: Second Story Press, 2018), p. 11.

'*Two more calls, one in tears ...*'   79

9   Quotation from Agnes Arnold Forster and Alison Mould, 'Introduction', in Agnes Arnold Forster and Alison Mould (eds), *Feelings and Work in Modern History: Emotional Labour and Emotions about Labour* (New York: Bloomsbury, 2022), p. 3. See also Barbara Brookes, Jane McCabe, and Angela Wanahalla, 'Introduction: care matters', in Barbara Brookes, Jane McCabe, and Angela Wanahalla (eds), *Past Caring? Women, Work, and Emotion* (Dunedin, OTA: Otago University Press, 2019), pp. 9–12.

10 Gemma Hartley, *Fed Up: Emotional Labour, Women, and the Way Forward* (New York: Harper One Press, 2018); Micaela de Leonardo, 'The female world of cards and holidays: women, families, and the work of kinship', *Signs: Journal of Women in Culture and Society*, 12:3 (1987); Thea Cacchioni, *Big Pharma, Women, and the Labour of Love* (Toronto, ON: University of Toronto Press, 2015).

11 Arlie Russel Hochschild, *The Managed Heart: Commercialization of Human Feeling* (Berkeley, CA: University of California Press, 1982, 2012), p. 5.

12 See, for example, Alicia Grandey, James Diefendorff, and Deborah E. Rupp, *Emotional Labor in the 21st Century: Diverse Perspectives in Emotion Regulation at Work* (New York: Routledge, 2013); Mckelvey Kelly, 'Seven Generations: Emotion Work, Women, and the Anderdon Wyndot Cemetery, 1790–1914' (Master's Thesis, University of Saskatchewan, 2019); Rebecca J. Erickson and Amy S. Warton, 'Managing emotions on the job and at home: understanding the consequences of multiple emotional roles', *Academy of Management Review*, 18:3 (1993).

13 Eileen Boris and Rachel Salazar Parreñas (eds), *Intimate Labors: Cultures Technologies, and the Politics of Care* (Redwood City, CA: Stanford University Press, 2010), pp. 5, 7.

14 Grace Clement, *Care, Autonomy, and Justice: Feminism and the Ethic of Care* (New York: Routledge, 1996, 2018), pp. 2, 6–7, 11–12.

15 Kline, *Bodies of Knowledge*, p. 2.

16 GBA, CBCA, M-7265-12, 'Notebook', c. 1970–72; GBA, CBCA, M-7265-185, 'History', c. 1978.

17 GBA, CBCA, M-7265-240, 'Newsletter', 17 July 1971.

18 GBA, CBCA, M-7265-240, 'Newsletter', July 1971; 'Newsletter', 21 March 1972; GBA, CBCA, M-7265-334 to M-7265-346, 'Questionnaires', 1972–78.

19 Shannon Stettner, *Without Apology: Writings on Abortion in Canada* (Edmonton, AB: Athabasca University Press, 2016), p. 43.

20 Galt Museum and Archives (hereafter GMA), Lethbridge, Alberta, transcript, 20171019, Terri Forbis, interview, 24 January 2013.

80   *Experiential expertise*

21 'Table A2-14 Population of Canada, by province, census dates, 1851 to 1976', Census of Canada, 1971, Vol. I, part 2, table 14; 'Table 3: Population for census divisions and subdivisions, 1971 and 1976', 1976 Census of Canada Volume I: Population, Geographic Distributions. Ottawa: Statistics Canada.

22 Patton, 'Con(tra)cepts of care'; see also GBA, CBCA, M-7265-79 to -95, 'Correspondence Files', 1971–79; GBA, CBCA, M-7265-99, 'Education Outreach', Local Initiatives Project, 1973.

23 GBA, CBCA, M-7265-65, 'Strategy Committee Files', 1977; Patton, 'Con(tra)cepts of care'; Paul Brunner (ed.), *Lougheed and The War with Ottawa*, Vol. 11 in *Alberta in the 20th Century: A Journalistic History of the Province* (Edmonton, AB: United Western Communications Ltd, 2002), pp. 17–18.

24 Katrina Ackerman and Shannon Stettner, '"The public is not ready for this": 1969 and the long road to abortion access', *Canadian Historical Review*, 100:2 (2019); Erika Dyck and Karissa Patton, 'Activists in the Bible Belt: conservatism, religion, and recognizing reproductive rights in 1970s Southern Alberta', in Sarah Carter and Nancy Langford (eds), *Compelled to Act: Histories of Women's Activism in Western Canada* (Winnipeg, MB: University of Manitoba Press, 2020); Nancy Janovicek, 'Protecting access to abortion services in rural Canada: a case study of the West Kootenays, British Columbia', *Women's History Magazine*, 73 (Autumn, 2013).

25 Palmer, '"Lonely, tragic but legally necessary pilgrimages"', 644, 663.

26 Nancy Janovicek, *No Place to Go: Local Histories of the Battered Women's Shelter Movement* (Vancouver, BC: University of British Columbia Press, 2007), p. 3; Tessa Jordan, *Feminist Acts: Branching Out Magazine and the Making of Canadian Feminism* (Edmonton, AB: University of Alberta Press, 2019), p. xxvii.

27 GMA, Forbis interview, 2013.

28 Patton, 'Con(tra)cepts of care'.

29 GBA, CBCA, M-7265-458, Proposal for the Women's Health Weekend Workshop, 1976.

30 GBA, CBCA, M-7265-99, 'Living with Sex'; GBA, CBCA, M-7265-100, Resource outline – Abortion, 1973.

31 Patton, 'Con(tra)cepts of care'.

32 GBA, CBCA, M-7265-458, Proposal for the Women's Health Weekend Workshop, 1976.

33 GBA, CBCA, M-7265-120, 4, 'Peer Education'.

34 Kline, *Bodies of Knowledge*, pp. 2–6; Whitney Wood, '"Put right under": obstetric violence in post-war Canada', *Social History of Medicine*, 31:4 (2018).

'Two more calls, one in tears ...' 81

35 Linda Nicholson, *The Second Wave: A Reader in Feminist Theory* (New York and London: Routledge, 1997), p. 3; Kline, *Bodies of Knowledge*, p. 1–3; Greaves, *Personal and Political*, pp. 10, 13.

36 GBA, CBCA, M-7265-191, 'Letter of appreciation', 1974.

37 GBA, CBCA, M-7265-192, 'Letter of appreciation', 1975.

38 GBA, CBCA, M-7265-193, 'Letter of appreciation', c. 1976–77.

39 GBA, CBCA, Phillips, 'Diary', 1972.

40 GBA, CBCA, Phillips, 'Diary', 1972.

41 GBA, CBCA, Phillips, 'Diary', 1972.

42 GBA, CBCA, Phillips, 'Diary', 1972.

43 GBA, CBCA, M-7265-282, Physician Information Cards. c. 1972–78.

44 Leonardo, 'The female world of cards and holidays', 441–2.

45 GBA, CBCA, M-7265-170, Newspaper clipping, periodical unknown, 'CBCA "prevention" defended by doctor', 14 February 1975.

46 GMA, transcript, 20171019, Rita Moir, interview, 13 December 2012.

47 GBA, CBCA, Physician Information Cards, c. 1972–78.

48 GBA, CBCA, Physician Information Cards, c. 1972–78.

49 Judy Rebick, *Ten Thousand Roses: The Making of a Feminist Revolution* (Toronto, ON: Penguin Canada, 2005).

50 Anon., 'For and Against Factions Don't Even Agree on Names', *Calgary Herald*, 2 August 1975, p. 25.

51 GBA, CBCA, Phillips, 'Diary', 1972.

52 GBA, CBCA, Physician Information Cards, c. 1972–78.

53 GBA, CBCA, Physician Information Cards, c. 1972–78.

54 GBA, CBCA, Physician Information Cards, c. 1972–78.

55 GBA, CBCA, M-7265-82, 'Letter from J.M. Dewart', 9 May 1973.

56 GBA, CBCA, Physician Information Cards, c. 1972–78.

57 GBA, CBCA, Phillips, 'Diary', 1972.

58 GBA, CBCA, Phillips, 'Diary', 1972.

59 GBA, CBCA, Phillips, 'Diary', 1972.

60 Erika Dyck, *Facing Eugenics: Reproduction, Sterilization, and the Politics of Choice* (Toronto, ON: University of Toronto Press, 2013), pp. 56–7; Maureen Lux, *Separate Beds: A History of Indian Hospitals in Canada, 1920s–1980s* (Toronto, ON: University of Toronto Press, 2016).

61 GBA, CBCA, Phillips, 'Diary', 1972.

62 GBA, CBCA, Phillips, 'Diary', 1972.

63 GBA, CBCA, M-7265-240, 'Newsletter', 15 September 1972, 3; GBA, CBCA, M-7265-99 to M-7265-101, Educational Outreach, 1968–79.

64 GBA, CBCA, Phillips, 'Diary', 1972.

65 GBA, CBCA, Phillips, 'Diary', 1972.

66 GBA, CBCA, Phillips, 'Diary', 1972.

67 GBA, CBCA, Phillips, 'Diary', 1972.

3

Expertise and experience in the Greek feminist birth control movement, c. 1974–86

Evangelia Chordaki

Introduction

The first feminist birth control movement emerged in Greece in 1974, after the fall of the dictatorial regime and in the era of Metapolitefsi, and ended in 1986 when the Greek constitution decriminalised abortion.[1] The Constitution of 1974 acknowledged the equal rights of Greek men and women for the first time, with important repercussions for matters of marriage, reproduction, family, and the role of women in society. In 1980, it became legal to disseminate family planning advice in state clinics, effectively making female-controlled forms of contraception accessible for the first time. Until this point, women had no access to contraceptives and so had to rely on their sexual partners to practise withdrawal or to use condoms. As a result, although abortion was illegal, it was also the only secure means of preventing birth. Gynaecologists who performed abortion under the pretence of treating medical conditions were not usually prosecuted. This led to an extremely high rate of abortion, with one study in the late 1960s suggesting that as many as one third of all pregnancies might end in termination.[2] The feminist birth control movement sought to change this situation.

The foundation of this movement demonstrates Greece's openness to wider European trends, including the liberalisation of sexual attitudes, in the era of democratic transition.[3] It was one of many social and political movements – including feminist, LGBT, ecological, anti-militarist, prison abolition, and HIV and AIDS pressure groups – that 'shaped the balances and priorities' of the period.[4] Like these

The Greek feminist birth control movement   83

other movements, it was linked to universities, the politicisation of young people, and the development of different types of public life, places, and spaces. Women's movement activists of the Metapolitefsi period struggled for political equality, bodily and sexual self-determination, to reclaim public space, and to politicise so-called private or personal experience. They recognised gender not only as a 'field of violent disciplinisation and traumatism but also as a space for collective action towards equality and liberty'.[5] In their political analysis and organisational structures, women's movement activists and feminists insisted on women's right to autonomy.

I use the terms 'women's movement activists' and 'feminists' because in the Greek context women's activism and action are not always best described simply as 'feminist'. Women's movement activists of this period rarely used the terms 'feminist' or 'feminism'. Instead, they often referred to the 'women's movement' (γυναικείο κίνημα) or to 'women's issues' (γυναικείο ζήτημα).[6] As Athena Athanasiou argues, in these contexts the term 'women' signified 'organisation against gender hierarchies, including the dominant feminine'.[7] This usage may correspond with a feminist politics (broadly defined), but it is important not to bracket all activists under that term, partly because we need to differentiate state feminists, who were linked to political parties, from those in grassroots organisations.

Although state feminists and those in the women's movement both actively participated in the Greek feminist birth control movement, they took very different approaches to experiential expertise. State feminists focused on women's participation in formal politics, prioritised medical expertise, and saw women's experiential expertise as, at best, merely additional to existing systems of knowledge. Women's movement activists focused on self-organisation, self-education, and self-determination, prioritising experiential expertise as a form of knowledge that could interact with medical expertise but was not inferior to it. This distinction is important for this chapter, which charts the development of approaches to experiential expertise in the feminist birth control movement, with particular focus on the women's movement.

The chapter examines the emergence of experience-centred philosophies of knowledge within the Greek feminist birth control movement. It shows how these concepts of experiential knowledge were firmly situated within national and international networks,

84   *Experiential expertise*

through which activists adopted and modified the aims and practices of other feminist movements to the Greek context. It makes extensive use of informal archives; items carefully preserved in private collections by Dr Eftychia Leontidou, a gynaecologist and founder member of the Autonomous Women's Movement, and by Anna Mihopoulou and other supporters of the Delfis Archival Center, established in the back room of the Women's Bookstore in Athens during the Metapolitefsi period. In drawing on material that exists beyond state-controlled archives, I work within the same tradition of looking beyond formal or professional expertise, and taking seriously women's experiential knowledge that inspired women's movement activists in the 1970s and 1980s.

I start by exploring different approaches to the concept of experiential expertise, including how we can draw on feminist methodologies to theorise experiential expertise. I then discuss the Greek feminist birth control movement as an example of a boundary movement that deconstructed demarcations between scientific and non-scientific knowledge and between experts and lay actors. The concept of boundary movements is useful because it situates social movements as 'cultural and analytical spaces' that 'move between social worlds and realms of knowledge'.[8] Here, I deploy the concept to show how women's movement activists blurred the lines between scientific and experiential expertise, developing a rival form of knowledge that illuminates aspects of women's 'everyday health' in a period of social and political transformation.

Approaches to experiential expertise

There are many different ways of approaching the concept of experiential expertise. Each involves judgements about the value of emotional, embodied, and subjective understandings as compared to more abstract, theorised, and formal knowledge, and whether it is possible to reconcile experiential and scientific forms of knowledge. Such judgements are inevitably perspectival, based in turn on different and often contested notions of 'expertise'. This section first examines current approaches to experiential expertise within the interdisciplinary fields of science and technology studies (STS) and health studies. It then considers how (following Sara Ahmed) a feminist

The Greek feminist birth control movement   85

positioning of experiential expertise as a 'sweaty concept' brings marginalised voices and perspectives into the picture, in this way challenging the blind spots of existing disciplinary notions. As will be seen in the remainder of the chapter, this approach also illuminates how and why the Greek birth control movement (a boundary movement) formulated and deployed sweaty concepts of experiential expertise within particular 'cultural and analytic spaces' as its participants moved between different 'social worlds and realms of knowledge'.

The traditional practice of science and technology rests on very formalised notions of expertise, and so STS scholars often wrestle with how to incorporate the concept of experiential expertise with existing understandings of scientific expertise.[9] Harry Collins and Robert Evans argue that the concept of experiential expertise itself derives from the perceived need to classify both 'science' and 'expertise', to understand the differentiation between scientific and other types of knowledge and expertise, and to reconfigure the relationship between experts (specialists) and the public (others).[10] STS scholars therefore often attempt to delineate under what circumstances experience might legitimately contribute to knowledge formation – looking at, for example, the perceived validity and potential wider applicability of specific types of experience (such as embodied or empathetic), as well as their compatibility with scientific expertise, which is always seen as primary.[11] Within STS, then, the concept of experiential expertise is always situated within a wider discourse about what kinds of knowledge are legitimate, what constitutes expertise and who can claim it, what kinds of knowledge *only* scientific experts can claim, and the relationship of knowledge and expertise to authority.

Approaches to experiential expertise within health studies usually start from a different premise. In this field, scholars are more concerned to bridge the gap between experiential and professional knowledge in order to democratise knowledge, empower patients, and improve both participation in healthcare and the quality of that care.[12] Health studies scholars are keen to understand how different aspects of identity affect health experience, and how subordinated groups create experiential expertise as a form of resistance to dominant knowledges and to domination.[13] In contrast to STS, the crucial question here is not whether experiential expertise is scientifically accurate or even

86 *Experiential expertise*

whether it can be reconciled with scientific knowledge but, rather, *how* people come to know in particular ways through their own, ultimately irreducible, experiences of the world.[14]

Scholars in both STS and health studies, therefore, tend to define experiential expertise as derived from lived experience rather than scientific knowledge. It is usually presented as a form of expertise that is highly situational and dependent on aspects of identity such as gender, race, class, and place, rather than on abstract concepts of objectivity, rationality, and truth.[15] The crucial difference is in the value (and purpose) assigned to experiential expertise within each field of study.[16] In STS, scientific expertise always holds primacy over other forms of knowledge. In its most rigid forms, STS tries to squeeze experiential expertise into categories created for analysing scientific expertise, and, unsurprisingly, finds it lacking in these terms. Health studies scholars, on the other hand, describe experience in more positive terms, emphasising the value of empathy, emotion, embodied experience, and co-production in healthcare. They are likely to emphasise the potential connections between experiential and scientific knowledge, but are also more overtly critical of the logic of 'otherness' that structures scientific knowledge and perpetuates discrimination against those groups and values deemed to be 'other'.[17] In essence, then, both fields position experiential and scientific expertise in opposition to each other.

But is this distinction justified when we think about how knowledge interacts with experience, and shapes how individuals understand these experiences? The concept of experiential expertise invokes the knowledge and understanding that individuals hold about their own bodies, but it is also reliant on their ideas and experiences of health and illness in general, as well as healthcare, medical services, and treatment.[18] This means that, as Stuart Blume argues, there is no necessary opposition between experiential and scientific expertise: experience and science can combine to form part of the same whole, as a kind of 'knowing in action'.[19] In this view, experiential expertise not only forms a vital part of how people make health decisions, but it is also associated with their abilities to understand illness within broader contexts, to make connections between their own experiences and those of others, and to use this shared knowledge to take action.[20] This interplay – perhaps even inseparability, in

The Greek feminist birth control movement 87

certain contexts – of experiential and scientific expertise is apparent in the history of the Greek birth control movement.

So far, so good. But we can go even further and employ feminist perspectives to illuminate how and why experiential expertise, as a distinctly gendered concept and/or way of knowing, has been devalued within both disciplinary subfields and wider systems of knowledge – and its potential power to subvert those systems of knowledge and empower marginalised groups. Here, Ahmed's theorisation of 'sweaty concepts' is useful.[21]

Influenced by Audre Lorde, Ahmed coined the term as a way of giving 'words to redescribe a situation' that dominant languages were not intended to analyse, and that do not fit the existing social order, such as 'how it feels to inhabit a black body in a world that assumes whiteness'. Ahmed argues that centring the difficult experiences of 'a body that is not at home in the world' can create new viewpoints and therefore new descriptions for the world. Her analysis aims not only to explore such difficult experiences but also to create a new language to describe these tough experiences that resist full comprehension within existing categories, and in this way to legitimise the experiences of marginalised and invisible groups.

Approaching experiential expertise as a sweaty concept, as in this chapter, means asking: how does it feel to produce and circulate knowledge in a world that denies your right to do so? How does it feel to relate the type of knowledge you produce to science – when science does not accept any different kind of knowledge? As Ahmed points out, in answering these questions, the difficulty appears both in experience and in the description of it. The women's movement activists and feminists in the Greek birth control movement were excluded from the production and circulation of knowledge, and therefore experienced difficulties in creating new networks, practices, and methods to communicate science themselves. A lasting effect of their exclusion, but also a testament to their creation of alternative forms of knowledge and channels of communication, is that the fullest history of this movement can be reconstructed only from informal archives in private collections, and is still incomplete. If experiential expertise is a sweaty concept, then piecing together how these women fought to demonstrate its value is likewise a sweaty act.

88   *Experiential expertise*

Expertise in feminist self-help health books

One of the main ways that women's movement activists and feminists articulated the value of experiential expertise was through their authorship and translation of self-help health books. These texts illustrate the interweaving of local, national, and international forms of knowledge, the transformation of this knowledge as it was reframed for different audiences, and the mechanisms of production and circulation of new concepts of experiential expertise. This section examines methods of communication, types of information about contraception, abortion, and sexuality, and approaches to scientific and experiential expertise within four feminist self-help health books that circulated within Greece.

At the global level, the most influential feminist self-help health book is the Boston Women's Health Collective's *Our Bodies, Ourselves*. First published under that title in 1973, nine new US editions have appeared since, as well as multiple translations, usually tailored to the contexts of local cultural and healthcare systems.[22] The first US edition in many ways provided the blueprint for the global feminist self-help health movement. It established a pattern for other texts, combining easy-to-understand explanations of scientific and medical information, practical guidance that emphasised women's capacities for action, political critique of patriarchal and misogynist structures that prevented women from understanding their own bodies or accessing necessary healthcare, and substantial use of first-person testimonies describing women's own experiences, thoughts, and emotions. Although the first Greek translation was not published until 1981, the influence of this feminist mode of communication is seen in all the other texts discussed here.

In order of publication in Greek, the first of these works is the Movement for the Liberation of Women's (MLW) *Methods of Contraception* (1977).[23] MLW was the first autonomous feminist organisation in Greece, and the book arose out of the education activities of its sexuality and contraception subgroup, which included staging a public exhibition about contraception. Collectively authored and textbook-like in appearance, it situated contraception within the political and historical context of Metapolitefsi, and portrayed women's access to medical knowledge as essential to their personal and sexual liberation.

The second text is the 1979 Greek translation of *Clémentine ou la contraception*, originally published in France the year before.[24] This is an illustrated history of contraception for all women, 'from virgins to women that experience menopause'.[25] The heroines of the story embody the experiences of teenage girls and their need to understand their bodies and sexual pleasure. Their stories illustrate the pressures of patriarchal ideology on women's lives in the 1970s, but the book also outlines a utopian vision of an alternative female-centred world. Third, we have the 1980 Greek translation of the Women's Group in Denmark's *Woman and Her Body* (originally published in 1975). This book explores multiple aspects of women's health, including reproduction, sexuality, and different illnesses, with strong emphasis on empowerment through bodily knowledge.[26] Last but not least is the 1984 Greek translation of *Our Bodies, Ourselves*, produced in close association with the Doctors Group, a women's collective that campaigned for better understanding of the female body.[27]

These texts were all explicitly feminist in orientation, with some providing short histories of women's oppression and explanations of the contemporary women's liberation movement.[28] They argued that women's lack of bodily autonomy both arose from and reinforced their political and social subordination, and that women could not achieve emancipation until they had control over their own bodies. The first step towards such control was women's understanding of their bodies and health, and these texts aimed to support readers in gaining this knowledge. They therefore sought to challenge dominant approaches to 'femininity', especially conceptions of female nature as determined by biology. In doing so, they simultaneously challenged patriarchal forms of knowledge and knowledge production, broke down silence and secrecy around the female body and sexuality, and put forward alternative feminist forms of expertise.

The multilayered approach of these feminist self-help health texts can be illustrated through discussion of the different types of expertise deployed in *Our Bodies, Ourselves*' chapter on the anatomy and physiology of sexuality and reproduction.[29] The authors use text and images to explain the structure and functions of the female and male reproductive systems while critiquing the standard scientific emphasis on difference and instead highlighting similarities in sexual organisation. Likewise, their discussions continually refuse standard

90 *Experiential expertise*

boundaries between body/mind and science/culture (a typical stance within these feminist self-help health texts).[30] Their account of the menstrual cycle blends the biological and the social, ranging across pain, flow, and desire, and highlighting that different women experience menstruation differently. This holistic view opens up space for different forms of management for menstrual pain, including massage, extraction (manual vacuum aspiration to pass the menses at once), and orgasm.

All the texts under discussion similarly interweaved different types of expertise, demonstrating the influence of approaches to feminist self-help health developed in the earlier US version of *Our Bodies, Ourselves*, and with it the existence of transnational feminist networks that exchanged knowledge and expertise. This is also seen in their coverage of contraception and abortion. All of these books provided an array of practical information on contraception, outlining how to use different methods (and whether they were female or male controlled and/or involved interaction with doctors) and considering the effectiveness, risks, side effects, and costs of each. They also discussed abortion, providing information on the status of abortion under different legal systems and what to expect when consulting a doctor, as well as the different techniques practised, potential risks and complications (including those resulting from medical mismanagement), and post-abortion care.[31]

In line with mainstream white western feminist movements, these texts usually presented access of safe abortion as essential to women's liberation.[32] They also, however, paid attention to the specificity of Greek conditions within this global context. *Methods of Contraception* delineates the central paradox of abortion in Greece: illegal, expensive, and dangerous, it is nevertheless often the only method of preventing birth that women kept in ignorance by a patriarchal society know about.[33] *Our Bodies, Ourselves*, meanwhile, focuses on two critical points about the local context: gynaecologists' frequent performance of curettage without a pregnancy test; and doctors' refusal to assist with contraceptive guidance or provision, related to their perception of abortion as one of the many contraceptive methods.[34]

These texts were often critical of existing healthcare systems, but they did not attempt to replace scientific and medical expertise. Indeed, *Methods of Contraception*, the most textbook-like of these works, makes extensive use of charts, tables, and statistics. However,

The Greek feminist birth control movement   91

they presented this information in ways that readers could easily understand, explaining technical terms in simple language.[35] Crucially, authors placed scientific and medical information alongside evidence that centred women's perspectives and their experiential expertise. *Clémentine ou la contraception* tells the story of a fictional heroine, but it also includes a glossary of medical terms.[36] The discussion of abortion in *Our Bodies, Ourselves* includes detailed information on every aspect of undergoing an abortion, but always accompanied by first-hand accounts of women's experiences, with attention to the diverse emotions that abortion might elicit.[37]

The introduction to *Our Bodies, Ourselves* elaborates on the authors' efforts to gather 'scientific knowledge' through talking to the medical community, but also their intention to present in parallel women's 'opinions, experiences, and emotions', and to provide political analysis of women's subordination and how this affects their physical and emotional health.[38] In places, they even privilege women's narratives, as in their claim that in sexual relationships, experience, reflection, and trust are often 'more educative' than scientific knowledge.[39] For the authors of *Woman and Her Body*, this approach was a means of challenging the dominant masculine language that had excluded women, and replacing it with a shared female voice that could speak of women's pleasures and pains.[40]

In such ways, feminist texts aimed to empower readers through education in scientific and medical languages, while also demonstrating the legitimacy of emotional and embodied knowledge. The information provided was intended to be put to use in all aspects of everyday life, including encounters with doctors. The MLW authorial collective included a list of questions that women should ask their doctors and/or vice versa.[41] The authors of *Our Bodies, Ourselves* emphasise that familiarity with medical terminology has enabled them to communicate with doctors as well as to deconstruct myths about the female body, and that readers can share these benefits.[42] As in *Woman and Her Body*, they insist that when women understand how their bodies work, they can not only manage health on their own terms but also more effectively manage their relationships with doctors (including action in the event of medical mistreatment). The texts consistently provided practical information on what to expect from medical encounters (for instance, a detailed description of how doctors fit intrauterine devices), and how to obtain the best results

92   *Experiential expertise*

from them (such as what questions to ask doctors when seeking an abortion, including around methods, location, and price).[43]

Although texts did not discourage the use of methods that required medical oversight, they were also often critical (implicitly or explicitly) of medical failures to fully support women, for example by not sharing information about contraception or the risks of abortion, or by not performing necessary examinations before recommending specific contraceptive methods.[44] At first glance, the one exception is *Clémentine ou la contraception*. Here, when the heroine visits a doctor to obtain the oral contraceptive pill, the doctor explains the risks and benefits of the different types of pill, performs an examination before issuing the prescription, and answers all Clémentine's questions. However, this is a deliberately idealistic vision. Its presentation of what medical encounters could look like – a friendly female doctor providing non-judgemental information and advice in a safe environment and treating the patient with respect at all times – simply underlines all that is wrong with patriarchal healthcare systems in reality.

These texts put forward alternative methods of bodily management, equipping women to take matters into their own hands. As part of its discussion of contraception, *Woman and Her Body* tells women how to chart ovulation by examining their cervical mucus and provided step-by-step guidance on fitting their own diaphragms.[45] It also provides a detailed discussion of cervical self-examination, a practice often undertaken by closed women's groups in Greece, including how to use a dilator, mirror, and light, what women should expect to see, and how to interpret differences in the consistency of mucus or odour of discharges.[46] This information was practical, but in redefining the possibilities of women's sexual knowledge, these texts also emphasise the expansion of their capacities for pleasure. *Our Bodies, Ourselves* explicitly positions itself in defiance of 'the traditional social and ethical order' by defining contraception in positive terms as enabling women to 'enjoy sexual relationships without the stress of a pregnancy'.[47] As an extension of its discussion of cervical self-examination, *Woman and Her Body* urges readers to know, love, and celebrate their bodies through masturbation.[48] In this way, feminist self-help health books centred a radical form of alternative self-knowledge that may have incorporated traditional

The Greek feminist birth control movement   93

scientific expertise but was far removed from it in aims, forms, and possibilities.

International networks: archival traces

These feminist self-help health texts were only one manifestation of Greek women's movement activists' involvement in transnational feminism. This section establishes the presence of an international network and channels of communication between Greek and other feminist birth control movements. Between 1974 and 1986, Greek women's movement activists and feminists drew on these sources to shape their practices. These sources testify to the transnational exchange of ideas, practices, and materials, building the development of a sense of 'belonging' to a global community that struggled for reproductive rights and empowerment. This shared knowledge constitutes another aspect of women's movement activists' and feminists' expertise. Tracing the contents of materials that formed part of this transnational exchange through the limited informal archives that remain is another sweaty act, but one that provides deeper understanding of how these women formulated their approach to experiential expertise, and how they put this expertise into practice.

Archival materials establish the existence of exchanges between the national and international feminist birth control movements. For example, one pamphlet provides information about Danish feminist group the Bookwomen (Bodveninderne), who ran a second-hand bookshop and organised exhibitions and meetings that addressed women's groups in Scandinavia and across the world.[49] The Greek feminist birth control movement hosted similar spaces, including the Women's Bookstore and the bookstore The Book/The Child.[50] Similarly, the newsletter of the Women's Reproductive Rights Campaign (WRRC), discussing news and actions around the world about abortion and contraception, indicates the multidirectional movement of knowledge. Its presence in Greek collections shows Greek women's involvement in global feminist networks, while the content of the newsletter shows that WRRC operated as a platform for feminists around the world to share their experiences and actions.[51]

94   *Experiential expertise*

Such examples depict not only the aims and content of feminist activism, but how knowledge circulated and therefore how expertise was constituted: the materials describe the global struggle for women's rights, including access to contraception and abortion, but their existence reveals skills in communication and organisation as essential forms of expertise for the women's movement. This point is reinforced by materials documenting Greek women's movement activists' and feminists' involvement in international conferences on women's health and reproductive rights. At the Women's International Information and Communication Service conference on Women and Health, held in Geneva in June 1981, Greek feminists contributed to discussions on diverse topics – contraception, abortion, sterilisation, and population control; pregnancy, childbirth, and breastfeeding; massage, natural medicine, yoga for birth control, the politics of self-help, and paramedical work; lesbian health and the relationship of poverty, racism, and health; and circumcision, violence against women, sexuality, menopause, madness, and the international feminist network.[52]

The eclecticism of topics under discussion at these major international conferences, and Greek women's movement activists' participation in the full range of debates, indicates their active efforts to combine different types of knowledge and move beyond the division between scientific and experiential expertise. At the International Tribunal and Meeting on Reproductive Rights in Amsterdam, held in July 1984, Greek women from the Autonomous Women's Movement and the Multinational Women's Liberation Group took their place among four hundred women from sixty-five countries to promote women's sexual and reproductive health.[53] Greek delegates organised tribunal sessions on multiple aspects of the personal and political struggle for contraception, abortion, and sterilisation: difficulties of access, issues of coercion and abuse, effects on health, and the consequences of illegal and dangerous abortions; the impact of pregnancy and childbirth on women's health; and the influence of religious ideologies, population control policies, and powerful pharmaceutical companies on women's lives. They also co-organised a session to exchange practical knowledge and skills on massage, diaphragm use, the menstrual cycle, herbs, family planning practices, and self-examination. As in feminist self-help health texts, feminist conferences on reproductive rights sought to foster new political,

The Greek feminist birth control movement 95

theoretical, and practical understandings through exchange of women's diverse knowledge, skills, and perspectives – in this way creating new experiential expertise.

These archival traces show that women's movement activists and feminists exchanged ideas about organisational issues and practices, shared their situated birth control experiences, and redefined knowledge and understanding of multiple issues through their collective actions. This redefinition constituted an important aspect of their experiential expertise, and was based on their ability to transform personal experience into collective experience. In doing so, these women's movement activists and feminists moved beyond the traditional divisions of centre/periphery, local/national/international, body/mind, theory/practice, and scientific/non-scientific knowledge. Their activities deny the rigid distinctions between different types of expertise that dominant approaches within STS and, to a lesser extent, health studies assume or attempt to impose on the world. The flow of knowledge and collaboration between feminist birth control movements across different parts of the globe broke down boundaries and created new forms of knowledge and expertise that cannot be measured, recorded, or understood through the inflexible definitions and sharp distinctions that originate out of the traditional scientific (and social) order. The sweaty concepts that these women evolved demand to be located within equally sweaty forms of knowledge generation and research practice.

Conclusion

The Greek feminist birth control movement was embedded in international communication channels. Archival material and translations of texts demonstrate the travel of knowledge across different national contexts, and the importance of multiple networks to the shaping of knowledge production and circulation. By viewing women's movement activism and feminist organisations as boundary movements, through which knowledge travels among different social realms, blurring the boundaries between science and society, we can better understand the content of knowledge and the type of experience-based expertise that women developed.

96   *Experiential expertise*

These women's movement activists and feminists employed numerous communication methods: formation of groups, meetings, courses, conferences, publications, translations, and exhibitions. Such practices focused on the mutual self-education of women, the infusion of medical knowledge with their own experiences, and the international exchange of knowledge. Out of both their own difficult existence in an oppressive society, and the materials exchanged within the global movement, they formed a concept of experiential expertise that emerged from the geographical and (bio)political margins but travelled along and to diverse social contexts.

In developing new, woman-centred approaches to contraception, they employed several tactics. First, they placed discussion of birth control in dialogue with multiple other topics and issues: women's anatomy, sex education, and sexuality, as well as abortion. Second, they located these discussions within a critique of the entire political and social order, and its manifestation in scientific and medical systems and orders of knowledge that replicated patriarchal assumptions and power dynamics. In doing so, they questioned established ways of knowing. Third, they explored different sources of knowledge and created different ways of knowing that combined scientific, medical, and experiential expertise, but did not assume the primacy of traditional, formal, and abstract expertise. They also infused medical science with their own knowledge and expertise, including alternative approaches, definitions, prioritisations, and categorisations. The notion of experience was crucial in this process. This validation of experiential expertise transformed access to contraception and the practice of birth control into political issues fundamental to women's bodily and sexual autonomy and their liberation.

In this chapter, I have theorised women's movement activists' and feminists' experiential expertise through Ahmed's prism of 'sweaty concepts'. This feminist methodology highlights the importance of bringing to the surface difficulties we encounter in our concepts, theories, and methods. Instead of 'tidying up' our theoretical schemes, this methodology incorporates these difficulties and makes them valuable in understanding the concept of experiential expertise. Archival materials show the transmission of multilayered bodies of knowledge that combined the practical and the utopian, the technical and the emotional, the abstract and the situational – in short, the scientific and the experiential. The concept of experiential expertise

The Greek feminist birth control movement 97

developed by women's movement activists and feminists was derived *from* and directed *to* the body. It was concerned with the body and its liquids – sweat, blood, discharges – but also how women experienced these bodies, their feelings of trauma, pain, and isolation, and their as-yet unrealised potential for pleasure. By further developing practices of communication, exchange, and education that placed this concept of experiential expertise in local, national, and international networks, these women transformed the private and personal into a public and collective good.

To trace the development of experiential expertise as a sweaty concept, I have followed the production and circulation of knowledge that derived from a marginalised social position, from an unfamiliar and invisible space, and from bodies that protested at their suffering. As Athanasiou has argued, Ahmed's work calls for making vulnerability and weakness our stepping stone rather than treating them like a collateral loss; for making concepts vulnerable and assailable by using language to expose the traumatic experiences that are part of their formation.[54] Unlike approaches that continuously multiply ever more specific categories of knowledge and expertise while still excluding some forms of understanding, this approach is fluid, flexible, and open, and can follow and reveal the complexities and transformations of knowledge in action. Women's movement activists and feminists sought to actively participate in making their own health, and their own liberation. To do this, they created knowledge based on women's needs, desires, and experiences. In a so-called peripheral country with an estimated 300,000–500,000 illegal abortions per year in the late 1970s and early 1980s, this marginalised and suppressed social group developed complex experiential expertise. The story of the Greek feminist birth control movement is a her-story of how women understood, shaped, and performed 'everyday health' as an issue of survival.

Acknowledgements

This chapter is based on Evangelia Chordaki, 'Science Communication in the Late 20th Century Greece: Public Intersections of Gender and Knowledge Circulation in the Feminist Birth Control Movement' (PhD thesis, Hellenic Open University, 2022). This research was

98   *Experiential expertise*

supported by the Hellenic Foundation for Research and Innovation under the HFRI PhD Fellowship Grant (Fellowship Number: 873). I am extremely grateful to Tracey Loughran and Hannah Froom for their valuable comments and suggestions.

Notes

1 Library of the Hellenic Parliament [Βιβλιοθήκη της Βουλής] (hereafter LHP), Athens, LHP 1: Law 1609/1986. Technical termination of pregnancy and protection of women's health and other regulations. [Τεχνητή διακοπή της εγκυμοσύνης και προστασία της γυναίκας και άλλες διατάξεις], 1986.

2 This overview is taken from Alexandra Barmpouti, 'Issues of biopolitics of reproduction in post-war Greece', *Studies in History and Philosophy of Science Part C: Studies in History and Philosophy of Biological and Biomedical Sciences*, 83 (2020), 1–8.

3 Antonis Liakos, *Ο ελληνικός 20ος αιώνας*, 3rd edn (Athens: Polis Publications, 2020); Stathis Pavlopoulos and Magda Fitili, Μεταπολίτευση: από την στιγμή στην διάρκεια. Τα χρόνια 1974–1989. Project: *Δημιουργία ιστοσελίδας για την ιστορία της Μεταπολίτευσης 1974–1989*, Contemporary Social History Archives (2017): http://metapolitefsi.com/%CE%A4%CE%B1%CF%85%CF%84%CF%8C%CF%84%CE%B7%CF%84%CE%B1 (accessed 26 June 2022); Manolis Avgeridis, Efi Gazi, and Kostis Kornetis (eds), *Μεταπολίτευση. Η Ελλάδα στο μεταίχμιο των δυο αιώνων* (Athens: Themelio Publications, 2015).

4 Vaggelis Karamanolakis and Kostis Karpozilos, Ενότητα: Κοινωνία και Κινήματα. Project: *Δημιουργία ιστοσελίδας για την ιστορία της Μεταπολίτευσης 1974–1989*, Contemporary Social History Archives (2017): http://metapolitefsi.com/%CE%95%CE%BD%CF%8C%CF%84%CE%B7%CF%84%CE%B5%CF%82/%CE%9A%CE%BF%CE%B9%CE%BD%CF%89%CE%BD%CE%AF%CE%B1 (accessed 25 June 2022).

5 Athena Athanasiou. Το να 'γίνεσαι φεμινίστρια' ως κριτική επιτελεστικότητα του πολιτικού', in Nt. Vaiou and A. Psarra (eds), *Εννοιολογήσεις και πρακτικές του φεμινισμού. Μεταπολίτευση και «μετά»*. Workshop Proceedings (Athens: Hellenic Parliament Foundation, 2018), p. 24.

6 Efi Avdela, 'Ο φεμινισμός ως κριτική της εξουσίας', in Nt. Vaiou and A. Psarra (eds), *Εννοιολογήσεις και πρακτικές του φεμινισμού. Μεταπολίτευση και «μετά»*. Workshop Proceedings (Athens: Hellenic Parliament Foundation, 2018), p. 11.

The Greek feminist birth control movement   99

7   Athanasiou, Το να 'γίνεσαι φεμινίστρια' ως κριτική επιτελεστηκότητα του πολιτικού', p. 29.

8   Sabrina McCormick, Phil Brown, and Stephen Zavestoski, 'The personal is scientific, the scientific is political: the public paradigm of the environmental breast cancer movement', *Sociological Review*, 18:4 (2003), 547; see also Phil Brown, Stephen Zavestoski, Sabrina McCormick, Brian Mayer, Rachel Morello-Frosch, and Rebecca Gasior Altman, 'Embodied health movements: new approaches to social movements in health', *Sociology of Health and Illness*, 26 (2004), 65.

9   Harry Collins and Robert Evans, *Rethinking Expertise* (Chicago, IL: University of Chicago Press, 2007); J. Francisca Flinterman, Rebecca Mesbah-Teclemariam, Jacqueline E.W. Broerse, and Joske F.G. Bunders, 'Transdisciplinarity: the new challenge for biomedical research', *Bulletin of Science, Technology & Society*, 21:4 (2001).

10 Harry Collins and Robert Evans, 'The third wave of science studies: studies of expertise and experience', *Social Studies of Science*, 32:2 (2002).

11 Brian Wynne and Michael Lynch, 'Science and technology studies: experts and expertise', in James D. Wright (ed.), *International Encyclopedia of the Social and Behavioral Sciences*, 2nd edn (London: Elsevier, 2015); Harry Kennedy, 'Rethinking expertise', *Journal of Forensic Psychiatry & Psychology*, 20:4 (2015); Reiner Grundmann, 'The problem of expertise in knowledge societies', *Minerva*, 55 (2016); Stuart Blume, 'In search of experiential knowledge', *Innovation: The European Journal of Social Science Research*, 30:1 (2017).

12 Eva M. Castro, Tine Van Regenmortal, Walter Sermeus, and Kris Vanhaecht, 'Patients' experiential knowledge and expertise in health care: a hybrid concept analysis', *Social Theory and Health*, 17:3 (2018).

13 Marcia C. Inhorn and K. Lisa Whittle, 'Feminism meets the "new" epidemiologies: towards an appraisal of antifeminist biases in epidemiological research on women's health', *Social Science & Medicine*, 53 (2001); O.D. Kolawole, 'Science, social scientization and hybridisation of knowledges', *Science as Culture*, 38:3 (2019).

14 Lori D'Agincourt-Canning, 'The effect of experiential knowledge on construction of risk perception in hereditary breast/ovarian cancer', *Journal of Genetic Counselling*, 14:1 (2005), 57.

15 Saul Halfon, 'Encountering birth: negotiating expertise, networks, and my STS self', *Science as Culture*, 19:1 (2010); Grundmann et al., 'The problem of expertise'; Erica Morrell, 'Localizing Detroit's food system: boundary-work and the politics of experiential expertise', *Science as Culture*, 28:3 (2019); A. Rip, 'Constructing expertise: in a third wave

100 *Experiential expertise*

of science studies?', *Social Studies of Science*, 33 (2003); D'Agincourt-Canning, 'The effect of experiential knowledge'.

16 For an extended discussion, see Evangelia Chordaki, 'Science Communication in the Late 20th Century Greece: Public Intersections of Gender and Knowledge Circulation in the Feminist Birth Control Movement' (PhD thesis, Hellenic Open University, 2022), pp. 303–20 [Part II, Section 8.3].

17 Inhorn and Whittle, 'Feminism meets the "new" epidemiologies'; D'Agincourt-Canning, 'The effect of experiential knowledge'.

18 Castro et al., 'Patients' experiential knowledge'; Flinterman et al., 'Transdisciplinarity'.

19 Blume, 'In search of experiential knowledge'.

20 Castro et al., 'Patients' experiential knowledge'.

21 Sara Ahmed, 'Sweaty concepts', *feministkilljoys* (22 February 2014): https://feministkilljoys.com/2014/02/22/sweaty-concepts/ (accessed 25 June 2022); Sara Ahmed, *Living a Feminist Life* (Durham, NC: Duke University Press, 2017), pp. 12–14, 94, 195.

22 See Kathy Davis, *The Making of Our Bodies, Ourselves: How Feminism Travels across Borders* (Durham, NC: Duke University Press, 2007).

23 Movement for the Liberation of Women [hereafter MLW], *Methods of Contraception* ([Unknown]: Movement for the Liberation of Women, 1977) [Κίνηση για την Απελευθέρωση των Γυναικών. Αντισυλληπτικά Μέσα].

24 Natalie Crinon, Cathrine Manes, Aurrelie Memmi, and Cathrine Revault, trans. R. Papadopoulou and illus. M. Papadopoulou, *Clémentine ou la contraception* ([Unknown]: Stohasmos Publications, 1979) [Κλημεντίνη ή τα Αντισυλληπτικά]. For further analysis see Evangelia Chordaki, 'Hidden paths – unconventional practices: a herstory of circulation of the medical knowledge in the late 20th century', in George N. Vlahakis, Kostas Tampakis (eds), and Evangelia Chordaki (language ed. and formatting), *Science and Literature. Poetry and Prose* (Athens: National Hellenic Research Foundation, 2020), pp. 103–10.

25 Crinon et al., *Clémentine ou la contraception*, unpaginated opening material.

26 Women's Group in Denmark [hereafter WGD], trans. M. Parashis, and Dr Alekou (scientific editor), *Woman and Her Body* (Athens: Odisseas (Kvinde kend din krop), 1980) [Ομάδα Γυναικών Δανίας. Η γυναίκα και το κορμί της].

27 Boston Women's Health Collective/M. Mitsou-Pappa [hereafter BWHC/MMP] (ed.), *Our Bodies, Ourselves*, 4th US edn [1979], trans. M. Magganari (Athens, 1984) [Ομάδα Γυναικών Βοστώνης. Εμείς και το σώμα μας].

The Greek feminist birth control movement   101

28 MLW, *Methods of Contraception*, pp. 3–24.
29 BWHC/MMP, *Our Bodies, Ourselves*, pp. 13–23.
30 See, for example, the discussion of sexual intercourse as both a biological and emotional act in MLW, *Methods of Contraception*, pp. 31–2.
31 BWHC/MMP, *Our Bodies, Ourselves*, pp. 136–40; WGD, *Woman and Her Body*, pp. 131–45; MLW, *Methods of Contraception*, pp. 71–9.
32 BWHC/MMP, *Our Bodies, Ourselves*, p. 125; WGD, *Woman and Her Body*, p. 131.
33 MLW, *Methods of Contraception*, pp. 18–24.
34 BWHC/MMP, *Our Bodies, Ourselves*, pp. 130–3.
35 MLW, *Methods of Contraception*, pp. 69–98, especially pp. 76–8.
36 Crinon et al., *Clémentine ou la contraception*, pp. 76–8.
37 BWHC/MMP, *Our Bodies, Ourselves*, p. 136.
38 BWHC/MMP, *Our Bodies, Ourselves*, p. 7.
39 BWHC/MMP, *Our Bodies, Ourselves*, p. 29.
40 WGD, *Woman and Her Body*, pp. 181–2.
41 MLW, *Methods of Contraception*, pp. 34–6.
42 BWHC/MMP, *Our Bodies, Ourselves*, p. 18.
43 BWHC/MMP, *Our Bodies, Ourselves*, pp. 93, 115–25; WGD, *Woman and Her Body*, pp. 95, 104–5.
44 BWHC/MMP, *Our Bodies, Ourselves*, p. 92; MLW, *Methods of Contraception*, pp. 40–1.
45 WGD, *Woman and Her Body*, pp. 240–1.
46 Mitra 2, Μήτρα 2η αναπαραγωγής ιδεών για την αθέατη πλευρά του ανταγωνισμού. Μια συζήτηση με την Γ.: Το βιβλιοπωλείο των Γυναικών και το γυναικείο κίνημα στην Ελλάδα ([Unknown]: No Woman's Land, 2005), pp. 1–24. See also WGD, *Woman and Her Body*, pp. 240–2.
47 BWHC/MMP, *Our Bodies, Ourselves*, p. 91.
48 WGD, *Woman and Her Body*, p. 189.
49 Delfis Archival Centre (hereafter DAC), The Bookwomen (Bodveninderne), File D, DEC 1.
50 A. Mihopoulou and M. Mpolota, 'Women's Bookstore', *City of Women*, 10 (1983) [Το βιβλιοπωλείο των γυναικών. Πόλη των γυναικών]; Mirto, Women's Bookstore in Athens, *The Earth* (1985) [Βιβλιοπωλείο γυναικών Αθήνας. Γαία]; Unknown author, 'A Brief History of Women's Bookstore The Book/The Child', *Bulletin of the Democratic Women's Movement*, 21 (1983) [Μικρό ιστορικό του γυναικείου βιβλιοπωλείου Το βιβλίο/Το παιδί. Δελτίο Κίνησης Δημοκρατικών Γυναικών].
51 E. Leontiduou Private Archival Collection (hereafter ELPAC), Newsletter of the Women's Reproductive Rights Campaign (April-May 1985), PACL 1.

52 DAC, Third ISIS Conference (Women's International Information and Communication Service), *Women and Health* (Geneva, 6–7 June 1981), File Health Issues, DEC 2.

53 ELPAC, Women's Global Network for Reproductive Rights, *Reproductive Rights International Tribunal. Divided in Culture United in Struggle* (Amsterdam, June 1986), PACL 2. The latter report was published by the Women's Global Network on Reproductive Rights in Amsterdam, in conjunction with the Women's Health Information Service and London Women and Manual Trades.

54 Athena Athanasiou, 'Θεωρία φτιαγμένη από ιδρώτα', *Feministiqa*, 3 (Autumn 2020): https://feministiqa.net/theoria-ftiagmenh-apo-idrwta/ (accessed 25 June 2022).

4

Migration, kinship, and 'everyday theorising': Black British women's narratives of genetic diagnosis in the postwar National Health Service

Grace Redhead

Introduction

In the 1980s, health visitor Lola Oni worked in the Lambeth Sickle Cell and Thalassaemia Centre. A key aspect of her role was the delivery of educational talks at local churches and community groups about sickle cell disease (SCD). After giving these talks, Oni remembered, many people would tell her about a cousin, a friend, or a schoolmate 'who used to have this pain and you know, and used to cry a lot, and we didn't know what was wrong with them'. Sometimes, Oni said, people 'started associating sickle with every kind of illness that exists' and linked it to every unexplained death they'd known, and she would try to emphasise its specificity. But many times, she said, 'a lot of people will actually describe it to you'.[1] This did not surprise Oni, who knew that western knowledge of SCD was pre-dated by West African knowledge, in which there are several names for an illness characterised by bone and joint pain bearing close resemblance to the symptoms of SCD observed in biomedicine.[2]

The diagnosis narrative, in both oral history and the history of medicine, is often understood as a moment of reconciliation, in which the individual finds an organising theory for their lives and experiences. Anne Hunsaker Hawkins has argued that diagnosis narratives are often framed around the 'epiphany' – a moment of realisation or recognition, as lifelong symptom patterns come into focus.[3] Lynn Abrams shows that epiphany in narrative can reflect a 'cathartic reconstruction of the self' as narrators seek to reconcile

104   *Experiential expertise*

changing social expectations in their experiences with the need for a 'coherent, acceptable and constantly revised life story'.[4] Susan Lindee has analysed these moments in the development of genetic medicine as 'moments of truth', which she describes as 'a moment of recognition or understanding, the moment when a given narrative can be classified or categorised and placed in a narrative that explains it'.[5] In her study of sickle cell anaemia in Senegal, Duana Fullwiley noticed that her interviewees often reinterpreted their early lives through their diagnosis, 'recounting their lives through the lens of sickle cell in an effort to make sense of the pain and fatigue that was only later given a name'.[6]

This chapter treats diagnosis as an entry point into how women with sickle cell trait or SCD theorised body, self, and family within the profoundly racialised social and political structures of postwar Britain. It foregrounds Black women's analysis of medical racism within the National Health Service (NHS), which often regarded them with suspicion or indifference.[7] The 'diagnosis' is understood as a narrative event in which women sought to reconcile multiple contrasting influences and narratives: memory and present experience, the healthcare environments of Britain and their (or their parents') home countries, traditional and biomedical medical systems, and the connections and divergences of first- and second-generation migrant identity.

SCD is a disorder which affects the structure and function of haemoglobin, in which blood cells become rigid and impede blood circulation. This can lead to a range of health issues, including chronic pain, strokes, ischaemia, fatigue, ulcers, and episodes of acute pain. SCD is a recessive genetic condition which is not sex linked and must be inherited from both parents. The mid-twentieth century saw the 'medicalization of family and kinship', beginning in western biomedicine following the 'blossoming' of molecular biology.[8] But advances in genetic knowledge were not matched by advances in treatments for genetic illness, and so, often the only available interventions were carrier screening and prenatal diagnosis – resulting in a medical focus on female bodies and reproduction as a site of genetic risk.[9] The focus on women was even starker in the case of the haemoglobinopathies – the set of interrelated genetic traits including sickle cell, thalassaemia, and haemoglobin C. The haemoglobinopathies have an evolutionary link to malaria and are

Migration, kinship, and 'everyday theorising' 105

more common among people with ancestors from West Africa, South Asia, and the Mediterranean. Institutional racism in Britain therefore inhibited the development of community neonatal and carrier screening programmes until the 1980s in many NHS districts.[10] Local health authorities' reluctance to extend carrier screening programmes to male partners, which sickle cell campaigners argued was rooted in racist assumptions about the stability of Black families, heightened focus on women's bodies.[11] This took place within a wider context of medical scrutiny of, and efforts to control, the fertility of racialised migrant women – as seen in scandals around the overprescription or unconsented use of the contraceptive injection Depo-Provera.[12]

In this context, many of the first cases of SCD identified in Britain came to light either as a result of the increased medical scrutiny of pregnant woman or as a result of mothers bringing sick children into hospital. As Beverley Bryan, Stella Dadzie, and Suzanne Scafe argued:

> because we are women, the Health Service is central to our lives. We cannot avoid using it. It is us who bear the brunt of the responsibility for our own and our families' health.[13]

Due to the hereditary nature of sickle cell, a diagnosis could have implications for both parent and child, with a child's diagnosis leading to a parent's, or a parent's to a child's. In the new age of genomic medicine, the individual – long responsible for the health of their own body – was placed in a network of responsibility to their genetic relatives, with the imperative to 'know and manage the implications of one's genome'.[14] Thus, women affected by the sickle cell trait or by SCD often took responsibility for familial health as well as for the implications of a familial genetic trait. Women were therefore on the front line of the medicalisation of family and kinship, and those diagnosed with SCD or with the sickle cell trait in postwar Britain often found themselves reframing kinship at the same time as dealing with familial change or separation after migration.

This chapter treats diagnosis narratives as a creative response to an external reframing of the meaning of body, self, and family. Carol Boyce Davies analyses Black women's writing as 'migrating' or 'boundary crossing' as the dismantling of empire redefined their identities and homes, and as they cross boundaries 'of space, time,

106   *Experiential expertise*

history, place, language, corporeality and restricted consciousness in order to make reconnections and mark or name absences'.[15] In this chapter's oral histories, women cross these boundaries as they remember family histories and situate themselves anew in their redefined identities. In doing so, they rework and reinscribe memories and meanings of health and family from 'homes' in the Caribbean or Africa within the new contexts of their lives in Britain.[16]

This chapter explores these diagnosis and illness narratives as creative enterprises that not only rework identity and kinship into new forms using a range of cultural, familial, and political influences but also undertake structural analysis of power relations within postwar British healthcare environments and within family units. Julia Chinyere Oparah has suggested that the positionality of Black British women meant they were engaged in 'everyday acts of theorising about their lives, experiences and struggles' and that motherhood and children were often central to this political work.[17] In line with this, and with the analysis of Umut Erel and Tracey Reynolds, this chapter treats intersectionality as 'connect[ing] the diverse and divergent parenting experiences and social histories of migrant mothers into claims of collective knowledge [...] interpreting the social world from a particular standpoint of gender and racialized subjugation'.[18] Diagnosis narratives are the product of everyday theorising about the relationship between Black British women, family, citizenship, and the NHS. Foregrounding Black women's analysis of their political and social circumstances in the 'postcolonial' NHS can refocus our attention on often overlooked practices of activism, resistance, and survival.

This chapter will explore the narratives of two women diagnosed with the sickle cell trait or SCD, as told in oral history interviews in 2018. Suzanne was born in the 1960s to Caribbean parents who had migrated to Britain, and has SCD, having inherited two copies of the 'S' gene from each parent. Julie was born in Nigeria during the 1960s and came to Britain in 2000, though some members of her extended family had migrated to Britain in the 1960s. These names are pseudonyms – both women asked for their identities to be protected, and both women reflected on periods in their lives when their sickle cell status was a closely kept secret, due to their anxieties about the social and professional consequences of disclosure.

Migration, kinship, and 'everyday theorising' 107

This oral history project began with the assistance of the Sickle Cell Society, who published a call for participants on their website and social media pages in the autumn of 2017, with the call, 'Tell Your Story'.

Biomedicine, family history, and revelation

This first section will discuss Suzanne and Julie's narratives of diagnosis or revelation of sickle cell status. In these stories, Suzanne and Julie articulated the different knowledges and experiences of SCD that they and their families had. They discussed these different frameworks of knowledge in their narratives, and often reflected on juxtapositions and overlaps between how they and their parents understood sickle cell. Their narratives reflect the opportunities and limitations of biomedicine as an explanatory framework for their experiences.

Suzanne

Suzanne's mother, Heather, migrated from Grenada to London in the mid-1950s. In London, Heather met Suzanne's father, who had arrived from Jamaica, in a shared boarding house. They had two children, but the pair eventually parted ways and Heather became the sole caregiver to their two daughters. Heather was diagnosed with SCD in the UK, when she became pregnant and experienced complications with her pregnancy. Suzanne explained that, when Heather was growing up in Grenada,

> S: She'd have recurrent episodes of pain, but she just learned to deal with it, cos in Grenada, you can't see a doctor, you can't afford it! So they didn't know about it, so and her mum, when my mum used to have – which I now realise she'd have recurrent crises, she said that when she was growing up she'd always have these really terrible pains, and her mum would always say you've been eating unripe mangoes. And her older brother would get the kerosene oil they used to light the lamps, and rub her belly with it. But they didn't know what it was.
>
> GR: Did she find that helpful?

Suzanne: Placebo effect. She was really close to her older brother. So it was only in childbirth when she was having complications that it really came to light. Because as I said she was anaemic so they gave her iron injections which is not going to do anything, and if anything makes things worse. At that time, when you have your blood tests for pregnancy, and they looked under the microscope and they saw it.

Travel from Grenada to Britain reframed the aches and pains that Heather had previously been told were related to her diet, while the physical distance separated Heather from a close relationship with her brother, which Suzanne described as physically soothing. Massage and close relationships between the healer and healed are a feature of SCD care in various parts of the world, framed often as alternative therapies.[19] Suzanne's account of her mother's early life linked the health environment of Grenada (where medical treatment was not free at the point of access) to her mother's approach to her illness and 'just learn[ing] to deal with it'.

Suzanne and her mother lived together for much of her adult life, and her testimony reflects many conversations between them. In her account, Suzanne editorialised her mother's diagnosis story with her own medical knowledge as a doctor. She noted that her mother's episodes of pain were 'recurrent crises', and places the soothing effect of Heather's brother's massage within a biomedical framework as 'placebo effect'. In her testimony, Suzanne imagined the moment in which Heather's blood was examined 'under the microscope', where, she says, 'they saw it'. This moment of discovery, of doctors viewing sickled blood cells under the microscope, is an epiphanic moment in which Suzanne reconciled her mother's early physical experience with her own experiences as a doctor and biomedical knowledge of SCD.

Suzanne explained that her interest in medicine stemmed from her own experience of SCD:

Oh, it was always science [my favourite subject]. It was science all the way along [...] when [my mum] went to work she used to leave us in the house on our own, me and my sister, and I just used to – she got us all these encyclopaedias and I just used to read them [...] I sucked it up like a sponge. The first time I said I want to do medicine, I was actually in hospital in Hoxton. And [my mum] came to visit me on the ward, cos in those days parents could only come like an hour in the evenings, and I said, mum, when I grow up I'm going to

Migration, kinship, and 'everyday theorising' 109

be like that man in a white coat and heal all the children in hospital [...] It was the paediatrician who looked after me. I suppose, I just, because I'd been in the NHS environment so long, in and out of hospital, all the time, it was just the natural environment for me.

Though Suzanne linked her biological interest and medical ambition with the doctors who treated her, she also observed that medical treatment of her illness could be far from healing. People with SCD in postwar Britain often found that their reported pain was dismissed or disbelieved by healthcare professionals making racist assumptions about drug addiction.[20] Both in her own experience as a child in the 1960s and in her observations as a junior doctor during the 1980s, Suzanne found healthcare professionals tended to underestimate the seriousness of SCD and the pain associated with crises. Suzanne recalled that as a child,

When I was really young [the doctors] didn't know about [sickle cell], so you'd be rolling in pain, you'd go to A&E [Accident and Emergency Department], they'd put you to sit in A&E, you'd be rolling in pain for hours, and then when you got seen you were just given like routine painkillers because they didn't realise how severe the pain was.

As a result, Suzanne and her mother shared a philosophy of treatment and care which prioritised home comforts and self-sufficiency over what the NHS offered. She recalled that during the long hours of 'rolling in pain' in hospital, Heather would usually take her home, 'because at least if you're home you're in a warm bed, instead of a wooden bench in A&E'.

Suzanne recalled that NHS disinterest in SCD meant that the education she received on her condition as a medical student was not only limited but inaccurate. She remembered a lecturer who confused SCD with chronic anaemia and claimed that people with the condition were often unaware that they had it. 'Did they ask us?' she said. As a junior doctor, she witnessed continued medical scepticism about the seriousness of sickle cell crises – during her paediatrics rotation in 1985, she saw children with SCD dying from pulmonary crisis in the waiting room. Suzanne saw institutional racism in the NHS operating at several levels – the overt racism of doctors who dismissed patients as drug addicts, and the structural indifference to the health of Black British people in the absence of education about the condition for healthcare providers. In asking,

110   *Experiential expertise*

'did they ask us?', Suzanne points to the limitations of medical 'expertise' as disconnected from the embodied reality of patients' experiences of SCD. Her experiential expertise sat in uncomfortable tension with that of the medical experts who taught her.

Suzanne's diagnosis narrative centres the explanatory power of biomedicine, and her own professional identity, and demonstrates a complex relationship to the NHS as an institution where she worked but (especially in her early life) was not cared for. Suzanne and Heather evolved their own familial culture of domestic care that was shaped by her mother's experience in Grenada. This section will now turn to Julie, who used biomedicine as a way to reinterpret charged social stories around family, marriage, reproduction, and infant mortality in 1960s Britain and Nigeria.

Julie

Julie was born in the late 1960s near Lagos in Nigeria, and moved to the UK in the early 1990s, where she married a British-Nigerian man and had four children before they later divorced. In her testimony, Julie retrospectively identified multiple instances of SCD within her family and extended social circle, which often centred upon the unexplained death of a young child being later revealed as due to SCD. In these anecdotes, there were two possible reasons for these late revelations: late or missed diagnosis of SCD by doctors, due to poor medical understanding of the condition in Britain, and the fear of stigma being attached to a family (and particularly to the mother) if the diagnosis of a hereditary illness was made public. In the interview, Julie offered analysis and reflection on why many families kept SCD diagnoses secret.

Julie remembered the day she was informed of her daughter's diagnosis, after neonatal screening in London, in 2000:

> J: Do you know in this country when you have a child, it is on the seventh day, you have a heel prick test [...] [it was] the morning of the christening, I had loads of people around me [when the nurse came]. So I took her into a room, away from people ... and then she said, 'oh I'm afraid, your daughter has got sickle cell' and I'm like – sickle what? I didn't even know my ex at the time had the trait! I knew I had the trait, I carried my card about, and I did mention to him when I met him that I've got the trait, and he said, 'oh I'm fine, I've never been ill, I'm fine'.

Migration, kinship, and 'everyday theorising'

GR: What's your ex's heritage? Is he from ...

J: Nigerian, born here, British born. Actually his sister died of sickle cell disease here in the UK, she was buried here [...] she was born in 1968 I think and she died at the age of two or so, she must have died in 1970 [...] I didn't know nothing [about that], until we had [our daughter], and he was telling me the story. No, he told his dad that [our daughter] had got sickle cell, and his dad had only told him that that was what his sister died of. You know, parents keep things from children. They don't really think it's important, so they never had that discussion [...] and it took him a long time because I told [my ex] not to tell them.

Julie's father-in-law revealed that his daughter had died suddenly, and that a post-mortem had indicated she had died from SCD. Several years had elapsed between Julie's daughter's diagnosis and her ex-husband's conversation with his father. Julie and her ex-husband kept their daughter's condition a secret from their extended families for years, for fear that their marriage would draw disapproval. Her mother had warned her against marrying her ex-husband. 'I said, no he is good for me, so [...] I ignored whatever she's got to say, so for me it was a case of "ooh I told you so".' When she did tell her mother, her mother discouraged her from telling other members of their family or social circle, for fear that they would interpret the illness as a mark of punishment from God.

Julie reflected on her experience of secrecy around diagnosis as part of a wider social practice and recounted and analysed multiple instances of this in her extended social circle. In one instance, Julie learned that a neighbour's son, who had died aged ten, had died from SCD. This was revealed only years later, when Julie's sister married into the family. Julie speculated that the family had kept the illness a secret to protect the child's mother, who might be ousted by her in-laws if they had learned the truth. 'They might think, oh she's not good enough for their son,' Julie said. She identified the gendered responsibility for genetic illness (as well as for the sex of children) as a source of stress for herself and other women with children with SCD. In her testimony, Julie contextualised the attribution of SCD to mothers within a broader gendered responsibility for childlessness, or failure to produce sons. She saw this as linked to women's disadvantaged position in society, because 'women are the weaker sex out of the two, it's easier to pick on the woman, as opposed to the man', and noted that in instances of separation and divorce, '[i]n Nigeria it is the woman who moves out' and suffers material consequences.

When discussing this sense of gendered responsibility and its financial impact, Julie editorialised her memories with her understanding of genetic inheritance. 'Even though it's both of [the parents] that would have carried the gene, the S gene, the woman gets blamed', Julie said. She recalled another neighbour who had thirteen daughters.

> What happened? Her husband left her. Because he wanted a male child. Now, it takes two of them! It is the man who actually produces the Y chromosome, and the woman is the X. So the two comes together, and then you have a male child [...] But again, the woman is blamed for that, and the husband can leave you for that.

Reflecting on a social context in which parental responsibility for reproductive outcomes was highly gendered, in our interview Julie deployed her knowledge of genetic inheritance to confront a patriarchal social code around marriage and separation.[21] But Julie also observed that secrecy around a diagnosis could be necessary to protect a couple from social disapproval or pressure to separate, and so technologies like sickle cell testing had the potential to both dispel unfair gendered responsibility for genetic conditions, and also break up happy marriages. Julie's testimony recalls Carole Boyce Davies's exploration of the concept of 'marking' within Black women's writing as a (sometimes inherited) multiple signifier of the physical marks of childbirth and motherhood, and also the societal inscriptions laid upon them in male-dominated and racially stratified societies.[22] In her observations on the social marking of mothers, and her empathic recollections of mothers she has known, Julie drew upon the science of heredity to redefine the meaning of motherhood.

Julie's story of her daughter's diagnosis, in which her daughter's christening was marred by news that the child had an illness that she understood as one 'that kills people', touches on another aspect of Julie's experience – that of early infant mortality. Many of Julie's experiences and stories of people she had known with SCD dealt with deaths of young children, in both Britain and Nigeria – one of her maternal cousins had died as a child after returning to Nigeria from Britain in the 1970s and was discovered to have had SCD when her brother looked up her NHS medical records decades later.

Migration, kinship, and 'everyday theorising' 113

She reported her first reaction to her daughter's diagnosis as one of grief, due to her understanding of SCD as an illness which killed children. She described lying awake at night to watch her daughter sleeping. '[I knew] that you could die at the age of two,' she said, 'and that was why I was so protective of her, throughout. I would wake up in the middle of the night, I would not sleep, I'd be looking at her, like I just wanna catch whatever is going to like, take her away from me.'

But Julie also expressed hope that biomedical advancements since many of her peers with SCD had died in the 1960s and 1970s would make a difference for her own daughter. She explained that when they learned this news from her father-in-law, he reassured them that 'she'll be fine, you know in those days, the kind of medicals you have now they didn't have back then'. She observed that when her ex-husband's young sister was born fifty years previously, 'there was little research, I don't think there were so many people with it, or people would have it and just didn't know they had it'.

In our interview, Julie detailed the social and familial networks she had grown up and lived in and distinguished between her experience of those events at the time, and her retrospective understanding of these past events. Throughout the interview, she reflected on the disparities between these two narratives. Julie's narrative draws on biomedicine as an explanatory framework that allowed her to refute gendered responsibility for genetic illness, and as a narrative of hope and progress that reframes SCD as a chronic illness that can be managed with treatment, rather than a death sentence. Both Suzanne and Julie's narratives were shaped by the context of growing up with SCD in the NHS in the 1960s – with poor treatment in Suzanne's instance and missed diagnosis and death in Julie's family.

Care, illness management, and living within the NHS

This section will discuss how Suzanne and Julie utilised these reinterpreted family histories and frameworks of biomedical knowledge and care experience in their everyday lives. Both women mobilised their understanding of SCD in their particular social and political contexts to advocate for themselves or for others in the structures of the NHS and the broader welfare state.

114   *Experiential expertise*

Suzanne

Suzanne and her mother, Heather, managed their symptoms at home, when they could, partly because of the ineffectiveness of NHS treatment and the ignorance of the healthcare professionals they encountered. Suzanne often described their methods of care and management of their shared condition in reference to bolstering mother and daughter for work. Heather worked in a range of cleaning and factory jobs for much of her life, and Suzanne described how her mother's example and lessons as a parent often centred on the importance of work. 'I always looked up to my mum because she brought me and my sister up on her own. She was working sixty hours a week, manual labour, she did it,' Suzanne remembered. Suzanne described pushing through her own career in spite of routine sexist, racist, and ableist harassment, including sexual assault and unequal treatment in comparison to less qualified white colleagues.

Suzanne kept her illness a secret from her fellow medical students and colleagues for years, never taking a day off sick, and broke her silence when she confided in the general practitioner (GP) who conducted a physical examination before she could start her clinical training in 1984. Suzanne recalled that 'he said "oh you should not have been allowed into medical school, you shouldn't be here, we'll have to tell the Dean, you're really not supposed to be here"'. She suggested that he was unaware of the variability of the disease, which could affect some people 'severely, but not everyone'. Although Suzanne was allowed to continue her training, years later she had an offer of a GP partnership withdrawn when her supervisor disclosed Suzanne's disease in her reference. Although the only impact of her disease on her work was one day off a month for a blood transfusion, she said that the image of the sickle cell patient as someone 'in and out of the hospital all the time' worried her would-be employers. Between these two events in 1984 and the late 1990s, the 1995 Disability Discrimination Act had made discrimination against people in respect to their disabilities in relation to their employment unlawful.[23]

Working long shifts as a trainee doctor, Suzanne said, 'no matter how bad the pain was during the night, my mum would just make the coffee extra strong and extra sweet and I'd put the matchsticks in [my eyes], so I never really had time off'. She rarely took painkillers,

Migration, kinship, and 'everyday theorising' 115

and today tries not to take morphine during her crises, because 'I wouldn't be able to function at work [...] I'll take co-codamol, drink fluids, just get through it'. That her mother, Heather, had managed her illness in Grenada without medical intervention had surely shaped her understanding of the illness and her approach to management of the condition – management which took place at home and within the comfort of family. But their refusal to take time off work or accept support or relief was also informed by their relationship to the British state and the stigmatisation of both immigrants and welfare benefits. In our interview, Suzanne moved rhetorically between speaking about analgesia and speaking about state benefits. She said that she and her mother were 'horrified' by the thought of accepting sickness benefits, saying 'My mum wouldn't accept state benefit for anything, it was work, you went to work!' In moving back and forth between discussing pain relief and state benefits, Suzanne observed how state stigmatisation of both disability and race intersected in her experience. She knew that both racism and NHS hostility to staff illness operated against her in British workplaces, and racist tropes of immigrants as 'benefit scroungers' were widespread in the 1960s and beyond. In her emphasis on the effort and physicality of managing her illness while working and not accepting welfare benefit, Suzanne both responded to Thatcherite rhetoric against 'dependency on the welfare state' and appropriated it as a defence against racist tropes.[24] But, in doing this, she also staked her claim to a place in the NHS, in defiance of white colleagues who had communicated that she could not, or should not, be there.

Speaking about her and her mother's shared experience of SCD, Suzanne said '[w]e got through it, we were like the people from world war times, they learned to make do and mend and get through it. And that's what we did.' Situating herself on the inside of the welfare state, as a doctor giving her care, and a worker paying her dues, rather than as a patient receiving its benefits, it is striking that Suzanne draws upon a founding myth of postwar British national identity, of 'Blitz spirit' and 'make do and mend'. Enoch Powell and others used national memories of the Blitz and the 'greatest sacrifice' of the Second World War to reify Britain and its welfare state as the inheritance solely of its white inhabitants, and to challenge the entitlement and citizenship of its Black subjects.[25] Suzanne and her mother's personal war was the internal and embodied one of working

116   *Experiential expertise*

as Black women, contending with exclusionary institutional racism that demanded perfection and self-reliance from them, whilst living with a painful chronic illness. Her use of 'make do and mend' in this context subverts it, for the 'Blitz' myth in part generated the conditions of Suzanne's own 'Blitz' – the 'exclusionary identity of "whiteness"' which underpinned notions of universal welfare in Britain.[26] This capaciousness of Second World War memory reflects the investment of West Indians in British national identity at the time – Kennetta Hammond Perry has shown that, of the many Caribbean men and women who served in the war, some who did so 'adopted a sense of Britishness that was both patriotic and capable of serving autonomous desires for social and economic mobility'.[27]

Suzanne's identity as primarily a doctor rather than a patient is felt in her distancing of herself from patient support groups when they were offered to her by consultants. 'I thought, well how is that going to help me, swapping cake recipes and knitting patterns,' she said. She felt that she would be a 'fraud' in a patient group as a doctor and was pessimistic about being 'welcomed' by laypeople who 'describe their symptoms in really odd ways' and repeat the 'myths' that she felt were common to SCD circles. Suzanne understood her status as a healthcare professional as dividing her from peer support. But in our interview she synthesised her own and her mother's experiences of work and health into 'everyday theorising' that analysed their positions as Black women in the postwar British workplace, and their responses to the sexism, racism, and ableism they experienced there.

Julie

Suzanne and Heather's approach to at-home management and their rejection of some forms of state 'care' or support, rooted in Heather's experience of having no access to biomedical treatment in Grenada, was, then, shaped by ableism in NHS employment practices and by discourses around immigrants and the state in Britain. Like Suzanne, Julie also participates in the health service, but as a layperson with experiential expertise. In working with a local support group, Julie listens to the stories of other mothers of children with SCD, generating a 'collective experiential knowledge' both of embodied experience of sickle cell trait and SCD and of the local healthcare structures.[28]

Migration, kinship, and 'everyday theorising' 117

Her narrative is shaped by a shift from paternalism to consumerism within the NHS since the 1960s, which enshrined in principle (if not in practice) the notion of the patient as a consumer whose feedback should influence NHS provision and incentives.[29]

As the mother of a child with SCD, Julie is active in a family support group in her local area. She has found that much of her supporting work is often done privately, through phone calls or messages, rather than the sometimes sparsely attended group meeting. 'It was working well, people were calling me, but they weren't attending the meeting. They didn't want to come [...] [because] families met, that have been hiding away from each other that they have kids with sickle cell.' Julie empathised, because she and her husband had kept their daughter's illness a secret from their families for many years out of fear that their marriage would be met with disapproval.

> I can understand these people not turning up for the meeting. I've been there, and I've come out of there, I am very open now I can talk about it, I was once upon a time not able to talk about my child with sickle cell disease openly. But I've got past that, and I think that was due to education, I educated myself, self-taught, read more about the disease, the management, and then researched what people had said and done around it.

One of the first books Julie read was produced in Britain by Nigerian-born nurse Lola Oni, *The Care and Management of Children with Sickle Cell Disease* (1997), as well as scholarly research articles from US medical journals. Through this research, and through building relationships with sickle cell specialist doctors and nurses in the NHS, she articulates the role that she, other parents, and people with SCD have in challenging NHS services for the condition. She has lodged complaints about the standards of SCD care in her local hospital and participated in events educating NHS staff about the condition.

> They need knowledge, they need education more. I was told by one nurse, we had these patient participatory days, like for parents of children with sickle cell, and the student nurses ... they want them to come and sit down with the parents so that we can share our experiences with them, so we had a day like that. So they were there, taking notes and all that [...] [The student nurses] have realised that

118   *Experiential expertise*

> throughout your nursing career, they don't mention sickle cell … Sickle cell goes under the carpet, just mentioned by the roadside. But now they're involving the new nurses, and they came to the meeting to hear from us, and they could ask questions from us or the haematologists, the specialists.

In our interview Julie detailed the different clinical standards and pathways for people with SCD in her local hospital in comparison with the services available in London. She described making official complaints about the services her daughter accesses. Julie combines her experience as the mother of a child with SCD, the research she has done, and the relationships she has built with healthcare professionals, into an expertise that she uses to inform NHS training and services. Her experience of this in the twenty-first-century NHS reflects a longer history of SCD patients and mothers advocating for their or their children's treatment in healthcare settings. Many accounts from the 1970s and 1980s describe difficult dynamics in which patients or their carers knew more about SCD than the attending nurse or physician. 'Doctors in Casualty do not like to be told your condition by you the patient,' one young sufferer commented in a survey.[30] One mother found that she was repeatedly required to give doctors instructions on emergency care for her son, and she sometimes turned to threats. Noticing that her son was dehydrated (a serious risk to a person with SCD), 'I said to this casualty officer "If you leave him to get more dehydrated and I lose this child, I will kill you." After about half an hour a drip was set up.'[31] Julie's experience reflects a changing approach to patient experience in the NHS, and also the patchwork nature of SCD services in England, which has continued well into the twenty-first century.

Julie articulated that her experience could educate trainee healthcare professionals, but also that her experience enables her to create a social and therapeutic space for other families in her position. She articulated a gradual change in her own thinking, moving away from a fear that her daughter would die young as many people from her own generation had, towards hope for the future and for biomedical promise.

> I started to change my thoughts, to that she was going to live, she wasn't going to die, that she's in capable hands […] I think it was

Migration, kinship, and 'everyday theorising' 119

because of that that I thought I could actually help other parents to come out of that and be open about it as well. Now look here, I know your pain [...] I have been through it, I'm going through it [...] the doctors will work on the medical side of things, but they can't actually fix the emotional side of things [...] The support group was set up to address that other aspect.

Julie's narrative of coming to terms with her daughter's diagnosis and moving beyond her familial experiences of early childhood mortality in SCD (in both Britain and Nigeria) is a therapeutic narrative for herself and for others. Her narrative reflects her resistance to the gendered assumptions about genetic responsibility that she grew up with, and her proactive advocacy for her daughter in a medical system that has neglected conditions like SCD, and where poor understanding of the condition is still widespread, particularly in A&E departments.[32] She affirms her trust in biomedical treatment and protocols for her daughter, which have given her hope for her daughter's future, and seeks to use her experiential expertise to hold the health system accountable as providers of that biomedical hope. Julie's experience aligns with broader histories of families using their 'emotional and technical knowledge [...] to foster networks of support from which activism may emerge'.[33] Her story also illustrates how this experiential expertise can be used for change at the level of family, community, and local state.[34]

Both Julie and Suzanne expressed in their testimonies that they feel they are different from those around them. Suzanne is self-reliant and sees herself as separate from others who might go to support group meetings because of her identification as a doctor, rather than a layperson. Julie notes that her unusual openness allows her to be a trusted social linchpin in, and representative for, her local sickle cell community. Both women perceived the gendered and racialised hierarchies of the NHS but seek to make the NHS into a place for them. Suzanne has configured her sense of belonging and citizenship through her identity as a worker in, rather than a claimant of, the NHS. Julie has sought to make the NHS into a place for SCD itself – she counters both social narratives of shame, fear, and silence around SCD, and instances of poor care for the condition in the NHS, by speaking about her experiences with her community and with medical staff.

Conclusion

The NHS was a critical site of labour for Commonwealth migrants to Britain in the postwar period, and a space which Black British women, whose own bodies were so scrutinised and who bore the responsibility for familial health, could not avoid entering.[35] Diagnosis narratives therefore foreground the relationships between health, 'race', gender, and anti-racist resistance which are rarely centred in traditional histories of Black British activism. Such stories illuminate the 'everyday theorising' that is a foundation for women's political organisation.[36] It also sheds light on the lives of Black women embedded in the health service as workers or patients, who observed and analysed the matrix of power operating within the NHS, and created everyday cultures of personal resistance beyond the spaces of organised political activism.[37] Denise Noble explores the 'untidy everyday tactics' deployed by Black women to confront systems that '[block] their path to autonomy, self-determination or freedom'.[38] Suzanne and Julie's situated experiences and narratives, as they examine and re-examine their identities and histories, reflect this resistance in different forms.

Suzanne described how her mother's understanding of her own health was reframed by her migration to Britain and her experiences of pregnancy. She articulated a personal identity in which she responded to sexism, racism, and ableism at work, and limited medical treatment for her illness, with self-sufficiency. For Julie's extended family, diagnosis and treatment of SCD in the 1960s and 1970s could be patchy or negligent, and children with the illness sometimes died young. But Julie used the insights of genetic medicine to construct a framework with which she could critique the gendered stigma around SCD that she had grown up with, challenge NHS underinvestment in the condition, and find hope for her own daughter's future. Both women differ in terms of how they view the changes in NHS care since the 1960s – Julie saw the changes as a hopeful sign that her daughter might have a different life to others she had known with the condition, while Suzanne worried that framing SCD as a disability might discourage people with SCD from achieving their potential. But both women had taken on roles within the NHS – Suzanne as a doctor who saw the NHS as a place where she could defy and refuse racist narratives about migrants and about

Migration, kinship, and 'everyday theorising' 121

SCD, Julie as an expert representing her community's interests to the NHS.[39]

Heidi Safia Mirza argues that '[i]t is only by attention to situated localised accounts of "marginalised lives" that we can reveal the ways of "being and becoming" a gendered, sexed, raced and classed subject of materialist discourse'.[40] Diagnosis narratives provide an entry point into how Black British women have navigated medical systems and structures of knowledge in twentieth- and twenty-first-century Britain. This chapter has shown how two women, as they navigate racism, sexism, and ableism in their personal and professional lives, bring a range of genetic, familial, and cultural frameworks to bear in analysing them. Biomedical knowledge, which often focused on Black women's bodies as a site of genetic risk, could also be repurposed by Black women to reject the gendered genetic responsibility they had been assigned. They perceived the limits of biomedical knowledge about SCD but were often constrained by racialised NHS professional hierarchies from correcting or challenging such 'expertise'. Their knowledge could sometimes be instrumentalised into the emerging role for patients of 'experiential expertise', as they used both their embodied experience and their understanding of health structures to seek to hold the NHS to account. Crucially, their 'think[ing] and know[ing]' produced narratives and strategies for forging relationships, coping with adversity, and surviving the NHS as a hostile space for Black women.[41]

Notes

1 Lola Oni, interviewed by Grace Redhead, 10 April 2018.

2 Felix Konotey-Ahulu, *The Sickle Cell Disease Patient* (London: The Macmillan Press, 1991), pp. 4, 115; Lola Oni, 'African and Caribbean People's Attitude to Sickle Cell and the Risk of Having a Child with Sickle Cell Anaemia' (PhD thesis, University of Surrey, 2007), pp. 48–9.

3 Anne Hunsaker Hawkins, 'Medical ethics and the epiphanic dimension of narrative', in Hilde Lindemann Nelson (ed.), *Stories and Their Limits: Narrative Approaches to Bioethics* (London: Routledge, 1997), p. 163.

4 Lynn Abrams, 'Liberating the female self: epiphanies, conflict and coherence in the life stories of post-war British Women', *Social History*, 39:1 (2014), 14–15.

122   *Experiential expertise*

5   Susan Lindee, *Moments of Truth in Genetic Medicine* (Baltimore, MD: Johns Hopkins University Press, 2005), p. 2.

6   Duana Fullwiley, *The Enculturated Gene: Sickle Cell Health Politics and Biological Difference in West Africa* (Princeton, NJ: Princeton University Press, 2012), p. 85.

7   Cecily Jones, '"Human weeds, not fit to breed?" African Caribbean women and reproductive disparities in Britain', *Critical Public Health*, 23:1 (2013).

8   Kaja Finkler, 'The kin in the gene: the medicalization of family and kinship in American society', *Current Anthropology*, 42:2 (April 2001).

9   Ilana Löwy, 'How genetics came to the unborn: 1960–2000', *Studies in History and Philosophy of Science Part C: Studies in History and Philosophy of Biological and Biomedical Sciences*, 47 (2015), 154–62; Finkler, 'The kin in the gene', 238.

10 Elizabeth Nneka Anionwu, 'Health Education and Community Development for Sickle Cell Disorders in Brent' (PhD thesis, University of London Institute of Education, 1988).

11 Grace Redhead, '"A British problem affecting British people": sickle cell anaemia, medical activism and race in the National Health Service, 1975–1993', *Twentieth Century British History*, 32:2 (2021), 205.

12 Caitlin Lambert, '"The objectable injectable": recovering the lost history of the WLM through the Campaign against Depo-Provera', *Women's History Review*, 29:3 (2020), 523–6.

13 Beverley Bryan, Stella Dadzie, and Suzanne Scafe, *Heart of the Race: Black Women's Lives in Britain* (London: Virago Press, 1985), p. 90.

14 Nikolas Rose and Carlos Novas, 'Biological citizenship', in Aiwha Ong and Stephen J. Collier (eds), *Global Assemblages: Technology, Politics and Ethics as Anthropological Problems* (Maldon, MA: Blackwell, 2007), p. 441.

15 Carole Boyce Davies, *Black Women, Writing and Identity: Migrations of the Subject* (London and New York: Routledge, 1994), p. 17.

16 Stuart Hall, 'Old and new identities, old and new ethnicities', in Anthony D. King (ed.), *Culture, Globalization and the World-System: Contemporary Conditions for the Representation of Identity* (Minneapolis, MN: University of Minnesota Press, 1991); Paul Gilroy, *The Black Atlantic: Modernity and Double Consciousness* (London: Verso, 1993), p. 4.

17 Julia Chinyere Oparah, *Other Kinds of Dreams: Black Women's Organisations and the Politics of Transformation* (London: Routledge, 1998), p. 3.

18 Umut Erel and Tracey Reynolds, 'Introduction: migrant mothers challenging racialized citizenship', *Ethnic and Racial Studies*, 41:1 (2018), 7.

Migration, kinship, and 'everyday theorising'   123

19 Carolyn Moxley Rouse shows that deep tissue massage has been used in alternative therapies for sickle cell pain in the United States, while in her study of SCD in Senegal Duana Fullwiley argues that the herbal therapies many employed 'often depend on the relationship between patient and healer'. Carolyn Moxley Rouse, *Uncertain Suffering: Racial Health Care Disparities and Sickle Cell Disease* (Berkeley and Los Angeles, CA: University of California Press, 2009), pp. 240–1; Fullwiley, *The Enculturated Gene*, pp. 18–19.

20 This continues to be a problem in NHS treatment of SCD. Redhead, '"A British problem affecting British people"'.

21 In other national contexts, women have used the technology of sickle cell testing to leave unhappy marriages. This technical liberation is not inherent to the technology – the technology is given this meaning and use by the 'wide-ranging lived experiences and personal biopolitics' of SCD. See Duana Fullwiley, 'Discriminate biopower and everyday biopolitics: views on sickle cell testing in Dakar', *Medical Anthropology*, 23:2 (2004), 186.

22 Davies, *Black Women, Writing and Identity*, pp. 137–9.

23 National Disability Council, *Disability Discrimination Act 1995: Code of Practice, Rights of Access, Goods, Facilities, Services and Premises* (London: Stationery Office, 1999).

24 Gary Craig, '"Cunning, unprincipled, loathsome": the racist tail wags the welfare dog', *Journal of Social Policy*, 36:4 (2007), 617; Emily Robinson, Camilla Schofield, Florence Sutcliffe-Braithwaite, and Natalie Thomlinson, 'Telling stories about post-war Britain: popular individualism and the "crisis" of the 1970s', *Twentieth Century British History*, 28:2 (2017), 15; Imogen Tyler, *Stigma: The Machine of Inequality* (London: Zed Books, 2020).

25 Camilla Schofield, *Enoch Powell and the Making of Postcolonial Britain* (Cambridge: Cambridge University Press, 2013), p. 15.

26 Des Fitzgerald, Amy Hinterberger, John Narayan, and Ros Williams, 'Brexit as heredity redux: imperialism, biomedicine and the NHS in Britain', *The Sociological Review*, 68:6 (November 2020), 1165.

27 Kennetta Hammond Perry, *London is the Place for Me: Black Britons, Citizenship, and the Politics of Race* (Oxford: Oxford University Press, 2018), p. 47.

28 Eva Marie Castro et al., 'Patients' experiential knowledge and expertise in health care: a hybrid concept analysis', *Social Theory & Health*, 17 (2019), 313.

29 Alex Mold, 'Repositioning the patient: patient organisations, consumerism, and autonomy in Britain during the 1960s and 1970s', *Bulletin of the History of Medicine*, 87 (2013), 226.

124   *Experiential expertise*

30 Sickle Cell Society, *Pain in Sickle Cell Disease: Proceedings of a Symposium Held at Central Middlesex Hospital, London, on 7 December 1983* (Cambridge: National Extension College, 1986), p. 63.

31 Janet Black and Sophie Laws, *Living with Sickle Cell Disease: An Enquiry into the Need for Health and Social Service Provision for Sickle Cell Sufferers in Newham* (London: East London Branch of the Sickle Cell Society, 1986), pp. 97–8.

32 Subarna Chakravorty et al., 'Patient reported experience measure in sickle cell disease', *Archives of Disease in Childhood*, 103 (2018).

33 Rayna Rapp and Faye Ginsburg, 'Enabling disability: rewriting kinship, reimagining citizenship', *Public Culture*, 13:3 (2001), 545.

34 Oparah, *Other Kinds of Dreams*, p. 60.

35 Christopher Kyriakides and Satnam Virdee, 'Migrant labour, racism and the British National Health Service', *Ethnicity and Health*, 8:4 (2003).

36 Oparah, *Other Kinds of Dreams*, p. 35.

37 Rob Waters, 'Thinking Black: Peter Fryer's *Staying Power* and the politics of writing Black British history in the 1980s', *History Workshop Journal*, 82 (2016), 116.

38 Denise Noble, 'Remembering bodies, healing histories: the emotional politics of everyday freedom', in Claire Alexander and Caroline Knowles (eds), *Making Race Matter: Bodies, Space and Identity* (Basingstoke: Palgrave Macmillan, 2005), p. 135.

39 Roberta Bivins, 'Commentary: Serving the nation, serving the people: echoes of war in the early NHS', *Medical Humanities,* 46:2 (2020), 154–6.

40 Heidi Safia Mirza, '"Harvesting our collective intelligence": Black British feminism in post-race times', *Women's Studies International Forum*, 51 (2015), 4.

41 Oparah, *Other Kinds of Dreams*, p. 35.

Part II

Sites and spaces

Part II: Introduction

Tracey Loughran

In 2019, exhausted from the long-term effects of bereavement, family illness, work stress, and separation from friends after moving to a new part of the country, I started to crack at the seams. I spoke to my line manager, who insisted that I take some time off. I went to my doctor, who prescribed anti-depressants as soon as I started crying and ushered me out not long after. I spent hours on the phone to family and friends. I tried to get endorphins to work their magic by running and swimming more and ended up with swimmer's ear (a bacterial infection), treated by antibiotics obtained at my local hospital walk-in clinic. I found a bereavement counsellor on the internet, and in our sessions spoke at length to her about all the different griefs that permeated my life. After four months, I was well enough to end these sessions. In early 2021, struggling with many lockdown-related problems, including more death and more illness, I contacted her again. In our first Zoom session I found myself puzzled by how difficult it was to hold her gaze, until I remembered: two years' earlier, sitting in the ground-floor consulting room of the converted residential townhouse she shared with other therapeutic practitioners, I had always faced the window and, as I tried to articulate the things that were hard to think, never mind speak, fixed my gaze on the upper window of the house opposite. On Zoom, there was nowhere else to look but at her or myself.

The workplace office, leisure centre, home, and Zoom call are sites of healthcare as important in this story as the GP surgery, hospital walk-in clinic, and private counsellor's consulting room. If understanding 'everyday health' involves shifting from a top-down

128   *Sites and spaces*

to bottom-up perspective, switching from the perspectives of medicine and science to those of 'ordinary' people, that also means looking at diverse sites and spaces of health/care. Traditional histories of medicine and health usually focus on institutional sites (hospitals, clinics, laboratories) and portray them as clearly demarcated from the spaces of everyday life (home, work, social venues).[1] This perceived division further implies the existence of firm boundaries between public and private life. The concept of 'everyday health' challenges these assumptions and collapses these divisions. Part II of this volume explores constructions and experiences of 'everyday health' in different spaces. It emphasises the porous boundaries between public and private realms; exposes the interaction between 'top-down' agencies, sites such as the mass media and community organisations, and individual subjectivities; and explores the challenges researchers face in seeking to understand intimate aspects of embodiment and selfhood and to communicate these understandings to different audiences, past and present.

Gareth Millward (chapter 5) examines the Housewife's Non-Contributory Invalidity Pension (HNCIP), a social security benefit payable to married and cohabiting women deemed incapable of fulfilling either 'normal household duties' or paid employment, and assessed through a 'household duties test' that determined whether women could perform 'everyday' activities. The story of HNCIP shows the reach of the state into the lives of disabled women. It also reveals that for a state tied to the model of nuclear families headed by male breadwinners, with an economy dependent on women's unpaid labour as housewives, it was not possible to square the circle of ending discrimination against disabled housewives, holding on to the key principles of National Insurance, and keeping costs down. The strange story of HNCIP underscores from an unexpected angle the truth of the contemporary feminist slogan 'the personal is political': through the claims of women who could no longer work in the home, it became evident that the division between public and private spheres, a founding assumption of the welfare state, simply did not exist for women who worked in the home – in the process throwing up questions about what defined not only 'work' but 'home' itself, and underlining the extent to which conventional answers to those questions depended on gendered assumptions.

Part II: Introduction

129

Where Millward uses the case study of HNCIP to unpick the unspoken beliefs about gender that governed British society and culture in the 1970s, Fleur MacInnes (chapter 6) explores the active remaking of gender in transfeminine spaces in the same period. If 'everyday health' is an underexplored concept in most contexts, it is virtually non-existent in trans history, a field still in its infancy but dominated by medicalised perspectives and narratives. MacInnes offers a counter-history of the role of friendship and mutual aid in building trans communities. They examine the newsletters and magazines of organisations including the Beaumont Society, the TV/ TS Group, and the Transsexual Action Group as spaces where transfeminine communities were forged. These organisations protected the identities of members, for example through measures to ensure anonymity and therefore privacy, but they also provided spaces in print, person, and the imagination for the quasi-public flourishing of their trans identities, as in the practice of all members using separate 'female' names to mark out their status within the Beaumont Society. MacInnes' chapter is a crucial first step towards moving the sites of trans history beyond medical spaces and into trans communities, where people are not case histories or medical records, but individuals who joke, bicker, and sometimes fight; where they are real people with real lives who exist outside the institutions that label and treat them (kindly or unkindly); in short, where they are exactly like the people who populate other histories.

Caroline Rusterholz (chapter 7) deals with young people, another group often positioned as the subject of discourse rather than its speakers, and their interactions with Brook Advisory Centres (BACs) between the 1960s and 1980s. Rusterholz explores BACs as semi-public, semi-private spaces that sought to help young people navigate sexual relationships against the backdrop of highly polarised public debates about the effects of 'permissiveness'. She also shows the many sites in which Brook supported young people to negotiate their emergent sexualities: adolescents traversed cities on public transport to access the deliberately home-like spaces of BACs; they watched BAC public education videos and read BAC leaflets in school, perhaps under the tutelage of teachers who had attended Brook training seminars; they consumed advice about Brook and from former Brook workers in teen magazines. In analysing BAC's

130 *Sites and spaces*

multiple techniques for positioning itself as a trusted interlocutor in young people's private lives, and its gradual transition from a controversial offshoot of Marie Stopes UK to an organisation promoted in the tabloid press for its responsible attitude to youthful sexuality, Rusterholz warns us against taking sensationalist public rhetoric at face value.

Finally, Daisy Payling (chapter 8) discusses her own experiences of moving historical materials from libraries and archives, often experienced as individual and private spaces during the process of research, into different arenas with the aim of engaging different publics. Payling created the quiz 'Could you be an agony aunt?' out of letters and responses from the 'semi-public, semi-private' space of the magazine problem page.[2] In repurposing problems and guidance to educate and entertain different audiences, she grappled with the specific needs and desires of each audience, as well as how to represent within a simplified format and to non-specialist audiences the past experiences of different groups, in ways that neither denied nor lingered on their oppression. The chapter argues for the value of remaining receptive to unexpected opportunities and trying out a range of creative practices when working with public audiences to use history to instigate social change.

Together, these chapters explore multiple sites and spaces for the making of 'everyday health': state bureaucracies, voluntary sector clinics, schools, community organisations, cultural institutions, magazines and newsletters, and the home. These particular sites are specific to postwar Britain, but healthcare has always taken place at multiple sites, the borders of public and private have always been porous, and similar processes can be traced at work across other modern polities. In welfare states, the government takes responsibility for the health of its populations, and people are simultaneously citizens, patients, and service users; but, paradoxically, direct interaction with the state in the form of medical care means that nationalised healthcare systems also become part of the backdrop of everyday life. In Britain, even at the height of the welfare state, voluntary organisations and other non-state actors still played a considerable part in the provision of formal and informal healthcare, while the ideologically driven dismantling of the welfare state since 1979 has expanded their role.[3] The reshaping of citizenship in the postwar period also involved redrawing the boundaries of public and private

Part II: Introduction 131

life as the state intervened to provide pensions for those in 'old age' and benefits for the sick and unemployed; to pass legislation to ensure married women's independence from their husbands, the rights of consenting gay men to sex in private places without fear of blackmail or prosecution, and the eradication of discrimination on grounds of 'race'; or, more ominously, to insist that teachers could not educate students about the full range of human sexualities.[4] At the same time, late capitalism's provocation of continuous and insatiable desire for bigger, better, more, has ensured the proliferating demand and supply of agencies for the perfectibility of body and self.

In tracing the operations and intersections of these trends at different sites, in different spaces, and at different times, the chapters in this section demonstrate the many agencies shaping experiences of 'everyday health' for individuals at any given place and time. But they also demonstrate the possibilities of implicit and explicit resistance, revealed here through creative engagement with different sources and the refusal to take a top-down perspective even when the sources seem to nudge in that direction. Millward uses state archives, but shows how pension tribunal documents open a window onto disabled women's needs and expectations of the welfare state; these sources need to be read with sensitivity to their limitations, but they still resonate with the words of women whose voices would otherwise be lost. MacInnes carefully reconstructs trans lives from archival traces. The catalogue entry for the Wellcome Library's 'Beaumont Society paper and publications' highlights the contingency of this material's survival: 'This collection comprises Beaumont Society membership materials belonging to the member Susan 176 [...] Anonymous donation received by recorded delivery Thursday 19th April 2018, addressed to "TG/TV Archivist, Wellcome Trust Library".[5] We are unlikely to ever know who Susan was. Rusterholz reminds us that investigating the history of the recent past, especially in relation to confidential services, involves negotiating restrictions to access that make it very difficult to hear young people's own voices; she picks out these voices, mediated as they are, from multiple sources including BAC annual reports, oral history interviews, newspaper articles, and teen magazines.

In placing herself in the history, Payling underscores another reason for the absence of certain voices: that Conservative politicians in the 1980s tried to intimidate, bully, and criminalise queer education,

132   *Sites and spaces*

to deny the validity of 'pretended family relationships', and to stop queer futures from coming into being. In public engagement, the embodied status of the researcher takes on a heightened dimension; unlike when we write an article or book, we are now talking to our audiences, aware of the aspects of identity we do or do not (apparently) share with them, and we are trying to provoke new thoughts and/or emotions with no knowledge of the backgrounds and histories they bring to this encounter. As a queer academic trying to work out what queer public history looks like at the same time as creating it, Payling had to grapple with aspects of selfhood and public presentation as well as representation. To claim belonging, to stand in a public space, to not only negotiate a site but to own it – that is an act of resistance, affirmation, and power.

Notes

1 For classic studies of institutional sites of healthcare, see Lindsay Granshaw and Roy Porter (eds), *Hospitals in History* (London: Routledge, 1990); Steven Cherry (ed.), *Medical Services and the Hospitals in Britain, 1860–1939* (Cambridge: Cambridge University Press, 1996); Steve Sturdy (ed.), *Medicine, Health and the Public Sphere in Britain, 1600–2000* (London: Routledge, 2002).
2 Fiona Hackney, 'Getting a living, getting a life: Leonora Eyles, employment and agony, 1925–1930', in Rachel Ritchie, Sue Hawkins, Nicola Phillips, and S. Jay Kleinberg (eds), *Women in Magazines: Research, Representation, Production and Consumption* (New York and London: Routledge, 2016), p. 108.
3 Geoffrey Finlayson, *Citizen, State and Social Welfare in Britain, 1830–1990* (Oxford: Oxford University Press, 1994); Jane Lewis, *The Voluntary Sector, the State and Social Work in Britain* (Aldershot: Edward Elgar, 1995); Nicholas Crowson, Matthew Hilton, and James McKay (eds), *NGOs in Contemporary Britain: Non-State Actors in Society and Politics since 1945* (Basingstoke: Palgrave Macmillan, 2009).
4 Frank Mort, 'The permissive society revisited', *Twentieth Century British History*, 22:2 (2011); Margherita Rendel, 'Legislating for equal pay and opportunity for women in Britain', *Signs*, 3:4 (1978); Nasar Meer, 'Race equality after Enoch Powell', *Political Quarterly*, 89:3 (2018); Jackie Stacey, 'Promoting normality: Section 28 and the regulation of sexuality', in Sarah Franklin, Celia Lury, and Jackie Stacey (eds), *Off-Centre: Feminism and Cultural Studies* (London: HarperCollines, 1991); Hannah

Part II: Introduction   133

Elizabeth, '"If it hadn't been for the doctor, I think I would have killed myself": ensuring adolescent knowledge and access to healthcare in the age of Gillick', in Jennifer Crane and Jane Hand (eds), *Posters, Protests, and Prescriptions: Cultural Histories of the National Health Service in Britain* (Manchester: Manchester University Press, 2022).

5 'Papers of Susan, Beaumont Society Member', Wellcome Collection Catalogue: https://wellcomecollection.org/works/hntza94x (accessed 22 June 2023).

5

Writing everyday life into law: the 'household duties test', disabled women, social security, and assumed normality

Gareth Millward

Introduction

The first payments of Housewife's Non-Contributory Invalidity Pension (HNCIP) were made in 1977. It was designed for married and cohabiting women who were '*continuously* incapable of [their] normal household duties for at least 28 weeks; and *continuously* incapable of paid work' over that same period.[1] It represented a landmark for the Disablement Income Group, a 'poverty lobby' organisation founded in the 1960s by two self-identifying housewives in Godalming, Surrey, to campaign for comprehensive social security benefits for all disabled people.[2] HNCIP represented the Group's peak and was the latest in a raft of benefits created after 1970 for 'the civilian disabled' – including Incapacity Benefit, Attendance Allowance, Mobility Allowance and Non-Contributory Invalidity Pension (NCIP). HNCIP was the first benefit to recognise the needs of disabled married women, a demographic that did not fit well with the insurance-based ethos of post-1948 Beveridgean welfare.

These other benefits evolved over time but essentially still exist through their descendants, Employment and Support Allowance and Personal Independence Payment. HNCIP, however, was withdrawn in 1984. In part, this was because the Department of Health and Social Security (DHSS) knew that it could face legal challenges. Britain was now subject to the terms of the 1978 European Council directive on equal treatment for men and women,[3] itself a result of growing acceptance legally and culturally across the European

Writing everyday life into law 135

Economic Community (a predecessor of the European Union) that welfare systems that prioritised male wage earners at the expense of other citizens were no longer acceptable.[4] Unlike NCIP – available to unemployed disabled single women and men – claimants had to show that they were incapable *both* of work *and* of their 'normal household duties'. To determine this, the DHSS made claimants undergo a 'household duties test'. This leads to the question: how did the state define 'normal household duties' for disabled women in the 1970s and 1980s?

This chapter interrogates the logic behind HNCIP and the 'household duties test' to show how the British social security authorities attempted to translate 'common sense' assumptions about domestic labour, women's lives, disability, and employment into coherent gatekeeping procedures. Or, rather, it is about the circulation of different common senses, visions of what the welfare state was or ought to be that were taken as 'true', but which differed among the various groups that had a stake in the development and implementation of policy.[5] For, while benefit authorities had one set of assumptions about the 'purpose' of disability benefits and what constituted 'a disabled person', people who identified as disabled – and may even have been identified as 'disabled' by other social services – had different expectations about what they needed, what they were entitled to, and what represented 'fair' treatment.

HNCIP's short life from 1977 to 1984 provides a fascinating window onto these issues. The welfare state underwent significant political turmoil in this period, leading to the end of what some historians refer to as Britain's 'classic welfare state'.[6] After the mid-1970s, social services had to contend with the oil crisis, restricted financial capacity, and ideological reforms under Margaret Thatcher's Conservative government. At the same time, pressure from 'the poverty lobby' on behalf of groups who had 'lost out' in the 1948 welfare state settlement stimulated demand for new benefits. The administrative machinery tried in vain to incorporate these demands with rights-based discourses from second-wave feminists, the nascent social-model disability movement, and equalities legislation in Westminster and Brussels. The tribunals and complaints initiated by various constituencies across the HNCIP period, as Jackie Gulland's research into 'incapacity' as a gendered concept has shown, provide historical evidence of multiple definitions of disabled womanhood.[7]

136 *Sites and spaces*

They also reveal articulations not just of how the welfare state *was* but of how it *ought to be*.[8]

What was 'HNCIP'?

Breaking down the initialisation shows the contradictions within HNCIP, the government's assumptions about women's lives, and its implications for claimants.

First is 'H', or 'housewife'. Explicitly, this was a benefit designed only for 'married or co-habiting' women.[9] The post-1948 welfare system was built on the assumption that citizens would normally form nuclear families headed by a male 'breadwinner'.[10] He would pay National Insurance contributions entitling the family to unemployment and sickness-related benefits if he could not work, and a pension for both him and his wife in retirement. The wife, meanwhile, would perform unpaid domestic labour. Ordinarily, then, the 'housewife' was not entitled to any form of disability benefit because household income should not be materially affected by her incapacity. Although rigidly gendered boundaries between domestic and paid labour were softening in many households around this time, the common sense of social security bureaucracy still worked on the 1940s assumptions of domestic economics.[11]

Under the 1948 system, married women automatically paid a lower rate of National Insurance (until this was equalised in 1977) on the assumption that they would retire earlier than their husbands and take more career breaks, so full-rate benefits were not as important to the family budget. If a wife worked, she could claim sickness benefit, though even here there were inequalities. Married women had the choice to pay the full rate of National Insurance (single women automatically paid the higher rate), but they were also much more likely to be ineligible for full-rate benefits because employment gaps to raise children or look after elderly relatives were common.[12] This was assumed to be the natural state of family affairs. While Britain, like other European states, had developed laws around equal pay and treatment (such as the 1970 Equal Pay Act), this did not overcome the other structural factors that led to discrepancies in wages.[13] If a wife did earn, that work was likely to be lower paid (even for the same labour performed by a man), of lower status, and considered

Writing everyday life into law 137

'extras' contra the 'meaningful' wage of the husband, regardless of the actual gross or relative value of that income.[14] In the late 1970s, the social security system had yet to fully respond to the significant changes in levels of women's paid employment over the second half of the twentieth century.[15] However, the Disablement Income Group and others pressured the government to both recognise and provide for the needs of disabled people whose assumed 'normal' earning patterns did not fit the National Insurance model of welfare, including married and cohabiting women.[16] By the 1970s, therefore, it was also common sense that disabled people, regardless of their gender or marital status, should receive support from the state. This created tensions within the system.

This leads us to 'NC': 'non-contributory'. HNCIP was among several new benefits emerging in the 1970s for disabled people without National Insurance contributions. This was a core demand of the Disablement Income Group and other poverty-lobby organisations, which argued that disabled people were much less likely to be able to maintain employment consistently enough to qualify for benefits. The Beveridgean model was designed to offer higher levels of sickness and injury benefits in return for weekly National Insurance contributions as a way of maintaining work ethic.[17] Those without consistent contributions were entitled to only a subsistence level of benefit, although the National Assistance Board (later the Supplementary Benefits Commission) could provide discretionary grants to disabled people when their expenses were clearly higher than those of non-disabled persons.[18]

The irony was that the very impairments affecting individuals' abilities to build National Insurance contributions were the reason they needed higher levels of financial support in the first place. Disabled people, especially those whose impairments began before adulthood, were discriminated against by employers, the education system, employment structures, and liberal capitalism's expectation of self-reliance through paid labour. They were less likely to be able to maintain regular employment (and therefore full National Insurance records). Yet they were also entitled to little statutory support unless they were injured at work or in the armed forces.[19] In 1971, Incapacity Benefit was introduced for unemployed disabled people with National Insurance contributions, while Attendance Allowance in 1971 and Mobility Allowance in 1975 provided non-means-tested benefits to

138   *Sites and spaces*

disabled people regardless of National Insurance status to cover the 'extra costs' associated with living with an impairment. NCIP (1975) was available to unemployed disabled men and single women without contributions. In this sense, HNCIP was also designed as a 'loss of earnings' benefit, though with some fundamental contradictions.[20] Housewives were not considered 'earners', at least not in a meaningful sense. Claimants had to prove they were incapable of work, but this was not enough to qualify. They also had to prove they were incapable of 'normal household duties', a double test that did not apply to single women or men. This hinterland between 'extra costs' and 'loss of earnings' was contradictory even within the common sense of the social security authorities. And while HNCIP met some of campaigners' expectations by providing support for disabled people, the double test left this definition of 'disabled housewife' open to challenge.

This leads to 'IP', or 'invalidity pension'. This benefit was designed to be paid over the long term. To access it, claimants were subject to gatekeeping procedures to determine 'invalidity'.[21] The combination of 'H' and 'NC' created problems for the DHSS. Tests of marriage (or cohabitation) and of ability to work were commonplace, the latter usually determined by a report from a doctor, or a secondary medical examination where the DHSS doubted the claim's medical legitimacy.[22] But the DHSS had no previous experience of measuring whether an individual could perform the tasks expected of a house-wife. Indeed, it had no experience of even defining what a 'housewife' was 'supposed' to do, and was attempting the task at precisely the same time that feminist writers and activists were challenging dominant assumptions about married women, 'housewifery', and domestic labour.[23] Applying the logic of 'invalidity' or 'incapacity' for paid work to domestic labour was inherently problematic. Doctors and benefit administrators made judgements on 'incapacity' based on the individual's past work experience, current medical conditions, and the likelihood of employers to offer the claimant work. Such judgements were subjective and open to challenge, but there was at least a century of bureaucratic machinery and precedent to lean upon.[24] Yet any test of domestic work had to make assumptions about the type of labour, frequency and length of performance, and extent of its necessity to the maintenance of a household – while simultaneously generalising this to *all* British families. How the

Writing everyday life into law 139

government chose to implement this test demonstrates its assumptions about everyday life for married women, disabled or not.

What was the 'household duties test'?

While a doctor's note was enough to satisfy the 'incapable of paid work' criterion, the DHSS felt the need to assess domestic labour differently. On top of the 'sick note', the DHSS asked a doctor, usually the claimant's general practitioner, to rate the claimant's capacities in four main areas: 'shopping', 'meals', 'washing and ironing', and 'cleaning'. Claimants were asked to evaluate themselves on the same criteria to determine where there might be disagreement. Within these categories, questions covered intellectual and physical disabilities. For example, under 'shopping' the DHSS asked about the claimant's ability to 'decide what to buy', 'get to the shops', 'collect what [they] want', and 'get the shopping home'.[25] In each case, claimant and doctor had to answer if the claimant was 'able to do it all', 'most of it', 'a little of it', or 'not able to do it at all'.

Such questions, however, were clearly dependent upon an individual's circumstances. Later generations of disability activists drew upon a social model of disability that emphasised the discriminatory effects of society upon people with impairments rather than locating disability as an inherent 'fault' within an individual.[26] The intellectual roots of this model were brewing at the same time as HNCIP was formulated. In 1975, Vic Finkelstein's seminal paper imploring readers to imagine how a society where the majority used wheelchairs would disable someone who could walk was published. (In this world, low ceilings and doors would constantly injure non-wheelchair users, but an unsympathetic medical establishment would do nothing for them and had no incentive to try.)[27] A year later, the Union of the Physically Impaired Against Segregation published its manifesto that formed the basis of the social model and laid bare this new rights-based movement's disagreements with organisations working on behalf of – rather than led by – disabled people.[28] These ideas became more mainstream at the end of the 1980s, but the underlying concept that built environments disabled people circulated widely in late-1970s Westminster, including in two committees launched under Prime Minister James Callaghan.[29]

140 *Sites and spaces*

Simply put, distance to the nearest shop, whether it was uphill or involved scaling flights of stairs, and how many public transport networks had to be navigated, affected a person's ability to 'get to the shops' just as much as any specific mobility or intellectual impairment; while the amount of shopping required depended upon the size of the family, and ability to accomplish any of these tasks also depended on the potential help that could be solicited from friends or other family members. The DHSS's assumptions about 'normal' domestic life in Britain could not account for such variety, leaving the eligibility criteria open to interpretation and challenge.

Challenging the system

The evidence from appeals tribunals deposited in The National Archives as part of the DHSS's policy files provides ample evidence of these inconsistences and protests. Tribunal decisions required the collection of many types of evidence, including the claimants' oral and written testimonies of their daily lives, familial relationships, and difficulties with paid and domestic labour. Gulland's insightful research has also demonstrated the wealth of information that can be traced through the archive from these sources, especially with regard to HNCIP.[30] Their gendered approach to the question of incapacity has further shown how these sources betray the prejudices of the social security authorities and how these fit within the longer history of exclusion in the welfare state.

We must be mindful, however, not to treat such sources as typical of all disabled experience. As Mike Oliver argues, the parsimony of the British benefits system required (and requires) disabled people to present themselves as helpless and vulnerable in order to meet incapacity criteria, a practice that ignores and obscures disabled people's capabilities, contributions, and rich lives that have nothing to do with medicine or impairment.[31] Gulland also emphasises 'the particular gendered humiliation of married women being forced to "admit" that they were unable to keep their houses clean or to feed their husbands and children to an imagined acceptable standard'.[32] These files further mediate the claimants' voices through official machinery, presenting issues as a dispute rather than as diversely organised individual reflections of the kind one might find in an

Writing everyday life into law 141

oral history or Mass Observation directive. Beckie Rutherford's research on Gemma, a network of disabled lesbians, explores these women's interactions and discussions of their multifaceted experiences; she shows that for these disabled women, disability was not a singular, all-encompassing identity that dominated their lives at the expense of all others.[33] This insight can get lost if we examine only those sources in which disability and impairment were the sole topics of conversation.

Furthermore, the DHSS explicitly retained copies of these tribunal documents because they exemplified 'edge cases' which fell into legal grey areas and tested the limits of gatekeeping criteria (either in the authorities' or the claimant's favour). They are therefore not even typical of HNCIP cases. Still, in treating these files as 'complaints' articulating perceived failings in HNCIP's systems and places where common-sense expectations about qualification had broken down, historians can read these records 'against the archival grain' to gain insights into different constituencies' assumptions about which disabled housewives 'deserved' access to benefit.[34] In these 'edge cases', claimants and authorities articulate what they considered *ought to be* 'normal'.

One of the more striking examples of the impossibility of generalising about women's experiences comes from Gulland's discussion of a South Asian woman awarded HNCIP (after appeal) on the grounds that preparing food and hand-laundering clothes was more difficult and time-consuming for her than for a white British housewife.[35] As noted in the previous section, the questionnaire-style appraisal of 'how much' a claimant could perform was entirely dependent upon what domestic tasks were considered 'typical', either for the individual or for some imagined 'average' woman. If living a 'typical' South Asian life made this woman 'atypical' in the eyes of the DHSS, this says something fundamental about the racialised 'normality' of British lives under the welfare state.[36]

In these tribunal records, insurance officers regularly made the point that they did not dispute the claimant's inability to work or that they were disabled according to common-sense cultural definitions – but officers did deny that claimants were 'substantially' incapable of housework according to the benefit criteria.[37] That was the sole definition of 'disabled' that mattered in these cases. A common objection focused on whether a claimant's condition was really

142　　　　　　　　　　*Sites and spaces*

'continuous'. Benefits relying on hard definitions of 'capable' or 'incapable' often display the 'snapshot' problem. A medical examination may give an indication of a person's capability on only that specific day. For those experiencing fluctuating or episodic conditions, it is difficult to 'prove' what is typical for that individual.[38] A Yorkshire woman in her early forties with Ménière's disease told her tribunal, 'I do not know when I will have an attack as there is no warning', but this was not considered acceptable evidence of incapacity. Yet a woman in Scotland in her mid-forties who had experienced a stroke was able to demonstrate that a 'typical' day left her unable to perform housework. 'It is absolutely illogical after eight years [...] not to realize that my general condition of health is not stable and that in fact I do not lead a normal housewife's life,' she argued. In South West England, a woman in her early fifties was denied benefit because her heart condition did not stop her from doing most housework, providing she could do it sitting down. The fact that her husband needed to help her prepare for these tasks was not considered strong enough evidence. As a woman from the English North West (early fifties) recounted: 'my doctor says you can't get a true picture from the little boxes you tick'.

In attempting to convince tribunals to award benefit, claimants expressed anger and disappointment. The claimants appear convinced of their moral entitlement to support from the welfare state on the grounds of disability. For, it should be noted, there was no denial in these cases as to whether the women were disabled. They all qualified on the 'incapacity for work' criterion and were clearly limited in their ability to perform 'domestic duties'. The question for the tribunal was whether they were incapable *enough* to qualify, based on the regulations.[39] Thus, being disabled by both social definitions and other welfare state agencies, yet somehow not disabled enough for HNCIP, created a common-sense paradox which left claimants frustrated.

A woman in her late fifties in the West Midlands wrote that the decision to deny her benefit was 'a Disappointment [...] it shows no one is Ready to help you when you are down'.[40] Another in her late forties in the East Midlands emphasised that her doctor's report 'proved that I am getting more <u>incapable of performing normal House hold duties</u>', while a Yorkshire woman stated 'if I am turned down again [...] my MP is taking it up'. There is also evidence of

Writing everyday life into law

the 'humiliation' that Gulland and Oliver identified. A husband wrote on behalf of his wife (mid-thirties, East Anglia) that 'she has a great deal of personal pride which seems to have been misplaced when answering the questions put to her' and that she 'tends to think about what she was able to do rather than her capabilities now'. Another claimant (East Midlands, mid-fifties) argued that the assessor had overestimated her abilities because her daughter had come round that morning to tidy the place up in preparation for receiving company.

This general sense of unfairness pervades the testimonies. The claimant from the West Midlands could not understand why the social services would give her a bus pass if she was not clearly disabled and in need of support. If this was a benefit for disabled housewives and she had been assessed as disabled and a housewife, it was common sense that she should qualify. Another, in Manchester (late fifties), had not heard about the benefit until she was hospitalised and complained in part at this injustice. Further, lack of access to the benefit worsened the problems that had caused some claimants to apply in the first place. A claimant in the East Midlands (mid-thirties) with two young children was known to social services and had been forced to flee her abusive husband. She claimed HNCIP would help her set up a new life, but she was deemed ineligible for benefit (regardless of her other social work needs) because the injuries sustained while rescuing her children from the husband were not deemed serious enough. Another in South East England in her mid-fifties with impaired vision found housework tasks very difficult in part because she did not have many modern appliances and aids that would allow her to live more independently. She won her appeal and stated that 'the pension will enable me to get [...] gadgets' not available through other health or social services. Meanwhile one doctor told the tribunal that a woman near London (mid-fifties) was disabled, but that part of her complaint was that she was dissatisfied with her council house and convinced her accommodation was making her condition worse. Claiming the benefit and appealing was, he considered, a way for her to draw attention to this fact.

In this last example, part of the claim was based on the claimant's depression. The DHSS officials in the tribunal files tended not to be sympathetic to people with such conditions. One commissioner argued that the London woman was physically capable of performing

144 *Sites and spaces*

household duties, but her general attitude – not clinical depression – was preventing her from doing so. A woman in Lancashire (mid-twenties) was also denied her claim based on a severe mental health condition, while another in Yorkshire (mid-fifties) was assessed as capable despite severe depression. The tribunal did not deny the diagnosis, though 'there is no medical evidence for it', but it was thought that her 'unwillingness' to perform housework 'may spring from her character'. The lack of physical incapacity in these cases was deemed to trump mental health conditions that, de facto, made it impossible for these women to perform housework. This demonstrates the lower priority given to mental health as a disabling factor in 1970s healthcare and welfare, but also suggests a rigid focus in the HNCIP on 'capacity' as a physical issue. A perceived lack of 'effort', regardless of any reasons backed up by psychological diagnoses, disqualified these women.

One of the reasons why these tribunals exist in the DHSS files in this form is that HNCIP was under heavy scrutiny. Disability organisations argued that HNCIP was fundamentally unfair because of the double test, while the DHSS felt that far more women were eligible for the benefit than originally intended. As with other disability benefits and policies in the 1970s – such as the fund established by Prime Minister Edward Heath's government in 1973 to provide support for the victims of the thalidomide scandal, or the Vaccine Damage Payments Scheme under Callaghan in 1979 – the DHSS worried that loose criteria would enable other interest groups to use legal precedent to expand schemes too far and cause financial problems for the Treasury.[41] For voluntary organisations, particularly the umbrella group Equal Rights for Disabled Women Campaign (ERDWC), the capacity to perform domestic work should have been supplementary evidence of incapacity and need for support, not an additional barrier to benefit. If incapacity for work was the primary issue in NCIP cases, so should it be for HNCIP. If a duties test were to exist at all, then assessors should focus on the claimant's limitations rather than dismissing appeals because the claimant was able to do some tasks without too much difficulty. The Disability Alliance on behalf of ERDWC supported one woman's case to test this looser interpretation of the law.[42] The DHSS strongly opposed this case. It estimated such an interpretation could triple expenditure on the benefit.[43] The Labour government changed the law in 1978 to enforce the stricter interpretation of 'substantial', and to ward

Writing everyday life into law 145

off bad publicity from campaign groups delayed making any further decisions by referring the matter to the National Insurance Advisory Committee and asking them to produce a report.[44] By the time it was published in 1980 there had been a change of government and the poverty-lobby coalitions that had succeeded in pushing for the expansion of disability benefits had lost much of their momentum.[45]

The end for HNCIP came from external sources rather than these direct pressures from claimants. In 1978, the European Economic Community passed a resolution that men and women must be equal under the law for social security purposes. Member states were given six years (or until December 1984) to reform their systems.[46] The UK anticipated a legal challenge against HNCIP, given that the double test applied only to married women. Although never tested in court, the DHSS was advised by its lawyers that the government would almost certainly lose in any action against it.[47]

'Severe Disablement Allowance'

The European position made things awkward for the Conservative government. It had, for the most part, wanted to leave disability benefits alone in its restructuring of the welfare state.[48] Maintaining coverage (even expanding it when finances allowed) had been part of the Conservative Party's 1979 election manifesto, with more social security cuts focused on stigmatised groups such as unemployed people and single parents.[49] For the Conservatives, it was common sense that disabled people as 'the deserving poor' ought to have access to some form of benefit.[50] Yet simply removing the household duties test would potentially increase the cost of the benefit to £275 million per annum, or 8 per cent of all disability benefit expenditure.[51]

The government responded by creating Severe Disablement Allowance (SDA), a new benefit payable to all men and women who could show they were incapable of working and were '80 per cent disabled'. This restricted who could make new SDA claims, affecting many disabled married women – but these restrictions, however unfair campaigners considered them, did not fall foul of gender discrimination rules.[52] There was still a second test that did not apply to National Insurance Incapacity Benefit claimants – but, based on gender, everyone was (in theory) equally disadvantaged.[53]

146 *Sites and spaces*

In the transition from HNCIP to SDA, all women who qualified for HNCIP (around 54,800 people) automatically qualified for the new benefit without having to go through new gatekeeping procedures.[54]

The concept of a percentage of disablement was borrowed from systems used in Industrial Injuries, War Pensions and Vaccine Damage Payments schemes. It leads to questions of how one can judge a specific percentage of disablement, especially as social models of disability were becoming more widely recognised in the 1980s. What is zero or 100 per cent disablement, and what normative assumptions necessarily underpin that judgement? Moreover, in practice such measures were linked to the ability to perform paid work, not the capacity to participate in wider society or to perform domestic work. They were designed to measure injuries to male breadwinners and did not necessarily work well for other impairments in other economic circumstances. Just like the 'household duties test', the '80 per cent disabled' criterion was full of subjective judgements dressed in the language of 'objective' medical testing.[55]

Still, the government did not escape the European Court unscathed. A 1987 case determined that 'it is not disputed that the transitionary provisions [from HNCIP to SDA] are contrary to the principle of equal treatment',[56] but because HNCIP was abolished before the six-year deadline no further action could be taken. There was, however, a twist. New applications to SDA were not accepted from all potential claimants until November 1985, meaning there was one year in which many married women who qualified for HNCIP on the 'incapable of work' criterion (as applied to single women and men) were denied SDA. The European Court ruled this discriminatory, meaning thousands of women became entitled to SDA. Though some of those women would have been able to claim SDA anyway through other criteria, other estimates of expenditure suggest that 3,000 to 4,000 new claimants now became eligible, costing the government around £4–5 million.[57]

Conclusions

HNCIP's demise reflected changing attitudes towards social security in Britain and Europe in the 1970s and 1980s. The idea that one group of people should be denied state support because of their

Writing everyday life into law 147

inability to perform 'household duties' was clearly discriminatory and against the principle of gender equality under the law. In an era when public attention and protest at the gendered burden of domestic labour coincided with high-profile legal scrutiny of equal pay and equal treatment, it is perhaps surprising that HNCIP was even created.[58] It was a benefit caught between two impulses: despite resistance from equal treatment campaigners, it at least finally acknowledged the discrimination against married women built into a 'breadwinner model' welfare state that had long neglected the economic effects of disability.[59] The crude nature of the Beveridgean National Insurance system meant that it was fundamentally incapable of resolving this tension.

It is this very tension that makes the benefit so interesting and provides historians with an opportunity to see these knotty debates playing out in public discourse. The tribunal documents show how disabled women understood their own disability and the unfairness of a system that ostensibly claimed to provide for them, and yet whose specific eligibility criteria denied them support. When it appeared that this common-sense tension might be resolved by the ERDWC's legal challenge, the government sought to restrict eligibility still further. The creation of the benefit suggests that the Labour government saw benefits for disabled housewives as 'a good thing'; but when the financial realities of providing that support became apparent, the need to protect the Treasury triumphed.

These tribunal cases provide rare testimony from disabled women themselves about this curious social security benefit. The range of medical conditions and personal circumstances described in these documents is notable. Across the UK there was no 'typical' life for a disabled housewife. Women had 'good days' and 'bad days' which crude medical assessments based on 'tick boxes' could never properly assess. At the same time, common experiences in life and through other arms of the welfare state bureaucracy allowed thousands of women to identify as housewives. Being unable to 'perform household duties' was self-evidently reason to need help. These claimants hoped to get that from the state, though it is notable how often other family members such as 'daughters' and 'husbands' come into their testimony to demonstrate their needs. As Gulland argues, if housewives were supposed to be able to look after the home, disabled women could see their inability to do so as a sign of failure.[60]

148   *Sites and spaces*

In the end, much like the 1990s decision to equalise the pension age for men and women, in removing one form of discrimination other forms emerged. Hugh Pemberton notes that one reason why women were entitled to a pension at sixty rather than sixty-five was because they tended to have more health issues than men and were more likely to have taken time away from work to raise children or care for elderly relatives. For much of their working lives, they had been unable to access full National Insurance benefits, unless they chose to pay a greater percentage of wages that were statistically likely to be lower than their husbands' in contributions.[61] A differentiated pension age was not equal under the law but did acknowledge and seek to redress other forms of gender and disability discrimination baked into the welfare state and capitalist economy. Thus, while the creation of HNCIP and the 'household duties test' was itself discriminatory, it was part of a wider acknowledgement of disabled women's disadvantages as identified by the Disablement Income Group and others. Similarly, its complete removal in 1984 complied with gender equality legislation on administrative grounds but left women at a disadvantage because of the focus of its replacement on paid, rather than domestic, labour. In failing to acknowledge this aspect of many British women's everyday experiences, the burden of discrimination simply shifted emphasis.

Acknowledgements

This research for this chapter was funded by the Wellcome Humanities Postdoctoral Fellowship 'Sick Note Britain', WT 208075/Z/17/Z at the University of Warwick. The author wishes to thank the editors of this volume, Martin Moore, and Hannah Elizabeth for their guidance in preparing the manuscript.

Notes

1 Original emphasis. The National Archives (hereafter TNA): PIN 15/4481, DHSS Leaflet NI 214, NCIP for Married Women, June 1977, pp. 1–2. Copy also consulted in Peter Townsend Collection, University of Essex (hereafter PTC): 78.19.

Writing everyday life into law 149

2 Jameel Hampton, *Disability and the Welfare State in Britain: Changes in Perception and Policy 1948–1979* (Bristol: Policy Press, 2016); Gareth Millward, 'Social security policy and the early disability movement – expertise, disability and the government, 1965–1977', *Twentieth Century British History*, 26:2 (2015); Paul Whiteley and Stephen Winyard, *Pressure for the Poor: The Poverty Lobby and Policy Making* (London: Methuen, 1987).

3 European Council, Council Directive 79/7/EEC, 19 December 1978.

4 Ann Shola Orloff and Marie Laperrière, 'Gender', in Daniel Béland, Kimberly J. Morgan, Herbert Obinger, and Christopher Pierson (eds), *The Oxford Handbook of the Welfare State*, 2nd edn (Oxford: Oxford University Press, 2021).

5 On how common senses circulate in policy discussions and can conflict between groups drawing on different forms of expertise, see Gareth Millward, '"A matter of commonsense": the Coventry poliomyelitis epidemic 1957 and the British public', *Contemporary British History*, 31:3 (2017).

6 Anne Digby, *British Welfare Policy: Workhouse to Workfare* (London: Faber, 1989); Rodney Lowe, *The Welfare State in Britain since 1945* (Basingstoke: Palgrave Macmillan, 2005); Hampton, *Disability and the Welfare State in Britain*.

7 Jackie Gulland, 'Extraordinary housework: women and sickness benefit in the early-twentieth century', *Women's History Magazine*, 71:1 (2013); Jackie Gulland, 'Conditionality in social security: lessons from the household duties test', *Journal of Social Security Law*, 26:2 (2019); Jackie Gulland, *Gender, Work and Social Control: A Century of Disability Benefits* (London: Palgrave Macmillan, 2019).

8 On the use of 'complaint' as a window onto these concepts, see Daisy Payling, '"The people who write to us are the people who don't like us": class, gender, and citizenship in the Survey of Sickness, 1943–1952', *Journal of British Studies*, 59:2 (2020).

9 Hereafter 'married' is used to reflect DHSS terminology, but the political significance and history of cohabitation must be remembered, while separated married women not living with their husbands were considered 'single' for benefit purposes. See Neville Harris, 'Unmarried cohabiting couples and Social Security in Great Britain', *Journal of Social Welfare and Family Law*, 18:2 (1996); Rebecca Probert, *The Changing Legal Regulation of Cohabitation: From Fornicators to Family, 1600–2010* (Cambridge: Cambridge University Press, 2012); Pat Thane and Tanya Evans, *Sinners? Scroungers? Saints? Unmarried Motherhood in Twentieth-Century England* (Oxford: Oxford University Press, 2012).

10 Jane Lewis, 'Gender and the development of welfare regimes', *Journal of European Social Policy*, 2:2 (1992); Ben Jackson, 'Free markets and feminism: the neo-liberal defence of the male breadwinner model in Britain, c. 1980–1997', *Women's History Review*, 28:2 (2019).

11 Laura King, '"Now you see a great many men pushing their pram proudly": family-orientated masculinity represented and experienced in mid-twentieth-century Britain', *Cultural and Social History*, 10:4 (2013); Jon Lawrence, *Me, Me, Me: The Search for Community in Post-war England* (Oxford: Oxford University Press: 2019), especially pp. 19–40.

12 Labour Party, *Towards Equality: Women and Social Security* (London: Labour Party, 1969); Hugh Pemberton, 'WASPI's is (mostly) a campaign for inequality', *The Political Quarterly*, 88:3 (2017); Jackson, 'Free markets and feminism'; Alice Hall and Hannah Tweed, 'Curating care: creativity, women's work, and the Carers UK Archive', *Journal of Contemporary Archive Studies*, 6 (2019).

13 Orloff and Laperrière, 'Gender'.

14 Dolly Smith Wilson, 'A new look at the affluent worker: the good working mother in post-war Britain', *Twentieth Century British History*, 17:2 (2006).

15 Helen McCarthy, *Double Lives: A History of Working Motherhood in Modern Britain* (London: Bloomsbury, 2020); Laura King, 'How men valued women's work: labour in and outside the home in post-war Britain', *Contemporary European History*, 28:4 (2019); Stephen Brooke, 'Gender and working class identity in Britain during the 1950s', *Journal of Social History*, 34:4 (2001).

16 Disablement Income Group, *Creating a National Disability Income* (London: DIG, 1972); Hampton, *Disability and the Welfare State in Britain*.

17 William Henry Beveridge, *Social Insurance and Allied Services (Cmd. 6404)* (London: HMSO, 1942); Deborah A. Stone, *The Disabled State* (Philadelphia, PA: Temple University Press, 1984); Deborah A. Stone, 'Physicians as gatekeepers', *Public Policy*, 27 (1979).

18 Hampton, *Disability and the Welfare State in Britain*.

19 Disablement Income Group, *Creating a National Disability Income*; Disability Alliance, *Poverty and Disability: The Case for a Comprehensive Income Scheme for Disabled People* (London: Disability Alliance, 1975); Michael Oliver and Colin Barnes, *The New Politics of Disablement* (Basingstoke: Palgrave Macmillan, 2012).

20 On this distinction see Tania Burchardt, *The Evolution of Disability Benefits in the UK: Re-Weighting the Basket* (London: Centre for Analysis of Social Exclusion, 1999).

Writing everyday life into law 151

21 Stone, *The Disabled State*; Gulland, *Gender, Work and Social Control*.

22 Gareth Millward, *Sick Note: A History of the British Welfare State* (Oxford: Oxford University Press, 2022).

23 Ina Zweiniger-Bargielowska, 'Housewifery', in I. Zweiniger-Bargielowska (ed.), *Women in Twentieth-Century Britain* (Harlow: Longman, 2001).

24 Gulland, *Gender, Work and Social Control*.

25 TNA: PIN 15/4481, DHSS Leaflet NI 214.

26 Michael Oliver, *The Politics of Disablement* (London: Macmillan Education, 1990); Jane Campbell and Michael Oliver, *Disability Politics: Understanding Our Past, Changing Our Future* (London: Routledge, 1996); Tom Shakespeare, 'The social model of disability', in Lennard J. Davis (ed.), *The Disability Studies Reader*, 2nd edn (London: Routledge, 2006).

27 Vic Finkelstein, 'Phase 2: discovering the person in "disability" and "rehabilitation"', *Magic Carpet*, 27 (1975).

28 The Disability Archive, University of Leeds: 'The Union of the Physically Impaired Against Segregation and the Disability Alliance discuss fundamental principles of disability' (1975).

29 Peter Large, *'Can Disabled People Go where You Go?' Report by the Silver Jubilee Committee on Improving Access for Disabled People* (London: HMSO, 1979); Committee on Restrictions Against Disabled People, *Report by the Committee on Restrictions Against Disabled People* (London: HMSO, 1982).

30 Gulland, 'Conditionality in social security'; Gulland, *Gender, Work and Social Control*.

31 Michael Oliver, 'Speaking out: disabled people and state welfare', in Gillian Dalley (ed.), *Disability and Social Policy* (London: Policy Studies Institute, 1991).

32 Gulland, 'Conditionality in social security'.

33 See chapter 10 in this volume, and Beckie Rutherford, 'Disabled women organising: feminism and disability rights activism', *British Library* (19 October 2020): www.bl.uk/womens-rights/articles/feminism-and-disability-rights-activism (accessed 17 November 2021).

34 Payling, '"The people who write to us"'; Ann Laura Stoler, *Along the Archival Grain: Epistemic Anxieties and Colonial Common Sense* (Princeton, NJ: Princeton University Press, 2010).

35 Gulland, 'Conditionality in social security'.

36 Nick Kimber, 'Race and equality', in Pat Thane (ed.), *Unequal Britain: Equalities in Britain since 1945* (Oxford: Oxford University Press, 2010); Satnam Virdee, *Racism, Class and the Racialized Outsider* (Basingstoke: Palgrave Macmillan, 2014); Millward, *Sick Note*.

152 *Sites and spaces*

37 All the cases quoted in this chapter come from TNA: PIN 19/514/4. They are anonymised here, but scholars interested in their provenance can consult the originals. This approach is taken from Roberta Bivins' treatment of sensitive medical information in the hinterland of the public domain in Roberta E. Bivins, *Contagious Communities: Medicine, Migration, and the NHS in Post-War Britain* (Oxford: Oxford University Press, 2015), p. 115, especially note 2.

38 Angela Hadjipateras and Marilyn Howard, *Worried Sick: Reactions to the Government's Plans for Invalidity Benefit* (London: Disability Benefits Consortium, 1993).

39 On this gatekeeping dilemma, see Gulland, *Gender, Work and Social Control*; Stone, 'Physicians as gatekeepers'.

40 In these documents, letters are typed but retain spelling and punctuation from the original handwritten testimonies.

41 Hampton, *Disability and the Welfare State in Britain*; Gareth Millward, 'A Disability Act? The Vaccine Damage Payments Act 1979 and the British government's response to the pertussis vaccine scare', *Social History of Medicine*, 30:2 (2017). On this concept in general see Stone, *The Disabled State*.

42 PTC: 77.02, Disability Alliance Steering Committee minutes, 18 October 1978.

43 TNA: PIN 35/495, Reference of the HNCIP question to NIAC [National Insurance Advisory Committee].

44 National Insurance Advisory Committee, *Report of the National Insurance Advisory Committee on a Question Relating to the Household Duties Test for Non-Contributory Invalidity Pension for Married Women (Cmnd. 7955)* (London: HMSO, 1980).

45 Gareth Millward, 'Invalid Definitions, Invalid Responses: Disability and the Welfare State, 1965–1995' (PhD thesis, London School of Hygiene and Tropical Medicine, 2014), pp. 161–4.

46 European Council, Council Directive 79/7/EEC, 19 December 1978.

47 TNA: PIN 35/96, Introduction of Severe Disablement Allowance, December 1983; Department of Health and Social Security, *Review of the Household Duties Test* (London: HMSO, 1983).

48 On expenditure policy see: Paul Pierson, *Dismantling the Welfare State? Reagan, Thatcher, and the Politics of Retrenchment* (Cambridge: Cambridge University Press, 1994).

49 Conservative Party, *Conservative Manifesto* (London: Conservative Central Office, 1979); Millward, *Sick Note*.

50 Clare Bambra and Katherine E. Smith, 'No longer deserving? Sickness benefit reform and the politics of (ill) health', *Critical Public Health*, 20 (2010).

Writing everyday life into law   153

51 TNA: PIN 35/96, Ministers' SDA Q&A briefing, attached to memorandum 1 December 1983.
52 Disability Alliance, *Severe Disablement Allowance – 'Hard to Claim, Impossible to Live On'* (London: Disability Alliance, 1988).
53 Gulland, 'Extraordinary housework'.
54 Parliamentary Debates (Commons), 18 July 1988, vol. 137, cc. 483–484W.
55 On this debate, see Disability Alliance, *Poverty and Disability*; Oliver, *The Politics of Disablement*; Gulland, *Gender, Work and Social Control*; Millward, *Sick Note*.
56 European Court, Case 384/85, Jean Borrie Clarke v Chief Adjudication Officer, [24 June 1987], ECR 1987-02865, para. 5.
57 Parliamentary Debates (Commons), 5 November 1987, vol. 121, cc. 859–860W; Parliamentary Debates (Commons), 22 April 1988, vol. 131, col. 602W.
58 Wilson, 'A new look at the affluent worker'; King, 'How men valued women's work'; McCarthy, *Double Lives*.
59 Lewis, 'Gender and the development of welfare regimes'; Hampton, *Disability and the Welfare State in Britain*.
60 Gulland, 'Conditionality in social security'.
61 Pemberton, 'WASPI's is (mostly) a campaign for inequality'.

6

Friendship, mutual aid, and activism in British transfeminine spaces, 1968–85

Fleur MacInnes

Introduction

In the social media age, as it becomes possible for networks to extend past geographical limitations, trans people are increasingly homogenised into the 'trans community'. Members of this community provide mutual aid for each other in the form of diverse resources and types of support. Such 'organised and spontaneous' actions constitute, in Chris Barcelos' words, 'collective co-ordination to meet each other's needs' after recognition that existing systems 'are not going to meet them'.[1] This form of mutual aid in trans spaces did not begin with the internet. As this chapter shows, in Britain the curation of trans resources and creation of communal spaces extends back at least to the 1970s.

The rich history of trans communities has barely been charted, while multiple factors have converged to present trans history along quite narrow lines. Trans narratives are still most often presented through medical and judicial lenses. Within this paradigm, medical transition, and especially '*the*' (sex change) operation, defines a universal trans identity and experience. This view of transness was encouraged by the medicalisation of trans identities in the 1960s and 1970s, wherein the concept of being 'born in the wrong body' permeated cultural understandings of gender transgression.[2] As a result, in historical and sociological scholarship trans care is most readily associated with medical interventions.[3] This approach marginalises the experiences of past trans people who did not, or could not, medically transition. It also sidelines the agency of gender-variant

British transfeminine spaces, 1968–85   155

people who were early advocates for sex reassignment surgery in favour of highlighting views from within the medical community.[4]

This tendency to think in medicalised terms is reinforced by the perennial lack of appropriate medical (and other) care services for trans people. Although there is an established National Health Service (NHS) gender identity service, some trans people in Britain endure waiting times of over sixty months for an initial appointment.[5] In this context, many look to the past to validate the necessity of medical interventions. The closure in 2024 of the Tavistock Clinic (Gender and Identity Development Service, also known as GIDS) exemplifies the uncertain cultural climate for trans identities in the UK. While current trans healthcare is not fit for purpose, the debate over trans people's right to transitioning treatments nevertheless requires a constant defence of this same system.[6] This political climate influences how trans history is understood, researched, and written.

In addition, because trans people can simultaneously hold multiple queer identities (for example, being both transgender and bisexual), the possibility of exposure to multiple intersections of oppression is constant. Although it is essential to chart past and present experiences of hostility and discrimination, these are not the only stories it is possible to tell. As geographer James Todd argues, to reflect the diverse realities of different people, research on transgender lives must also explore 'affirming and even mundane experiences'.[7] Trauma is a common aspect in trans experiences, but it is not the foundation of trans identities. It is essential to explore trans narratives from a position outside trauma to fully comprehend the multitudes of experiences that these identities encompass.

Looking to the histories of trans communities is essential in order to nuance understandings of trans experiences and to challenge these individualised, medicalised, and isolated narratives. This chapter, which explores mutual aid in transfeminine spaces in 1970s and 1980s Britain, is a first step in tracing this history. In trans spaces, the exchange of resources and services was (and is) a crucial aspect of community building.[8] Here, I trace textual evidence of community organising among trans groups including the Beaumont Society, the Transvestite/Transsexual Group (TV/TS Group), the Transsexual Action Group (TAG), and smaller, locally based support groups. The archival records of these groups bear witness to the creation of information leaflets, social groups, helplines, pen-pal services,

156   *Sites and spaces*

newsletters, and medical advice, and other forms of mutual aid.[9] They demonstrate that in Britain, the 1970s was a crucial decade for community building in transfeminine spaces. The transfeminine mutual aid created and shared in this period was foundational in the development towards stronger, well-established transfeminine communities.

A new focus on mutual aid in community spaces therefore enables us to view transfeminine histories through the lens of belonging, shared values, and friendship. One way into understanding these histories from this alternative perspective is through analysing humour as a tool in community building. Humour can be an expression of defiance against oppression, but it can also establish common ground that 'enable[s] parties to begin a relationship based on shared values', to foster intergenerational integration, and to facilitate plural identities.[10] The use of humour in contemporary trans newsletters and information sheets illustrates the complexities in gendered mentalities that transfeminine people navigated as part of trans multiplicity. Looking at trans humour therefore simultaneously defies standard narratives of transfeminine experiences as negative, reframes aspects of trans identities previously viewed through a cis-normative lens, and highlights an overlooked aspect of trans activism.

Finally, a note on language is necessary. In transgender studies, terminology is constantly evolving.[11] In writing trans histories, it can be difficult to find terms that both respect the agency of past peoples and their own descriptions of their worlds and are intelligible, meaningful, and appropriate in trans communities now. Here, I use trans to refer to anyone, past or present, holding a gender identity that does not align with the one assigned at birth. I also cite historical materials that use terms such as 'transsexual', 'transvestite', and 'cross-dresser', and employ those terms where it is appropriate. I follow Lauren Fried in utilising 'trans' to point 'to the multitude of terms and ways of living and being in the world' that include 'the terms transvestite, transsexual and transgender'.[12] I use 'transfeminine', with accompanying she/her pronouns, to discuss people who were assigned male at birth and whose gender identities align with femininity.[13] The blanket use of she/her does not assume a cohesive, unified gender experience for transfeminine individuals or communities but, rather, clearly signals when transfeminine subjects are under discussion.

British transfeminine spaces, 1968–85   157

There are no easy answers when trying to convey the complexities of identities at a historical moment when languages were fluid and shifting, and in a moment now, when language holds such deep political resonances; but if my solutions are imperfect, they also stem from recognition of these difficulties and respect for the identities of past and present trans people.

Early organisation: the Beaumont Society

The Beaumont Society, still operational today, was one of the first groups in Britain established specifically to provide support to (some) trans people. It originated in 1966 as a UK chapter of the secret American organisation Full Personality Expression (FPE), and in 1969 established itself as an independent society (while still affiliated to FPE). By 1970 it had 140 members, and by 1973 this had grown to 233.[14] By 1975, membership numbers extended 'well beyond' 1,000.[15] It produced a regular publication, the *Beaumont Bulletin*, which encouraged members to write in, and which allows us to trace the dominant concerns and changing relationships among members of the Society.

Alice Purnell, one of the Society's founding members, has since reflected on the initial conditions of the Society and the position of transvestites in late 1960s Britain, recalling that it was not illegal to 'dress' in public but you 'could and probably would be arrested for disturbing the peace, importuning or worse'.[16] The need for self-preservation may help to explain why an organisation for gender-variant people reinforced strong heteronormative values. These values are repeated in the Society's constitution from 1979, which articulated the following purposes (first established in the late 1960s):

i. To promote and assist by all possible means the study of gender role differences.

ii. To form an association of heterosexual transvestites, whose motivation for cross-dressing is primarily of a gender, rather than a sexual nature. Through this association to provide a means of help and communication between members in order to reduce emotional stress and eliminate the sense of guilt, and to aid in gaining the understanding of their families and relations.[17]

158 *Sites and spaces*

The continued emphasis on 'motivation for cross-dressing' as 'primarily of a *gender*, rather than a *sexual* nature' provides insight into contemporary misinformation and preconceptions around trans identities.

Founding members of the Society have explained that, while existing in a society where gender transgression was not tolerated by the public, law, or police, it was necessary to enforce an explicit separation from homosexuals.[18] This position was challenged by some at the time. In May 1979, a member named Hazel wrote to the *Beaumont Bulletin* to say that she found 'it remarkable that gays should be deterred from joining the B.S [Beaumont Society]' and speculating that 'there must be plenty of gays in the B.S anyway'. Sceptical of the heteronormative membership conditions employed for over a decade, Hazel argued that 'the phoney veneer of respectability which the B.S attempts to foster kills off any chance of making any real breakthrough in public opinion'. Although this letter was published, the response of editor Alice Purnell did not invite further discussion, simply asserting that, 'The B.S is a society for heterosexual TVs and TSs. It is not a gay organisation, and for that reason has excluded gays.'[19]

This heteronormative emphasis perhaps formed part of a strategy to ease conflict between 'cross-dressing' individuals and their families and relations, with recognition of the effects that gender nonconformity or transgression could have on the people around them. The 'help and communication' that Beaumont Society members provided to each other in negotiating these problems within their personal networks was an important form of mutual aid. This is clear when we look at how members discussed guilt, an emotion highlighted in the 1979 constitution.

Guilt was perceived as an important shared experience, particularly guilt stemming from open gender transgression. The preface of one 1979 letter to the *Beaumont Bulletin*, titled 'This Is Your Dad', addressed to the member's children, and signed 'Tanya', explained:

> I joined the B.S after some time in the wilderness of despair and guilt. And I told my children, now aged 33, 31 and 29, of the fact that their father was a transvestite. They accepted the fact and said it would make no difference in their attitude to me. However, I felt that I owed it to them to explain what made me tick.

British transfeminine spaces, 1968–85   159

In the letter itself, Tanya wrote:

> The Beaumont Society showed me that a sense of guilt was irrelevant – I was a victim of my own personality and no shame was attached. As a result, I now dress as often as I please and I think I have learned a very great deal about being a woman and perhaps even more about being myself.[20]

Below the letter were three cartoons (Figure 6.1). One depicts a young boy wearing a long dress with stuffed breasts, high-heeled shoes, flowered hat, and holding a handbag. A woman (presumably his mother) instructs him 'Junior – go to your room and take off your father's clothes!' Here, humour provided relief from an emotionally tumultuous situation.

In a later issue, Tanya's daughter wrote to the *Beaumont Bulletin*, referencing the earlier letter from her Dad. She stated that, 'Once the initial relief that it was nothing worse was over, I have found that I have adjusted to the situation well, even with humour. I have always been close with my father, and this has brought us closer.'[21] Humour functioned not only to foster community between members, but also to ease tensions in relationships between members and their families.

The Society also facilitated members' self-acceptance and growth by ensuring that they received regular communications and had outlets for sharing their concerns, questions, and successes. June, the regional representative for the North of England, wrote to her 'girls' approximately every quarter, in a bulletin titled the *Northern T.V. Newsletter*. When first assigned in 1970, June wrote to each member of her area, introducing herself and requesting similar information from her group: 'Many of you "Northern Girls" are already known to me, either through letters or from personal contact, but I felt that this introductory letter should be sent to all members in the area, as an obvious first step to broadening our knowledge of one another.'[22] This first posting included twenty introductory letters, with four members not contacted because of failure to pay the Society's subscription fee or because they had 'expressed a wish for no correspondence'.[23] In April 1971, June reported that twelve new members had joined in the area, and a few months later wrote that she had met 'nearly all the new girls', that 'there has been an

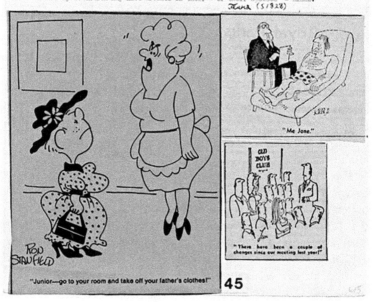

Figure 6.1 Final page of Tanya S1828's letter to the *Beaumont Bulletin*, May 1979, including cartoons. Photograph courtesy of Special Collections and Archives, Bishopsgate Institute. All rights reserved and permission to use the figure must be obtained from the copyright holder.

encouraging influx of new members' since the last newsletter, and briefly introduced some of the new members.[24]

This impressive rate of growth, even in areas of Britain not known for their accommodation of LGBTQ+ identities, shows that word

British transfeminine spaces, 1968–85 161

was spreading about the Society. June's efforts to make members feel welcome and connect them to each other were doubtless invaluable. These practices likely created a sense of community and belonging to the Society before members had even attended a social or party. The June 1973 newsletter further underlined committee members' dedication to fostering a strong sense of community. This issue described 'acquisition of a suitable premise in Leeds' as a 'dream come true', as it would allow the hosting of social events in a safe environment. It also reported on a 'Welcome North Dinner and Dance' in Doncaster that seventy-one members and their wives attended, summarising that 'it is fair to say a good time was had by all', and discussed more intimate house parties.[25] The newsletters therefore reveal the Society's creation of a social world for members, and how this was facilitated by print communications. Even in the early days of the Society, away from cities like London with a more established transgressive scene, members of the Society fostered a strong sense of community.

Defining trans identities

Members also united through the experience of gender transgression and exploration, including attempts to define and work out different categories of experience. In late 1973, the *Beaumont Bulletin* included an article in which an unnamed area representative drew distinctions between 'transvestites' and 'transsexuals'. The author expressed frustration with a recent *Guardian* article that 'poorly understood' the 'condition of transvestism':

> Transsexualism is a rare but much dramatized state in which a person, genetically, structurally and hormonally male, persistently believes and behaves as though he were a woman [...] Transvestism shares with transsexualism the compulsion to dress and appear like the other sex but in other respects it is quite different. Whereas the transsexual is firmly convinced that he is not a 'he' at all but a 'she' who has been given the wrong body, the transvestite finds that he is both a 'he' AND a 'she' together, at one and the same time or alternating from one to the other as the opportunity permits or the desire compels.[26]

This distinction did not necessarily reflect the Society's own definition of transvestism as predominately concerned with cross-dressing.

162   *Sites and spaces*

The Beaumont Society's conventions assumed that members were bonded in their identification with transvestism (a condition of membership). The Society built connections for members specifically while they embodied a transgressive feminine gender identity, as emphasised by the assumption from its inception that all members would have separate 'female' names to distinguish their trans identity. The frustration of this anonymous author suggests that some members did not identify with such rigid gender categorisation. The sense of duality evoked in the author's description ('both a "he" AND a "she" together, at one and the same time') is in some ways closer to current definitions of non-binary or genderfluid people that emphasise mutability rather than gender as a fixed state.

In 1975, Rosemary King wrote about her experience of transvestism in the *Beaumont Bulletin*, asking 'Why Two Genders?' Rosemary suggested that transvestites were 'obsessive or compulsive personalities' driven by 'a compulsive desire' to 'adopt the personal and social role, to a lesser or greater extent, normally thought appropriate to the other sex'. Radically, she went on to question the concept of gender itself as a form of categorisation:

> If there were no boundary between the genders, then one could neither wish to cross it, nor could the stress that caused the wish ever have arisen. How do we bring such a society into existence? Is it, in fact, generally desirable? I don't know the answer to the first of these questions, but have argued repeatedly in favour of 'yes' to the second.[27]

The gender experiences of members of the Beaumont Society were varied. Some viewed transvestism as a compulsion, a trait that 'is probably inborn'.[28] Others, situated transvestism as a fluid, permeable, and sometimes plural gendered experience. Members debated how transvestism encompassed their transgressive gender experiences. Nevertheless, bonds and friendships were formed in the shared community of transfeminine transvestites. Allison Miller writes that transgender history allows us freedom to imagine different possibilities of gender across all of history.[29] If so, perhaps we can situate the Beaumont Society as a community that transcends the need for a mutually agreed category. Shared transfeminine gender experiences, however varied, rather than specific categories themselves, enabled the growth of the community across the 1960s and 1970s.

British transfeminine spaces, 1968–85   163

Sociability, community, and transfeminine organising

The Beaumont Society was successful in many ways, building a strong sense of community for members from its inception. Yet, in the early 1970s it also faced criticism from those dissatisfied with its exclusionary membership policy. Carol Steele argues that the 'explosion of groups beginning to form in the mid-seventies' that 'catered for all transgender people' was partly a reaction against the 'restricted membership' of the Beaumont Society.[30] An early example of one such group is the Transvestite/Transsexual Social Group (the TV/TS Group), which began organising in the late 1960s.[31]

Speaking directly to the community, an initial TV/TS Group leaflet asked:

> How would you like to know that there is a house where you can come and go freely, where you can indulge yourself in an agreeable environment and where you can be welcomed by understanding like-minded persons? This is the dream of all T.V's isn't it? And it can now be realised! This is one of the major long-term objectives of the [group]. Meanwhile, we are pursuing more modest, but equally useful goals. We are concerned with a dignified, helpful approach to the whole field of transvestism and aim to give expression to the special needs arising out of their situation.[32]

By 1970, the Group was firmly established. It included anyone assigned male at birth who identified with gender transgression, rather than solely transvestites. In an October 1970 members' newsletter, Della asked, 'Has it ever occurred to you that, unlike similar groups, [our group] creates no barriers between transvestites and tran-sexuals [sic], or even sex changes.' She continued, undoubtedly referencing the strict membership conditions of the Beaumont Society, 'Nobody trying to join this group will ever be asked about his private sex life, what pills he takes, his mental history or how he removes his beard.'[33] Evidently, the goals and beliefs of the TV/TS Group as an organisation were far more fluid than those of the Beaumont Society.

In the same letter, Della argued that the distinction between transsexualism and transvestism was meaningless: 'according to Dr. Benjamin of New York, probably the world's leading authority, both points are on the same gradient scale, so all transvestites are

164   *Sites and spaces*

potential tran-sexuals'. She concluded that, 'Along the gradient scale of one sex to the other, we all find our own level the best we can', once again emphasising that it is not the specific identity that bonds members as a community but, rather, their inherent transness.[34] Della referred here to the Sex Orientation Scale developed by the sexologist Harry Benjamin, which was based on Kinsey's sexual behaviour rating system and included seven categories of 'sex and gender role disorientation'. Della's interpretation of this scale provided a very distinct, progressive view of trans identities that was not Benjamin's own intention.[35] The contrast between Della's identification with the scale as an expression of her fluidity and Benjamin's motivations to medically categorise trans people shows how trans people could resist attempts to pathologise trans identities, putting such categorisations to uses unintended by their creators.

The growth of the TV/TS Group indicates the importance of community for transfeminine people in the 1970s. By the middle of the decade, there were multiple TV/TS Groups catering to different regions of Britain.[36] The Manchester TV/TS Group began in late 1973, shortly followed by the Leeds TV/TS Group, which started the magazine *Gemini* in 1975.[37] A leaflet advertising *Gemini* was then distributed across TV/TS Groups, citing the necessity to further strengthen their regional communities, in the belief that 'there is a very real need for some sort of publication to co-ordinate and record the various activities that are happening nationwide', to help other TV/TS Groups to 'know what other groups are doing and where they operate from', and to provide information so that 'counsellors and social workers' would know 'who, in their area, they can contact if they come across any TVs or TSs'. This undertaking shows mutual aid in action, as local transfeminine communities recognised and addressed the needs of the wider trans community as well as their own members. The leaflet concluded, 'IT CAN SUCCEED IF YOU WANT IT TO', reminding readers of their own role in the success of *Gemini* as a community endeavour.[38] A separate sheet was provided for any individual or organisation who wanted their details to be published in the magazine.

By its second issue, *Gemini* was well on the way to achieving the goals set out in the introductory leaflet. It commented on national newspaper articles which addressed (and often criticised) transness, provided information about transitioning treatments, and filled three

British transfeminine spaces, 1968–85   165

pages with details about '*your* local groups' across the country. It included a commentary, 'THE SUNDAY TIMES SAYS/ WE SAY', on the newspaper's article 'Scandal of the sex change "surgeons"', originally published on 25 May 1975. This discussion illustrates how this process of organising socially in turn encouraged trans activism. The *Sunday Times* article examined 'backstreet' gender-confirming surgeries, focusing on how people without medical qualifications could carry out these surgeries, so long as the patient gave consent. The unnamed *Gemini* author found this report 'unsettling', and asked:

> Are we seeing here the same kind of situation which existed in this country a few years ago, before abortions were taken out of the back streets into the hospitals? Are we seeing the true picture or is this just the iceberg? How do we know that people have not died undergoing this sort of 'operation'?

The author stressed that 'whatever the reasons for their actions, these people are not criminals' and should not be punished. They worried that doctors would refuse to perform corrective surgery 'because it might be "encouraging the back street trade"', and that in the short term this refusal would cause further suffering for those who needed surgery, while 'these operations will continue regardless since nothing effective will have been done to stop them happening'. They set out three demands, each prefaced with a strident 'WE SAY': 'find the people who are doing the operations and stop them!', 'all those people who have had these operations should be helped as much as possible', and 'doctors and psychiatrists should find out what drives people to operations like these, and learn from what they find out. And adapt their approach to help prevent this sort of thing re-occurring!'[39]

This author's confident use of 'we' assumed a collective identity in some ways at odds with *Gemini*'s insistence that any views expressed were only those of the authors. One highlighted text box titled 'WHAT WE WANT' read: 'You may think, after reading this issue, that this magazine does not represent your views. If so, this is your fault and you are the only person who is able to remedy the situation [...] This magazine belongs to YOU.'[40] Yet it is evident that the Group assumed a sense of communal responsibility at a very early stage. This difficulty in balancing out individual views with collective

166 *Sites and spaces*

identities is often found in radical activist movements, and can result in permanent splits or factions.[41] In the mid-1970s, alongside bodies such as the Beaumont Society and the TV/TS Groups, publications like *Gemini* gave power and strength to those looking to organise. Although initially concerned primarily with creating links between trans people and organisations, by providing both community and anonymity, a space was made that fostered the growth and development of transfeminine identities. In these transfeminine communities, the creation, influx, and eventual partition of support groups reflects the shifting nature of the shared values and goals of the members. These changing goals can now be charted to identify the different forms of activism that took place within these communities.

Transfeminine activisms

In the second half of the 1970s and into the 1980s, division developed between those who favoured and prioritised friendship, and those who saw groups as a tool for organising and activism. In activism of this period divisions often occurred after a change or disagreement in values. The Women's Liberation Movement (WLM), for example, fragmented as the result of a concept of 'sisterhood' which only really included white, middle-class women.[42] The formation and activities of the Transsexual Action Group (TAG), founded in 1979 by members of existing TV/TS Groups who wanted to concentrate their activism through a feminist lens, illustrate how and why such splits could occur.

TAG, remembered by contemporaries as 'more activist' than other associations, set out its early aims as being to 'increase mutual awareness' among transsexuals, to 'liaise with other groups fighting against sexism', to 'increase public awareness of transsexualism', and to 'campaign for equal rights, and particularly the right to change birth certificates'.[43] The group took off, and the TAG newsletter was well established by the early 1980s. It usually consisted of around ten pages and featured regular columns from contributors and contact lists of members who opted in. The contact list in the summer 1982 issue included details for more than forty people. To contact someone on the list, members had to 'write the name and membership number in the top right hand corner of the envelope

British transfeminine spaces, 1968–85   167

(to be covered by the stamp) and place this envelope and the correct number of stamps inside a 2nd envelope', and send this to a business box in London.[44] As with other groups, the reassurance of anonymity, while simultaneously encouraging communication and correspondence among members, allowed this community to develop and for friendships to grow outside of official meetings.

In the early 1980s there were around two or three meetings between each new edition of the newsletter. The meetings centred on different topics related to the group's activist aims, with some social meetings. The forthcoming meetings listed in the January/February 1982 issue included a 'problem workshop', discussion on 'can we actually have paternal or maternal feelings', and 'Easter Social'.[45] There is evidence of crossover between newsletter content and group discussion topics. For example, the previous newsletter, dated November 1981, featured an article on the implications of parenting as a trans person as part of member Cheryl's regular 'Alternatives' column, intended to spark controversy and discussion.[46] A disclaimer above the article stated: 'Last month's first contribution carried my name though I asked that it should not, because I was expressing views I felt TSs might like to consider and ought to debate and which were not necessarily my own. The same applies to this month.'[47] This devil's advocate-adjacent approach was clearly effective in encouraging debate in both the newsletter and group meetings – hence trans parents becoming a meeting topic a couple of months after publication of Cheryl's article.

However, this approach could also sow (or reveal) discord. At one point in the article on trans parenting, Cheryl queried whether 'TSs in such cases really consider the problems they may be causing their children and the harm they may do'. She pointed to 'how seriously the law and the medical, social-work and child-care specialists view the effect of a changed gender role on children' and said she had been 'appalled to meet a TS recently who said arily [sic] that she and her wife had decided to tell the children and change over fully when they were ready'.[48] Several members responded to this claim. Tracy drew on personal experiences to counter Cheryl's claims, laying out the realities of parenting while navigating a transfeminine identity. She stated that, 'My wife and I both believe in truth and honesty as the foundation for our relationship with our fellows. This belief is fundamental to how we raise our daughter.'

168 *Sites and spaces*

She went on to explain that while she might 'decide that after all the best thing to do is to remove myself from my Daughter's [sic] life', if her daughter did not understand the reasons for this withdrawal, 'such apparent desertion' might 'have a worse effect on her'. Angrily, Tracy insisted:

> No Cheryl I have thought a lot about my daughter. Though I don't know what the future holds for her, for my wife or for myself. I'll do all that I can to ensure my existence does not cause her life to be any less full of happiness than it would otherwise be. I believe my present course to be that which offers the best chance.[49]

This interaction exemplifies the emotionally pressing discussions of these decades. It shows that members felt personal responsibility for representations of their community. But, crucially, such heated interactions about personal topics also speak to members' confidence in expressing their views in a safe environment. The newsletter was sent only to members and tried to ensure anonymity for contributing members. These discussions were not viewed by members of the general public who had not made up their minds on the legitimacy of trans identities. The fact that so many members wrote in response to articles like these, even with Cheryl's disclaimer, illustrates how trans activism was a fundamental part of community building at this time.

Although vigorous internal debate is often a sign of a strong community, TAG increasingly fragmented over time. In summer 1982, Hazel, a regular newsletter editor, announced that she was leaving the Group. She lamented that 'TAG has never quite worked out as I had wanted. There just aren't enough TSs around who agree with feminism. (If you remember, TAG was originally called the Feminist Transsexual Discussion Group – less ambitious, more justifiable, doomed to a tiny membership!)'[50] Hazel departed after Cheryl accused some TAG members of acting like 'Queen Bees'. In the previous issue Cheryl had written, 'It seems that every TS wants to be Queen Bee in the hive [...] the TS is often a rather a vain creature as she flits around dispensing advice & attacking others that do not match her image of what a TS ought to be.'[51] This portrait, suggestive of internalised misogyny and transmisogyny, conflicts with the original anti-sexist foundations of the Group.[52] Arguably, TAG experienced so much 'in-fighting' because of inconsistencies in what members

British transfeminine spaces, 1968–85   169

wanted from the Group. The Group provided contact lists, hosted socials, and encouraged friendship across members. But it was also founded as a feminist organisation, and so it is unsurprising that members voiced their grievances or even left when the newsletter published (trans)misogynistic views.

After almost a year of heated discussions, the last newsletter issue appeared in October 1982, with the title 'TAG LIVES: OFFICIAL'. Diane reassured members that 'TAG is not dead' and set out how the Group planned to go forward even though the newsletter would no longer be produced. Diane restated the original feminist intentions of the Group, and explained that it would try to continue 'in a way which will reflect the basic feminist viewpoint of the group', as an association of 'like-minded individuals interested in feminism and having a common background of TSism – instead of being a group catering for all TSs'.[53] This example of formation, development, and then refragmentation illustrates the rapid evolution of communities within transfeminine spaces. TAG's decision to refocus on its feminist roots, despite awareness that some members would leave the Group, contrasts with the ethos of early 1970s groups, where members were often just happy for opportunities to interact with other transfeminine people. In this instance, we can see how transfeminine groups became divided. Conflicts arose between those whose primary interest was making social connections, and those who had developed activist identities while participating in community building.

In this context, it is especially significant that even at the height of TAG's conflict, contributors consistently used humour. For example, Cheryl's 'Alternatives' column that accused some members of acting like 'Queen Bees', opened: 'Buzz! Buzz! Buzz! Do you know I reckon SHAFT [the Self-Help Association For Transsexuals] is run by middle-class middle-aged matrons? Of course TAG is just a bunch of disorganised adolescent left-wing pre-ops! Cheryl's stirring things up again.'[54] This excerpt illustrates the dual function of humour in these transfeminine spaces; it facilitated community building and allowed shared experiences to be critically considered in complete separation from trauma. SHAFT and TAG were two trans communities which predominately focused on transfeminine people. Cheryl, an active member of both groups, was able to satirically summarise their functions, suggesting that the sense of community

170   *Sites and spaces*

within transfeminine spaces had strengthened enormously by the early 1980s.

Simone Murray argues that feminist publishing identified that 'the production of the printed word and its interpretation constitute forms of *political* power'.[55] Conflict and debate within these publications show transfeminine communities gaining political power. A person who can mock their community space usually has confidence in their acceptance within that space. If humour established community through shared values, it also shaped how these shared values were perceived. The use of humour in these political expressions allowed transfeminine communities to resituate their position and develop identities away from individual experiences of trauma.

Conclusion

This chapter has shown that the 1970s in Britain was a crucial moment of community building in transfeminine spaces. The 1970s saw an explosion of trans activism, with dozens of groups established both nationally and locally. Within these spaces, members sought to organise, defend and improve the position of trans people in Britain – and they did so partly through internal debate and discussion that was part of working out trans identities, as well as through practical support and social networks. These support networks constituted a form of mutual aid. Personal investments in these shared spaces, despite disagreements on some issues, strengthened the overall position of these communities. A middle-aged matron in SHAFT and a left-wing adolescent in TAG might be totally divided in their politics, their values, and even their trans experiences, but they could both cherish and draw strength from the sense of friendship, support, and community offered in these spaces.

Not all of the groups lasted very long, and this raises the question of how we define success within communities. The Beaumont Society was the first of its kind and continues to this day, while the TV/TS Group was revolutionary in its flexible membership policy and unapologetic criticism of the former's exclusionary conditions. Yet, these two groups certainly had overlap in membership.[56] All of the groups discussed provided a foundation for friendships to be formed on mutual transfeminine experiences – but friendship was not the defining factor of their success. Members' desires to organise for trans activism spurred on the growth, but also the eventual division, of many transfeminine groups. Should these divisions be seen as evidence of the transfeminine community's failure to come together? On the contrary, they suggest how strong the community had become in the short span of a few years. The groups of the late 1960s relied solely on a shared transfeminine experience. By the early 1980s, there was such a personal investment in transfeminine spaces that members were willing to hash it out on a monthly basis to help guide the future direction of their community – and they were secure enough in the eventual survival of this community, and these spaces, to allow discord.

A similar reframing occurs when we think about the development of trans support networks, from the formation of the Beaumont Society to the explosion of trans activism in the 1970s, as mutual aid. The humour explored (albeit briefly) in these transfeminine spaces indicates how these communities thought about their own experiences. Thinking about friendship and humour as central aspects of transfeminine communities reframes the trans experience away from trauma and isolation, and also gives a further insight to just how strong these communities had grown in just over a decade. This chapter has resituated the 'difficult decades' of the 1970s and 1980s. Certainly, transfeminine people endured trauma during this time as a result of their gender expression, and this should never be forgotten or denied. But when we view trans experiences solely through the lenses of medicine or trauma, we overlook the complexities of these experiences and the development of trans communities – as well as the laughter and joy of trans lives.

Notes

1   Chris Barcelos, 'The affective politics of care in trans crowdfunding', *Transgender Studies Quarterly*, 9:1 (2022), 32. On mutual aid as a community response to structural inaction, see Dean Spade, *Mutual Aid: Building Solidarity during This Crisis (and the Next)* (London: Verso, 2020).
2   Kinnon Ross Mackinnon, 'Pathologising trans people: exploring the roles of patients and medical personnel', *Theory in Action*, 11:4 (2018), 76.

3 Jamison Green, Dallas Denny, and Jason Cromwell, '"What *do* you want us to call you?": respectful language', *Transgender Studies Quarterly*, 5:1 (2018), 102.

4 Mackinnon, 'Pathologising trans people', 76, 84.

5 'NHS waiting lists force trans people to leave the UK', *GenderGP* (16 March 2021): www.gendergp.com/nhs-waiting-lists-forcing-trans-people-to-leave-the-uk/ (accessed 1 July 2022).

6 Jasmine Andersson and Andre Rhoden-Paul, 'NHS to close Tavistock child gender identity clinic', *BBC News* (28 July 2022): www.bbc.co.uk/news/uk-62335665 (accessed 25 May 2023).

7 James D. Todd, 'Exploring trans people's lives in Britain, trans studies, geography and beyond: a review of research progress', *Geography Compass*, 15:4 (April 2021), 2.

8 Amira Lundy-Harris, '"Necessary bonding": on Black trans studies, kinship and Black feminist genealogies', *Transgender Studies Quarterly*, 9:1 (2022), 95.

9 The sources for this chapter illuminate trans experiences in different regions of postwar Britain. It therefore joins recent scholarship centring queer and activist experiences beyond London. See Matt Cook, 'Local turns: queer histories and Brighton's queer communities', *History Compass*, 17:10 (2019); Sue Bruley, 'Women's liberation at the grass roots: a view from some English towns, c. 1968–1990', *Women's History Review*, 25:5 (2016).

10 Marty Branagan, 'The last laugh: humour in community activism', *Community Development Journal*, 42:10 (2007); Umut Korkut et al., 'Looking for truth in absurdity: humour as community-building and dissidence against authoritarianism', *International Political Science Review*, 43:5 (January 2021), 2; Margaret Galvan, 'Making space: Jennifer Camper, LGBTQ anthologies, and queer comics communities', *Journal of Lesbian Studies*, 22:4 (2018), 385; Meg-John Barker, 'Plural selves, queer, and comics', *Journal of Graphic Novels and Comics*, 11:4 (2020), 472.

11 Green, Denny, and Cromwell, '"What *do* you want us to call you?"', 100.

12 Lauren Fried, 'A Material History of Trans Identities in UK Performance (1967–1990)' (PhD thesis, Royal College of Art, 2019), 32.

13 See Nat Raha, 'Transfeminine brokenness, radical transfeminism', *South Atlantic Quarterly*, 116:3 (2017).

14 Alice [Purnell], 'A history of the Beaumont Society', *Beaumont Magazine*, 13:4 (2005).

15 Wellcome Library, London (hereafter WL), PP/SUS/A/7, Papers of Susan, Beaumont Society member, Beaumont Society Papers and Publications, *Northern T.V. Newsletter*, 11 June 1975.

British transfeminine spaces, 1968–85   173

16 [Purnell], 'A history of the Beaumont Society'.
17 WL, PP/SUS/A/3, Papers of Susan, Beaumont Society member, Beaumont Society Papers and Publications, Beaumont Society Governance Papers, Beaumont Society Constitution, July 1979.
18 [Purnell], 'A history of the Beaumont Society'.
19 Bishopsgate Institute, London (hereafter BI), Box 3/1/1, Purnell Collection, letter to Editor of the Beaumont Bulletin from Hazel S1503, June 1979, pp. 42–4.
20 BI, Box 3/1/1, Purnell Collection, letter to *Beaumont Bulletin* from Tanya S1828, May 1979, pp. 43–5.
21 BI, Box 3/1/1, Purnell Collection, letter to *Beaumont Bulletin* from 'Daughter of Tanya S1828', June 1979, pp. 47–8.
22 WL, PP/SUS/A/7, Papers of Susan, Beaumont Society member, Beaumont Society Papers and Publications, *Northern T.V. Newsletter*, 1970.
23 WL, PP/SUS/A/7, Papers of Susan, Beaumont Society member, Beaumont Society Papers and Publications, *Northern T.V. Newsletter*, April 1971.
24 WL, PP/SUS/A/7, Papers of Susan, Beaumont Society member, Beaumont Society Papers and Publications, *Northern T.V. Newsletter*, July 1971.
25 WL, PP/SUS/A/7, Papers of Susan, Beaumont Society member, Beaumont Society Papers and Publications, *Northern T.V. Newsletter*, June 1973.
26 WL, PP/SUS/A/9/2, Papers of Susan, Beaumont Society member, Beaumont Society Papers and Publications, *Beaumont Bulletin*, 5:6 (November/December 1973), p. 23.
27 WL, PP/SUS/A/7/3/4, Papers of Susan, Beaumont Society member, Beaumont Society Papers and Publications, Rosemary King, 'Why two genders?', *Beaumont Bulletin*, 7:5 (September/October 1975), p. 52.
28 WL, PP/SUS/A/7/3/4, King, 'Why two genders?', p. 52.
29 Allison Miller, 'Beyond binaries: how transgender history advances discourse on identity', *Perspectives on History* (20 July 2015): www.historians.org/publications-and-directories/perspectives-on-history/summer-2015/beyond-binaries-how-transgender-history-advances-discourse-on-identity (accessed 29 May 2023).
30 Carol Steele, 'The formative years', in Christine Burns (ed.), *Trans Britain: Our Journey from the Shadows* (London: Unbound, 2018), p. 59.
31 The TV/TS Group incorporated multiple groups with slightly differing names, including the TV/TS Social Group. For ease of reference, I have used TV/TS Group throughout this chapter.
32 Women's Library, London School of Economics (hereafter WL-LSE), Hall-Carpenter Archives (hereafter HCA), Box 1412, Ephemera 572: The TV/TS Group, Information Sheet about the TV Social Group, 1970.
33 WL-LSE, HCA, Box 1412, Ephemera 572: The TV/TS Group, TV Social Group Newsletter, October 1970.

34 WL-LSE, HCA, Box 1412, Ephemera 572: The TV/TS Group, TV Social Group Newsletter, November 1970.

35 Beans Velocci, 'Standards of care: uncertainty and risk in Harry Benjamin's transsexual classifications', *Transgender Studies Quarterly*, 8:4 (2021), 473.

36 As well as the English examples given here, groups existed in Belfast, Cardiff, and north-west Scotland: WL-LSE, HCA, Box 1412, Ephemera 572: The TV/TS Group, 'Your local groups', *Gemini*, 2 (1975).

37 Steele, 'The formative years', p. 59.

38 WL-LSE, HCA, Box 1412, Ephemera 572: The TV/TS Group, Introductory leaflet about *Gemini* magazine, c. 1975.

39 WL-LSE, HCA, Box 1412, Ephemera 572: The TV/TS Group, letter on 'Scandal of sex change surgeons', *Gemini*, 2 (1975).

40 WL-LSE, HCA, Box 1412, Ephemera 572: The TV/TS Group, letters from readers, *Gemini*, 2 (1975), p. 15.

41 Jonathan Horowitz, 'Who is this "we" you speak of? Grounding activist identity in social psychology', *Socius*, 3 (2017).

42 George Stevenson, *The Women's Liberation Movement, and the Politics of Class in Britain* (London: Bloomsbury, 2019).

43 WL-LSE, HCA, Box 1411, Ephemera 566, Transsexual Action Group Leaflet, c. 1979; Steele, 'The formative years', p. 59.

44 WL-LSE, HCA, Box 1411, Ephemera 566, Transsexual Action Group Newsletter, 3:5 (June 1982), pp. 7–8.

45 WL-LSE, HCA, Box 1411, Ephemera 566, Transsexual Action Group Newsletter, 3:1 (January/February 1982), p. 1.

46 WL-LSE, HCA, Box 1411, Ephemera 566, Transsexual Action Group Newsletter (December 1981), p. 1.

47 WL-LSE, HCA, Box 1411, Ephemera 566, Transsexual Action Group Newsletter (December 1981), p. 4.

48 WL-LSE, HCA, Box 1411, Ephemera 566, Transsexual Action Group Newsletter (December 1981), p. 4.

49 WL-LSE, HCA, Box 1411, Ephemera 566, Transsexual Action Group Newsletter, 3:1 (January/February 1982), pp. 6–7.

50 WL-LSE, HCA, Box 1411, Ephemera 566, Transsexual Action Group Newsletter, 3:6 (c. 1982), p. 1.

51 WL-LSE, HCA, Box 1411, Ephemera 566, Transsexual Action Group Newsletter, 3:5 (March/April 1982), p. 1.

52 I use transmisogyny to describe sexism directed towards transfeminine people. See Pelagia Goulimari, 'Genders', in John Frow (ed.), *Oxford Encyclopedia of Literary Theory* (Oxford University Press Online, 2022): https://doi.org/10.1093/acrefore/9780190201098.013.1123 (accessed 29 May 2023).

British transfeminine spaces, 1968–85   175

53 WL-LSE, HCA, Box 1411, Ephemera 566, Transsexual Action Group Newsletter, 3:7 (October 1982), p. 1.
54 WL-LSE, HCA, Box 1411, Ephemera 566, Transsexual Action Group Newsletter, 3:5 (March/April 1982), p. 2.
55 Simone Murray, *Mixed Media: Feminist Presses and Publishing Politics* (London: Pluto Press, 2004), p. 27.
56 Simone Murray, *Mixed Media: Feminist Presses and Publishing Politics* (London: Pluto Press, 2004), p. 27.

7

A private matter? The Brook Advisory Centre and young people's everyday sexual and reproductive health in the 1960s–80s

Caroline Rusterholz

Introduction

In 1994, Jenny reflected on her experience in the 1960s as a teenage Brook Advisory Centre client. She recalled how patchy her sexual knowledge was. She did not have sex education at school and did not discuss the subject with her parents; she mainly received information from her friends, but it was very unreliable. As she put it: 'it was rather King's suit of clothes, we all presumed that or tried to make out that we knew more than we did so what we did learn along the lines was very hit and miss and whether at the end of it we cobbled anything together like the truth or any framework was pretty accidental'.[1] As a result, she turned to Brook for information and advice. Jenny's experience was not unusual, although it does not match public perceptions of sex in the 1960s.

Young women's (apparent) independence and sexual precocity generated much anxious commentary in the press and on television in these years.[2] Girls reached menarche earlier (thirteen and a half years in the 1960s, compared with sixteen to seventeen years a century before); women married younger and in greater numbers; more young women undertook higher education, with a wider range of professional opportunities open to them; and they reached maturity in a relatively affluent society. From the late 1950s, increasing recognition of premarital intercourse led to new anxieties around illegitimacy, while the prescription of new contraceptive technologies from the early 1960s (the oral contraceptive pill for married women from 1961, and new forms of intrauterine device [IUD] from 1963) fuelled

A *private matter? The Brook Advisory Centre* 177

fears of sexual promiscuity. The wave of liberalising legislation at the end of the 1960s generated further fierce public debates that pitted partisans of 'permissiveness' against traditional moralists who advocated premarital chastity as the only acceptable solution to these problems.[3]

Despite this prominent public discourse on sexuality, sexual knowledge, information, and contraceptives were still difficult to obtain in the late 1960s. 'Permissiveness' was more apparent than real.[4] Teenagers remained fairly traditional in their expectations, valuing marriage, and still lacked reliable birth control information.[5] Hormonal and mechanical methods of birth control remained difficult to obtain for young people prior to the 1967 Family Planning Act, which encouraged local authorities to provide contraception to all women, regardless of their marital status. Condoms had to be bought in pharmacies, which did not place them on display; purchasers had to request them. The barber shop was another option, but not all young people had the financial means to go to the barber regularly. Advertisements did become less coded after the introduction of the Pill, but the public nature of buying condoms still caused young people much embarrassment.[6]

In this context of increasing sexual activity amongst young people, the possibilities offered by new contraceptive methods, media panic about morality, and fierce debates about the boundaries of public and private life, Helen Brook opened the Brook Advisory Centre (BAC) in 1964. This was the first charity specifically dedicated to providing contraception to young people. BAC played a central role in the development and transfer of knowledge and information about young people's sexual and reproductive health. They believed that lack of sexual knowledge had negative outcomes for young people, ranging from unwanted teenage pregnancies and abortions to sexually transmitted diseases. To mitigate these risks, BAC developed ways of reaching out to young people: offering contraceptive and advice services at their clinics; working with schools by giving talks and creating sex education materials; developing more inclusive forms of sex education, including for disabled young people; and working closely with teenage magazines.

This chapter situates BAC as an organisation that operated at the intersection of the private and public realms. It explores BAC's tactics for intervening in young people's intimate lives, their activities

178   *Sites and spaces*

in public forums from schools to magazines, and their success in shaping the everyday sexual and reproductive health of young people between 1964 and the outset of the AIDS crisis in the mid-1980s – including attempts to make sex education more inclusive and so to reshape concepts of 'everyday sex'. Operating at the cusp of private and public life, BAC constituted a key channel of information on everyday sexual and reproductive health in postwar Britain and helped to foster a more inclusive view of sex education, where information on contraception was not limited to able-bodied young women.

Researchers investigating BAC have to negotiate the boundaries of public and private statements on sexuality. BAC's policy about the confidentiality of services and data protection means that clients' records are either completely protected, under restricted access, or simply absent in the archives of welfare organisations. This makes it difficult to document young people's own views on sexual and reproductive health services. By combining oral history interviews, anonymised case studies in BAC's annual reports, newspaper articles, and teenage magazines, we can gain some insight into how young people responded to BAC's attempts to expand sexual and reproductive health information.[7] Nevertheless, the difficulties in accessing information about young people's actual sexual behaviour in the past further warn us not to take sensationalist public rhetoric about moral breakdown at face value.

BAC services for young people

The first Brook Advisory Centre, targeted towards young unmarried people, was opened in 1964 in London by Helen Brook. A former Family Planning Association (FPA) volunteer and director of the Marie Stopes clinic, Brook was convinced that a centre for young people would prevent unwanted pregnancies, especially for young women at university, for whom pregnancy usually meant the end to a potential career. She believed that in order to reach true equality, young women needed to be free from the fears and risks of unwanted pregnancies.

Prior to the opening of the BAC, contraceptive information and products were provided only in Family Planning Centres and Marie Stopes clinics for married or about-to-be-married women, or discreetly

A private matter? The Brook Advisory Centre 179

in private practice. From 1962 onwards, Brook, as director of the Marie Stopes clinic, used a loophole in the organisation's constitution to hold secret contraceptive advice sessions for unmarried women. In 1963, the board of the Marie Stopes clinic officially approved these sessions, but it was a controversial decision. In 1964, the FPA, the main charity providing contraception to the married and about-to-be-married, refused to broaden the scope of its work by including the unmarried in its clientele. This prompted the official creation of the Brook Advisory Centre charity.[8]

The Centre's aims were 'the prevention and the mitigation of the suffering caused by unwanted pregnancy and illegal abortion by educating young persons in matters of sex and contraception and developing among them a sense of responsibility in regard to sexual behaviours'.[9] The Centre was the first of its kind to cater specifically and openly for young unmarried people. To help young people access information on contraception, the Brook charity encouraged and financially supported the setting up of similar centres in various cities, including Birmingham (1966), Bristol (1967), Edinburgh (1968), and Liverpool (1974). The number of BAC clients increased from 1,056 in 1965 to 59,265 in 1980.[10]

At first, only young people over sixteen, the age of consent, were seen in centres; however, in 1969, Helen Brook decided to allow under-sixteens to benefit from BAC services. The clients were mainly young women, though some young couples came together. By catering mainly for young women, BAC contributed to assigning contraceptive responsibility to this population. This emphasis was recognised by BAC. As a result, they tried to encourage young women to bring their boyfriends with them and in the mid-1980s, when there was a push from both the FPA and BAC to make birth control a shared responsibility, designed special sessions for boys.[11]

The centres functioned as hubs for information on contraception, pregnancy testing and abortion referrals, psychosexual difficulties, and access to testing for various sexually transmitted diseases. Most clients came to clinics for contraception (prescribed after contraceptive counselling and smear tests to check for infection or abnormality). Contraception was always the mainstay of BAC's work. The teenage birth rate in England and Wales had risen steadily until, at its peak in the early 1970s, 'it was three times the rate in the early 1940s'. The rate then decreased until 1977, rose again for three years, then reduced again. In 1981, the birth rate amongst teenagers in Britain

180   *Sites and spaces*

was the lowest for more than twenty years.[12] BAC's annual reports drew on newspaper headlines about rates of teen pregnancy and abortion and presented case histories, stressing the necessity of contraception as a preventive measure against unwanted pregnancy and abortion and their dramatic outcomes.

Counselling and referrals for abortion were also a key service. The Abortion Act 1967 made abortion legal up until twenty-eight weeks of pregnancy. The Act required women to obtain the signatures of two doctors, and young people under sixteen also needed the approval of their parents. In 1989, it was estimated that since the mid-1970s, about 40 per cent of conceptions outside marriage had ended in legal abortions.[13] The percentage of legal abortions for under-sixteens remained stable at about 3 per cent of the abortions for unmarried women. For instance, in 1978, 89,226 single, divorced, widowed, or separated women had an abortion, 2.6 per cent of whom were under sixteen (3,724).[14] The data showed that the highest proportion of abortions were in the age group fifteen to twenty-four.[15] In the context of the rising pregnancy and abortion rates among young women, BAC developed pregnancy counselling to help these women make informed choices.

Finally, BAC also provided emotional support and psychosexual counselling for young people. Psychosexual counselling dealt mainly with anxiety; as clinic doctor Fay Hutchinson noted, 'the younger the client the more areas of anxiety she is likely to have'.[16] According to Hutchinson, clients presented with a wide range of psychosexual problems, including lack of orgasm, fear of intercourse, impotence, anxieties related to the body, sexual abuse, same-sex attraction, and difficulty with parental relations. Clinics also received a constant stream of telephone calls and letters from anxious young people asking for advice about contraception and their sexual lives. BAC's services filled a gap in sexual and reproductive health provision for young people, helping them with their everyday challenges.

BACs as semi-public, semi-private spaces

The location and layout of clinics were key in attracting young people. They needed to be located in city centres, with good public transport links, or close to universities and schools, so that students

A private matter? The Brook Advisory Centre   181

could attend easily during daily life. BAC counsellor Dorothy van Heeswyk, who opened the first Brook centre in the multiracial neighbourhood of Brixton in 1980, home to a vibrant Caribbean community, explained that the centre needed to be 'accessible but not visible. It could be reached by passing buses, be anonymous enough looking so that young women could come without friends of their parents identifying where they were going'.[17] She added that Brixton Brook was on the top floor of a building 'in a very accessible street but you wouldn't know that Brook was there since there was only a small notice'. Brook centres also paid particular attention to their atmosphere. They were welcoming and informal, with low seating, a children's play area, coffee, tea and biscuits, plants, youth magazines, and leaflets about sexual health designed especially for young people. Some centres played background music. These factors created a relaxing and warm ambience where clients could feel comfortable and at ease.

This unclinical environment, designed to create a feeling of trust to allow young people to share their questions and emotions, was particularly valued by clients. Jenny, who attended a London Brook clinic in the 1970s, remembered the discreet location of the centre and her feelings on first entering the clinic:

> It was in East Street so we went to the market and pretended to buy a few vegetables and then just slipped in the door to find this very nice professional, not clinical but not unfriendly but professional feel about the place and masses of other women in the waiting room who'd come from all corners of the country, from Ireland, from Scotland, I was astonished that people had to travel so far to get any advice.[18]

Similarly, Lesley, who visited a Brook clinic in Edinburgh in the mid-1970s – brought by a friend who was horrified that Lesley had started a sexual relationship without using any method of contraception – remembered that the centre was located in the city centre, 'just a street off the main street'.[19] She noticed lots of plants when she entered the room and some tea and coffee on the side, creating a relaxed atmosphere. The spatial dynamics of the city and the contrast with entry into a welcoming, intimate, or almost homely space were key in both women's recollections.

This attention to location and décor encouraged young people into BACs, while the thoughtful management of care ensured that

182 *Sites and spaces*

many returned. One anonymous woman who used Brook in her teens in the late 1980s recalled that, 'It felt like my whole year at school (it wasn't, just felt like it) [I] went up to Brook on Tottenham Ct Rd to get the pill.' Travelling through the urban environment to BAC offered the comfort, reassurance, and understanding lacking from her domestic life. Brook provided a crucial service at a pivotal moment in her sexual and reproductive health journey:

> It was my first foray into an adult world of looking after myself really. I didn't want to go to the GP [general practitioner], I'd had a disastrous discussion with my mum about my sex life. I was nearly 16, it was love, I was with him until I was 19, we were both virgins but she did not approve at all, which I now understand. I felt like my mum and I went from being 'best friends' (in retrospect I'm not sure how healthy that was) to child and disapproving authority figure overnight. I'm not sure our relationship has ever recovered. However, her extreme reaction to my burgeoning sexuality was if anything, entrenching me in my decision: I needed contraception. Brook were kind, friendly, extremely respectful of me and of my wish for confidentiality. They didn't just hand me over the pill as I think my GP might have (and subsequently has!). They took time, asked me how I felt in my relationship, talked to me about the bigger picture in terms of starting to have sex. I felt listened to, and valued.[20]

This testimony points to elements prevalent in clients' experience and in the staff narrative around the clinic: young people needed special confidential services, since they did not want to go to their GPs, or their GPs had refused to provide birth control; they did not feel confident discussing sex and contraception with their parents; and they needed a place to feel listened to, and where they could confidentially express their emotions and needs around sexual and reproductive health.[21]

As this testimony suggests, young people received little information while growing up and were often discouraged when they tried to seek contraceptive advice from other avenues. In 1976, the Liverpool BAC's annual report stressed the number of young people who had come to them after being turned down somewhere else:

> we had repeated instances of responsible young people having been refused birth control even though they were at risk of unwanted pregnancy. While some of this group were far-sighted and persistent enough to seek our help and receive the advice they sorely needed,

A private matter? The Brook Advisory Centre   183

we had reason to ponder on the fact that no doubt many others less persistent inevitably must have been discouraged from pursuing a responsible course of action.[22]

In this context, BAC services were unique. Joanne Brien, who worked in the London BAC in the 1980s, highlighted that BAC offered young people the opportunity 'to talk to someone in a non-judgemental space'. She had joined BAC 'to provide young people with a level of understanding and respect that young people did not have', since the majority could not talk with their parents or their friends about their sexual life: 'Brook wasn't moralistic, it was sort of saying, yes, this is enjoyable activity, but you need to do it as safely as you can.'[23] BAC was a much-needed service that became key in young people's everyday management of their sexual health.

This service was recognised and promoted in the national press as abortion became (relatively) more accepted, and moral panics about sexual promiscuity shifted to public concerns about teenage pregnancy. From the late 1970s, against the backdrop of the rising birth rate among teenagers, the press hotly debated teenage pregnancies; headlines about teenagers who abandoned their babies or died while giving birth were common.[24]

In 1978, the *Daily Mirror* tackled this topic through an article on BAC's work.[25] It related the journey of one teenager from unprotected sexual intercourse through to pregnancy and abortion. Jill had been going out with David for two years but started to 'make love' only a few months before she visited BAC. One night, David refused to wear a condom, and since Jill's period had ended only a few days before, she believed she would be safe. When her period was late, David initially refused to believe that Jill was pregnant. Jill did not want to go to her own doctor, and a friend encouraged her to visit BAC instead. By the time of the visit, David had got over his reluctance to discuss the subject, and they had decided that it would be best for Jill to have an abortion. At the BAC, a test confirmed Jill's pregnancy. A doctor examined her, asked about her feelings and why she wanted an abortion, and explained the different contraceptive options available after termination of the pregnancy; Jill opted for the Pill. A 'friendly and kind' counsellor then advised on the assistance available for girls who decided to keep their babies, talked Jill through the termination procedure,

184 *Sites and spaces*

and finally discussed her contraceptive options again, emphasising the importance of a reliable method. After gaining the approval of two doctors, Jill had the abortion.

This example is heavily mediated, but believable; it illustrates that young people often struggled to find support and BAC was a lifesaver for some. The *Daily Mirror*'s decision to run this story also illustrates BAC's success in establishing its vision of responsible sex within the mainstream of British life by the end of the 1970s as young people's sexual decision making became entrenched as a matter of public concern.

Sex education in schools

BAC also moved into semi-public, semi-private spaces beyond the clinic to provide information about sex and contraception to young people. Their most important work outside the centres was around the contentious topic of sex education in schools. After the Second World War, responsibility for sex education was shared between the Departments of Health and Education and sub-contracted to the Central Council for Health Education (from 1968, this became the Health Education Council), which worked with independent voluntary agencies such as BAC to train, and provide resources for, teachers.[26] By the 1970s, many schools offered sex education classes with content on relationships instead of a narrow focus on the 'facts of life'. However, as Hannah Charnock's work on teenagers and sexual knowledge between 1950 and 1980 has illustrated, the sort of sex education provided at school was nevertheless deemed inadequate by young people.[27]

From the 1960s, BAC became involved in providing teaching resources and speakers for sex education in schools. This work stemmed from their commitment to 'educate young people in matters of sex and contraception'.[28] BAC workers were well aware that the clinics attracted only a comparatively small number of young people, and that the majority were young girls. Other means had to be found to broaden the scope of BAC's work, including sex education in schools and training for individuals working with young people.

This work started in the Birmingham BAC, which set up a 'talks and sex education group' in 1969.[29] That year, nine evening lectures

A private matter? The Brook Advisory Centre 185

on sex education for teachers were given, followed by a similar course in 1970.[30] In Bristol too, BAC members were increasingly called upon to provide 'factual information on birth control and talks on personal relations'. As a result, in 1970 they ran a seminar on 'Sex education and the role of Brook' at Bristol University, attended by Brook workers from London, Birmingham, Edinburgh, and Coventry, as well as many social workers, teachers, and individuals involved in education.[31] Each BAC branch regularly received requests for members to give talks in schools or to train teachers, and this work expanded over the course of the 1970s. In 1974, Brook members participated in more than 150 speaking engagements to over 10,000 people, from small groups in schools and youth clubs to large public meetings of women's organisations.[32] In 1982, again, more than 150 talks were given in schools and to youth groups.[33]

The provision of sex education talks in a wide range of educational settings was complemented by the production of teaching materials. Again, the Birmingham BAC pioneered this work. In 1969 they examined the material and visual aids available to teachers and soon decided to create their own educational materials to meet teachers' needs. In 1972 they produced video interviews as teaching resources on sexual knowledge. For instance, *Hello Gorgeous* was a series of seven interviews with young girls and mothers about sexual relationships and sex education, while *Boys Talking* was a series of interviews with boys aged fourteen to eighteen to promote group discussion on the issues 'they are all after the same thing', 'boys talk about it more than girls', 'who makes the first move' and 'I suppose I was really a bit of a fool'.[34] These tapes placed young people's lived sexual experiences at the centre of the narrative, allowing connection with young audiences by tapping into an emotional community. Moreover, by integrating the voices of young men, BAC subtly spread the idea that boys also had to play a role in using contraception, and that both sexes shared emotional struggles and anxieties around sexual relations.

Throughout the 1970s and 1980s, BAC developed a clear style for their educational materials on sex and contraception, combining simple vocabulary with graphic illustrations. This approach is seen in Birmingham BAC's 1973 eight-page leaflet 'Safe Sex, Contraception', created to answer the questions clients most frequently asked. It presented all available methods of birth control, and the advantages

186   *Sites and spaces*

and effectiveness of each, with drawings of the different methods. In 1976, they produced the 'Safe Sex' kit, a teaching tool that showed a young couple's visit to a doctor and contained the 'Safe Sex' leaflet as well as contraceptive samples including a pill packet, IUDs, sheaths, caps, cream foams, and pessaries.[35] They also developed more sophisticated materials in the form of role-play activities to foster group discussion on diverse topics including sexual experimentation, relationship, consent, and intergenerational discussion.[36]

The opening of BAC's Education and Publication Unit in 1978, funded partly through an annual grant from the Department of Health and Social Security, formalised this production of educational material. This unit created new materials for teachers. In 1980, four new teaching aids were produced: a booklet, 'Abortion', presenting ways to obtain an abortion and describing the procedure; a discussion tape, 'Girls Talking about Sex Education'; a set of slides on 'Gynaecological Examination'; and a 'Contraception' teaching pack. The pack covered the biology of sex, methods of contraception, and use of contraception, and included visual materials designed to help young people grasp complex matters more easily. For instance, the leaflet 'A Look at Your Body' combined frontal depiction of the male and female genitals with identification of the different anatomical parts and cut-side views of the same genitals.[37] Adopting a similar style, the 1981 BAC leaflet for boys 'What You Need to Know about the Sheath' depicted the correct way to put on a condom.[38] As in other BAC education materials for young people, this leaflet espoused direct, down-to-earth vocabulary and visuals.

From the 1960s to the 1980s, BAC's educational work gradually expanded and was formalised through different arms. BAC had always dealt with client letters and telephone calls, but this was a central plank of the work of the Education and Publication Unit. In 1981, the Unit replied to 1,800 letters from young people, youth workers, and parents asking for information about contraception. In 1982, it sent out more than 30,000 educational materials. The same year, with the help of the Department of Education and Science, a School Publication Advisory panel, made up of BAC members and experts in the field of education, was set up to advise BAC on their educational material.[39] Through this multilayered work, BAC played a key role in shaping school pupils' sexual knowledge and fostering discussion on sex and relationships.

A private matter? The Brook Advisory Centre 187

Inclusive sex education

These educational initiatives included efforts to make sex education more inclusive. BAC's pioneering work to improve access to sexual health information and services for 'physically handicapped and mentally sub-normal young people', to use the terminology of the time, further demonstrates how they promoted sexual knowledge among young people and their involvement in public debates on sex and sexuality. In the early 1970s, following the rediscovery of poverty and the subsequent push towards a reduction of inequality, disabled people finally became a new 'worthy target for state-funded provision'.[40] The Chronically Sick and Disabled Person Act of 1970 gave people with disabilities the right to equal access to recreational and educational facilities. In the context of growing recognition of the rights and needs of disabled people, BAC developed a new dimension to their work.

The first efforts occurred in Birmingham. From July 1970, a team of doctors, nurses, and social workers with a special local authority grant made special visits to a hostel for 'young adult spastics', reporting that 'the young people are relieved to have their sexual needs recognised and discussed and contraceptives prescribed when needed'.[41] In 1974, Birmingham BAC participated in a working group on the sexual needs of blind and/or deaf young people. In addition, the Birmingham BAC imported and created films and tapes as teaching resources to use with young people with disabilities. 'Touching' (US import, 1973) was part of a series of films encouraging children to explore ways to heighten sensory awareness, and 'Just What Can You Do' (Birmingham BAC, 1976) talked about contraception for blind people.

These activities were followed in 1978 by the Education and Publication Unit's 'Look at Safe Sex' leaflet for young people with learning and reading difficulties. As in other BAC leaflets, this depicted different methods of birth control, and ways to insert them, including images of young women and men's naked bodies. It included language used by young people to describe genitalia alongside scientific homonyms and was deliberately simple and factual, so that young people with disability could understand it.[42] The nature of the information and the depiction of naked bodies, however, proved controversial. BAC was attacked by conservative lobbies such as the Responsible Society

188 *Sites and spaces*

who accused BAC of pornography and criticised it for not situating sexual relationships within a moral framework.

BAC continued to feel that physically disabled young people's need for sexual information was not being met. In 1983, they made the video *Why Is It for Them and Not Me?*, featuring four young adults with 'congenital or derived disability' discussing their lack of sex education and their sexual needs. BAC worked in tandem with the Spastics Society and SPOD (Association to Aid the Sexual and Personal Relationships of the Disabled) to create this video. At its launch, the secretary of the All Party Disablement Group recognised BAC's role in enabling disabled young people to live fulfilling lives:

> In our efforts to integrate disabled people into the community and enable them to lead fuller lives, we have sadly neglected to give sufficient understanding and attention to their emotional and sexual needs. Attitudes run deep and there is a tremendous need for education. I welcome this film as a step forward in that direction.[43]

BAC also started to provide materials for young people with learning disabilities. In 1983, the Sex Education Resources Centre in Avon (set up in 1978), worked with Avon Health Office to arrange three training days for carers and to develop a syllabus for a twelve-session course with 'mentally handicapped people' aged eighteen and over. Social worker Dorothy Keeping created Daisy, a felt cut-out doll mounted on stiff cardboard and dressed in removable clothes, to explain sex education to young people with learning disabilities. The 1983 annual report pictured Keeping using the Daisy doll with disabled teenagers who were listening attentively. This picture illustrated BAC's commitment to providing sexual and contraceptive information to disabled teenagers. BAC pioneered this approach and recognised for the first time the sexual needs of young disabled people.

Teenage magazines

Brook also contributed to providing information and advice on sexual and reproductive health in teenage magazines, particularly in the 'semi-public, semi-private' space of the problem page.[44] As much recent historical work has shown, problem pages are excellent

A *private matter? The Brook Advisory Centre*   189

sources for understanding the everyday sexual problems and anxieties of ordinary people.[45] Hannah J. Elizabeth has demonstrated the crucial role that teenage magazines played in the sex education of young people.[46] This chapter argues that Brook capitalised on the good relationships they built with agony aunts to provide information on BAC services. In doing so, they recognised that problem pages in teenage magazines functioned as a key resource for young people to learn about sex.

In their 1972 annual report, Brook referred for the first time to the role of teenage magazines in publicising their services. They reported nineteen mentions of BAC in *Petticoat*, a weekly magazine for young women. To BAC, the misery and suffering expressed by young people in letters sent to women's and teenage magazines suggested that they lacked people to turn to for personal advice. In particular, young people did not discuss sex in the private sphere of the home, underlying the need for BAC services.[47] Magazines frequently directed readers to BAC, reflecting the efforts of, first, BAC's Public Relations Officer Valerie Gilbert (1969–74), and then Press and Information Officer Suzie Hayman (1975–84) to encourage such referrals.[48] Hayman described this work as 'send[ing] a letter to all the papers saying I'm Suzie Hayman and I'm now Brook advisor you know, if you want any information or any questions you've got on any of these subjects, please do come, call me. Mainly what I was doing was trying to raise the profile.'[49]

In 1981 it was estimated that an average of two advice columns a month recommended Brook to their readers.[50] One example among many is a sixteen-year-old who in 1978 wrote to *She*, a monthly magazine that targeted younger adult women, for help with her lack of sexual experience. The girl felt pressured into having sex by her friends, who teased her because she was still a virgin; the girl wanted to 'keep herself for the man she [would] marry' but was tempted to 'give way'. Agony aunt Denise Robins emphasised in her reply that the girl herself had to freely decide to have sex and recommended a visit to BAC: 'It's your life and your conscience. Whatever you decide don't risk pregnancy. You could go to the nearest Brook Advisory Centre. Women counsellors will talk things over with you and give you advice.'[51]

The relationship between BAC and teenage magazines was reciprocal. Magazines referred readers to BAC, including in special feature

190 *Sites and spaces*

articles. In 1987, the UK's market-leading teen girl magazine *Just Seventeen* provided vignettes of clients visiting the centre for different reasons; male and female teenagers were represented, as well as clients of different ages.[52] Sixteen-year-old Jackie had unprotected sex and wanted the morning-after pill; seventeen-year-old Jane, accompanied by her boyfriend, had a late period; and eighteen-year-old John had just started dating a new girl and wanted information about AIDS. This article was aimed at reassuring teenagers about the prospect of a visit to BAC. Some agony aunts even co-produced educational materials with BAC; *Just Seventeen*'s agony aunt Melanie McFadyean wrote the leaflet 'Love Carefully', about AIDS, in tandem with BAC and the FPA.[53]

BAC members, in turn, wrote informative pieces for teenage magazines and some acted as agony aunts. Brook Press Officer Suzie Hayman penned several articles on sexual and reproductive health for *Just Seventeen* in the 1980s.[54] These included a 1985 explanation of the Gillick ruling, which raised great fears that under-sixteens would not be able to obtain contraceptives without their parents' permission.[55] Hayman subsequently published *It's More than Sex! A Survival Guide to the Teenage Years*, a book based on her *Just Seventeen* articles and aimed at a broader audience.[56] From 1980, BAC clinic doctor Fay Hutchinson answered letters for *19* magazine, a monthly magazine for teen girls with an estimated readership of 175,000. She undertook this work because Brook acknowledged that the clinics could not fully meet young people's need for information. Hayman, who was instrumental in getting Hutchinson the role at *19*, reflected: 'that was a tremendous link because the demographic of the magazine was actually 15, 16, 17. Yeah. Um, so we got a fair number of people, I think through that, you know, they'd read that.'[57]

Other agony aunts were also closely involved with the charity, either before or after their careers as journalists. Anne Lovell was the administrative manager for BAC in the late 1960s and early 1970s before she became an agony aunt at women's magazine *Bella*.[58] Tricia Kreitman, agony aunt for *Mizz* teen magazine, became a BAC board member in 1993, and its chair in 2001. Nick Fisher, agony uncle for *Just Seventeen*, first turned to BAC for expert information on teenage sexual health. He explained in a private interview:

A private matter? The Brook Advisory Centre   191

I wasn't a psychotherapist, I wasn't a doctor, I, you know, I was a journalist who wrote a lot of features about boyfriends (laughs) and this sort of thing, and so that made me do a lot of research and get involved with the Brook Advisory Service, and all sorts of, different, erm, charities and agencies that dealt with teenagers, to kind of get as much input and information and kind of right, er, right points of view that I could get.[59]

This close collaboration between agony aunts and BAC ensured a wide advertisement to readers of teenage magazines whilst allowing it to lend its credentials and expertise to agony aunts.[60]

Teenage magazines enabled the charity to reach out to millions of sexually active young people who would not visit a Brook centre. This seemed to work, as some BAC clients later reported visiting a centre after having read about it. Jane, who attended a Brook clinic in 1970s London, vaguely remembered having learned about it in a magazine: 'I think there was something about, it might have been in the papers, or it might have been in one of those magazines, like *Honey* or *Nova* mm-hmm, you know, it was kind of in the air.'[61]

Conclusion

At a time when sex education was still relatively absent or focused mainly on the 'facts of life', and when young people became sexually active earlier than previous generations, BAC took up the mission of providing contraceptive information to young people, helping them to deal with their everyday sexual and reproductive health. In doing so, BAC operated on the edges of the public and private domains: starting up at a moment when the boundaries of public and private life were being debated and redrawn, it provided guidance on intimate areas of life within semi-public settings (the clinic, schools, and magazines), in order to counteract the lack of information provided within the home, and against the backdrop of very public concerns about sexual morality, teenage pregnancy, and abortion.

BAC recognised that the best way to prevent unwanted pregnancies and abortions was to educate young people about contraception. They adopted three main strategies to do so, each of which shows their tactics for negotiating the complicated status of sex as simultaneously

192 *Sites and spaces*

deeply private and a matter of intense public concern: they opened clinics in urban centres, conveniently located for young people, that fostered a relaxed atmosphere in order to make discussion of sex less scary; they collaborated with schools and produced educational materials, in the process making sex education more inclusive (as in their work with young people with disabilities, as well as attempts to involve young men in contraceptive decision making); and they worked in tandem with teenage magazines to disseminate guidance on sexual and reproductive health. Using these tactics, BAC reached an increasing number of young people. By the 1980s, the charity had not only become an authoritative provider of everyday sexual knowledge for young people but had contributed to shifting the boundaries of public debate on young people's sexuality.

Acknowledgements

This research was funded by the Wellcome Trust, WT 209726/Z/17/Z.

Notes

1 Wellcome Library, London (hereafter WL), PP/MEW/C/4/4, John McEwan Collection, Brook Advisory Centres: Research for History: Transcripts of BBC Interviews on Brook for *Everyman*, interview with Jenny, 1994.
2 Carole Dyhouse, *Girl Trouble: Panic and Progress in the History of Young Women* (London: Zed Books Ltd, 2014), pp. 105–74; Melanie Tebbutt, *Making Youth: A History of Youth in Modern Britain* (London: Palgrave Macmillan, 2016), p. 127. On anxieties regarding young women see also Callum G. Brown, 'Sex, religion and the single woman c. 1950–75: the importance of a "short" sexual revolution to the English religious crisis of the sixties', *Twentieth Century British History*, 22:2 (2011); Hera Cook, *The Long Sexual Revolution: English Women, Sex, and Contraception 1800–1975* (Oxford: Oxford University Press, 2004), pp. 282–92.
3 Caroline Rusterholz, 'Youth sexuality, responsibility, and the opening of the Brook advisory centres in London and Birmingham in the 1960s', *Journal of British Studies*, 61:2 (2022); Jeffrey Weeks, *Sex, Politics and Society: The Regulation of Sexuality since 1800*, 4th edn (London: Routledge, 2017); Stuart Hall, 'Reformism and the legislation of consent',

A private matter? The Brook Advisory Centre   193

in National Deviancy Conference (ed.), *Permissiveness and Control: The Fate of the Sixties Legislation* (London: Macmillan, 1980), pp. 1–43.

4 Frank Mort, 'The permissive society revisited', *Twentieth Century British History*, 22:2 (2011).

5 Michael Schofield, *The Sexual Behaviour of Young People* (London: Little Brown, 1965).

6 Claire L. Jones, *The Business of Birth Control: Contraception and Commerce in Britain Before the Sexual Revolution* (Manchester: Manchester University Press, 2020), pp. 356–76.

7 For more information about the difficulties in documenting young people's sexual and reproductive health experience see Caroline Rusterholz, 'Teenagers, sex and the Brook Advisory Centres (1964–1985)', in Sian Pooley and Jono Taylor (eds), *Children's Experiences of Welfare in Modern Britain* (London: Institute of Historical Research, 2021).

8 Rusterholz, 'Youth sexuality, responsibility, and the opening of the Brook advisory centres'.

9 WL, SA/FPA/A13/13, Family Planning Association, Organisations: Brook Advisory Centres (formerly Youth Advisory Centres), 'Brook Advisory Centre, Aims and Principles, July 1964'.

10 WL, SA/ALR/F.1, Abortion Law Reform Association, Annual Reports of the Brook Advisory Centres, National Brook Advisory Centre Annual Reports, 1965 and 1980.

11 On the campaign to encourage men to become more involved in birth control see Katherine Jones, '"Men too": masculinities and contraceptive politics in late twentieth century Britain', *Contemporary British History*, 34 (2019).

12 Judith Bury, *Teenage Pregnancy in Britain* (London: Birth Control Trust, 1984), p. 7.

13 Diane Munday, Colin Francome, and Wendy Savage, 'Twenty one years of legal abortion', *British Medical Journal*, 298:6682 (1989), 1231.

14 T.L. Lewis, 'Legal abortion in England and Wales 1968–78', *British Medical Journal*, 280:6210 (1980), 295.

15 John R. Ashton et al., 'Trends in induced abortion in England and Wales', *Journal of Epidemiology & Community Health*, 37.2 (1983).

16 WL, SA/BRO/E11, Brook: Archives, Brook: Publications: Conference Papers, Fay Hutchinson, 'The Brook Clinic, the doctor's view point'.

17 Dorothy van Heeswyk, interviewed by Caroline Rusterholz, November 2022.

18 WL, PP/MEW/C/4/4, John McEwan Collection, Brook Advisory Centres: Research for History: Transcripts of BBC Interviews on Brook for *Everyman*, interview with Jenny, 1994.

194 *Sites and spaces*

19 WL, PP/MEW/C/4/4, John McEwan Collection, Brook Advisory Centres: Research for History: Transcripts of BBC Interviews on Brook for *Everyman*, interview with Lesley, 1994.

20 This testimony is from a Mumsnet thread that answered a call for testimonies to celebrate the fiftieth anniversary of Brook. Of course, testimonies published on an open platform to celebrate a charity were more likely to be positive (though some negative recollections were also published): RowanMumsnet, 'Ever used a Brook clinic of service?' (28 October 2013): www.mumsnet.com/talk/site_stuff/1895087-Ever-used-a-Brook-clinic-or-service-Are-you-willing-to-share-your-stories-to-celebrate-Brooks-fiftieth-birthday (accessed 29 May 2023).

21 Caroline Rusterholz, '"If we can show that we are helping adolescents to understand themselves, their feelings and their needs, then we are doing [a] valuable job": counselling young people on sexual health in the Brook Advisory Centre (1965–1985)', *Medical Humanities*, 49:2 (2023).

22 WL, SA/BRO/D12/1/1/, Brook: Archives, Brook: Local Centres: Merseyside, Merseyside Annual Report, 1976.

23 Joanne Brien, interviewed by Caroline Rusterholz, 29 March 2020.

24 See, for instance, 'Girl smothered secret baby', *Daily Telegraph*, 26 June 1981; 'Anguish of mum who dumped a baby', *Sun*, 14 September 1981; 'Baby killer hunt', *The Times*, 22 May 1982.

25 Sue Tranter, 'A sad story that statistics cannot tell', *Daily Mirror*, 27 November 1978, p. 8.

26 Lesley Hall, 'Birds, bees and general embarrassment: sex education in Britain from social purity to Section 28', in Richard Aldrich (ed.), *Public or Private Education? Lessons from History* (London: Woburn Press, 2004); Rachel Thomson, 'Prevention, promotion and adolescent sexuality: the politics of school sex education in England and Wales', *Sexual and Marital Therapy*, 9:2 (1994); James Hampshire and Jane Lewis, '"The ravages of permissiveness": sex education and the permissive society', *Twentieth Century British History*, 15:3 (2004).

27 Hannah Charnock, 'Girlhood, Sexuality and Identity in England, 1950–1980' (PhD thesis, University of Exeter, 2017); Hannah Charnock, 'Teenage girls, female friendship and the making of the sexual revolution in England, 1950–1980', *The Historical Journal*, 63:4 (2019).

28 WL, SA/FPA/A13/13, Wellcome Library. Family Planning Association, Organisations: Brook Advisory Centres (formerly Youth Advisory Centres), 'Brook Advisory Centre, Aims and Principles, July 1964'.

29 WL, SA/ALR/F.3, Abortion Law Reform Association, Annual Reports of the Brook Advisory Centres: Birmingham, Annual Report 1969.

A private matter? The Brook Advisory Centre   195

30 WL, SA/ALR/F.1, Abortion Law Reform Association, Annual Reports of the Brook Advisory Centres, National Brook Advisory Centre Annual Reports, 1969.

31 WL, SA/BRO/D/1/1/1, Brook: Archives, Brook: Local Centres, Brook: Avon (formerly Wessex): Annual Reports, 1971.

32 WL, SA/ALR/F.1, Abortion Law Reform Association, Annual Reports of the Brook Advisory Centres, National Brook Advisory Centre Annual Reports, 1974.

33 WL, SA/ALR/F.1, Abortion Law Reform Association, Annual Reports of the Brook Advisory Centres, National Brook Advisory Centre Annual Reports, 1982.

34 WL, SA/ALR/F.1, Abortion Law Reform Association, Annual Reports of the Brook Advisory Centres, National Brook Advisory Centre Annual Reports, 1974.

35 WL, SA/ALR/F.1, Abortion Law Reform Association, Annual Reports of the Brook Advisory Centres, National Brook Advisory Centre Annual Reports, 1976.

36 WL, SA/BRO/J/4/1, Brook: Archives, Brook: History and Memorabilia, Dilys Cossey's material relating to Brook, 'Safe Sex' kit.

37 WL, SA/BRO/J/4/1, Brook: Archives, Brook: History and Memorabilia, Dilys Cossey's material relating to Brook, teaching pack, in SA/BRO/J4/1.

38 WL, SA/BRO/J/4/1, Brook: Archives, Brook: History and Memorabilia, Dilys Cossey's material relating to Brook, 'What You Need to Know about the Sheath'.

39 On BAC's creation of sex education material during the AIDS crises, see Hannah J. Elizabeth, '*Love Carefully* and without "over-bearing fears": the persuasive power of authenticity in late 1980s British AIDS education material for adolescents', *Social History of Medicine*, 34:4 (2021).

40 Jameel Hampton, *Disability and the Welfare State in Britain* (Bristol: Policy Press, 2016), p. 82.

41 WL, SA/ALR/F.1, Abortion Law Reform Association, Annual Reports of the Brook Advisory Centres, National Brook Advisory Centre Annual Reports, 1972.

42 On this issue see Caroline Rusterholz, '"A mechanical view of sex outside the context of love and the family": contraception, censorship and the Brook Advisory Centre in Britain (1964–1985)', *Journal of the History of Sexuality*, 33:1 (2024).

43 WL, SA/ALR/F.1, Abortion Law Reform Association, Annual Reports of the Brook Advisory Centres, National Brook Advisory Centre Annual Reports, 1981.

196 *Sites and spaces*

44 Fiona Hackney, 'Getting a living, getting a life: Leonora Eyles, employment and agony, 1925–1930', in Rachel Ritchie, Sue Hawkins, Nicola Phillips, and S. Jay Kleinberg (eds), *Women in Magazines: Research, Representation, Production and Consumption* (New York and London: Routledge, 2016), p. 108.

45 Adrian Bingham, 'Newspaper problem pages and British sexual culture since 1918', *Media History*, 18:1 (2012); Claire Langhamer, 'Everyday advice on everyday love: romantic expertise in mid-twentieth century Britain', *L'Homme: Zeitschrift für Feministische Geschichtswissenschaft*, 1 (2013); Tracey Loughran, 'Sex, relationships, and "everyday psychology" on British magazine problem pages, c. 1960–1990', *Medical Humanities*, 49:2 (2023); Laura Kelly, '"Please help me, I am so miserable!": sexual health, emotions and counselling in teen and young adult problem pages in late 1980s Ireland', *Medical Humanities*, 49:2 (2023).

46 Hannah J. Elizabeth, '[Re]inventing Childhood in the Age of AIDS: The Representation of HIV Positive Identities to Children and Adolescents in Britain, 1983–1997' (PhD thesis, University of Manchester, 2016), pp. 111–49.

47 WL, SA/ALR/F.1, Abortion Law Reform Association, Annual Reports of the Brook Advisory Centres, National Brook Advisory Centre Annual Reports, 1972.

48 WL, SA/ALR/F.1, Abortion Law Reform Association, Annual Reports of the Brook Advisory Centres, National Brook Advisory Centre Annual Reports, 1974.

49 Suzie Hayman, interviewed by Caroline Rusterholz, September 2018.

50 WL, SA/ALR/F.1, Abortion Law Reform Association, Annual Reports of the Brook Advisory Centres, National Brook Advisory Centre Annual Reports, 1981.

51 'What's your problem?', *She*, October 1978.

52 'A visit to Brook', *Just Seventeen*, 22 April 1987, p. 19.

53 Elizabeth, '*Love Carefully* and without "over-bearing fears"'.

54 Suzie Hayman, '"What boys think" about love, sex and birth control', *Just Seventeen*, 6 March 1985, p. 18; Suzie Hayman, 'Teenage mothers', *Just Seventeen*, 4 October 1984, pp. 20–1.

55 Suzie Hayman, 'The effects of the Gillick case', *Just Seventeen*, 20 March 1985, p. 61. In the early 1980s the activist Victoria Gillick, a Roman Catholic mother of ten children, launched a case against the Department of Health and Social Security (DHSS) in England and Wales. The case challenged the authority of the DHSS to enable doctors to prescribe contraception to under-16s without parental consent. Although Gillick lost the case, the publicity surrounding it heightened tensions around the provision of sex education. It contributed to an atmosphere in

A *private matter? The Brook Advisory Centre* 197

which many people with responsibility for the wellbeing of children and adolescents felt anxious about the potential legal consequences of their actions.

56 Suzie Hayman, interviewed by Caroline Rusterholz, September 2018. See Suzie Hayman, *It's More than Sex! A Survival Guide to the Teenage Years* (Aldershot: Wildwood House, 1986).

57 Suzie Hayman, interviewed by Caroline Rusterholz, September 2018.

58 Anne Lovell, interviewed by Tracey Loughran, 24 September 2018. I would like to thank Tracey Loughran who kindly shared the transcript of her interview with me.

59 Nick Fisher, interviewed by Tracey Loughran, 1 September 2018.

60 See Loughran, 'Sex, relationships, and "everyday psychology"'.

61 'Jane', interviewed by Caroline Rusterholz, July 2021.

8

Queering the agony aunt: reusing and adapting a public engagement activity for different audiences

Daisy Payling

Introduction

'There is no such thing as the general public.' Almost a cliché among public engagement professionals, this statement encourages researchers to consider *who* they are aiming to engage with and to tailor their public engagement activities accordingly.[1] Indeed, for the National Co-ordinating Centre for Public Engagement, 'People' – the *who* – are one of the three pillars of public engagement: 'Purpose, People, Process', or the 'Why', 'Who', and 'How' to consider when planning activities.[2] Public engagement was an important part of the Wellcome Trust-funded project 'Body, Self, and Family: Women's Psychological, Emotional and Bodily Health in Britain, c. 1960–1990', on which I worked from January 2018 until March 2022. As well as exploring the histories of women's everyday experiences of health, the project aimed to use historical resources to improve the emotional health and wellbeing of adolescents.[3] From the start, I and my colleagues (Tracey Loughran, Kate Mahoney, and Hannah Froom) were considering how to engage young people with the themes of the research so that they might better understand the structural problems within society whilst also seeing how individuals and communities have agency to affect change. We wanted to create a resource, a toolkit, which would engage young people with the histories of women's 'everyday health', encourage them to take control of their wellbeing in the present, and help them to build better futures.

While this was the overarching aim with a clear 'purpose' and 'people' in mind, in the early stages of the project there was not a

Queering the agony aunt   199

clear 'process'. We had a general sense that we would need to create activities and gather feedback on them, but no clear roadmap. Throughout the course of the project, we sought out public engagement opportunities for which to design and gather feedback on activities, but we also often accepted invitations that came our way in an ad hoc fashion. The toolkit was always the end goal, but on the way to it our engagement activities picked up other purposes. They provided fun opportunities to tell people about the project and to recruit oral history participants – women born between 1940 and 1970 – to contribute to the research and an archive of interviews to be held in the British Library; another integral aim of the project.[4] Some of these public engagement opportunities required a whole new activity, but sometimes it was easier and much more time-efficient to tweak a pre-existing activity for a new audience.

In this chapter I discuss how I created and adapted a public engagement activity called 'Could you be an agony aunt?' for different audiences; from the original audience of school pupils aged fourteen to fifteen, to attendees at two LGBTQ+ history fairs, to a sixteen+ audience attending a Valentine's Day Late at the Royal College of Nursing, before finally returning to an adolescent audience when shaping the activity for our toolkit 'Bodies, hearts, and minds: using the past to empower the future'.[5] This chapter details how I adapted the activity to suit these different audiences and how they responded to it differently. It explores the complexities of using magazine sources to do this work and discusses how the activity changed as my research evolved; as I explored titles aimed at diverse readers and my knowledge of women's magazines broadened and deepened, prompting new research questions and points of discussion. I reflect on my attempts to include diverse experiences in the activity and how people responded to this representation in the context of different events, exploring the difficulties of framing public engagement activities for marginalised groups that neither ignore nor replicate the terms of that marginalisation.

Taking a reflexive approach, the chapter also discusses my own grappling with the question of what queer public engagement looks like to me as a queer academic and how the conversations I had with people at these events influenced my perspective. In documenting our ad hoc approach to public engagement, the chapter demonstrates the value in remaining receptive to unexpected opportunities and

200 *Sites and spaces*

conversations. However, it also highlights the importance of attending to the 'who' not just in terms of identity but also within the wider context of the event and those individuals' likely experiences. A discussion of public engagement 'on the ground' rather than an idealised account, this chapter demonstrates some of the messiness that shifts in research and encounters with different publics can bring to public engagement projects.

Could you be an agony aunt?

The public engagement activity 'Could you be an agony aunt?' used letters and responses from problem pages in 1970s magazines for teenagers and adult women. Women's magazines have been sites of advice and support for women for centuries, but in postwar Britain problem pages and advice columns in women's magazines had 'enormous potential reach and influence' through the sheer size of their readership.[6] In the early 1960s, over fifty million British women read a women's weekly and thirty-four million read a monthly. By 1987, the number of readers of women's weeklies had declined to nearly twenty-four million, whilst readers of monthlies had risen to nearly forty million – still a substantial reach.[7] The letter-response format of agony aunt advice columns fostered a 'supportive community' within the magazines' pages.[8] Agony aunts, as emotional advisors, played an especially important role in creating this 'fiction of friendship and trusted relationship', and held 'considerable power to shape popular understandings' of gender, sex, and relationships.[9] Crucially, however, agony aunts fulfilled a dual role: they offered both 'serious emotional advice and voyeuristic entertainment'.[10] As an activity, 'Could you be an agony aunt?' embraced the dual role of problem pages. In showing participants glimpses of the letter writers' lives it aimed to provoke empathetic responses to these voices from the past while allowing for the baser pleasures of prurience and *Schadenfreude*.

The premise of the activity was simple. It reproduced questions and answers from problem pages but presented them separately from each other. Questions were scattered on one half of a table and responses on the other half (see Figure 8.1). Participants were asked to match questions with responses. Some responses could plausibly match more than one problem, so participants had to be aware of tone and content. To a certain extent they had to imagine themselves as 1970s agony aunts – as the magazine-quiz-style title immediately challenged them to do: 'Could you be an agony aunt?' Magazine quizzes encourage readers to imagine new selves and can direct the nature those selves take.[11] In this activity, the newly imagined self was an agony aunt, but the quiz-style title also transported adult participants to the playful spaces of their teenage years, with the challenge of the task reinforcing the sense of play for participants of all ages. It drew on the recognised role of play and creative engagement in supporting learning.[12] Throughout the activity, participants were encouraged to empathise with the letter writers and the agony aunt, paying attention to both in identifying the real-life advice.

During and after the activity, I asked follow-up questions, including 'What do you think of this advice?', 'What advice would you give to this person if they were your friend?', 'Do these problems resonate with you?', and 'How do you think teenagers or women's lives have changed since the 1970s?' These questions aimed to draw out the historical context behind the problems posed and the advice given, prompting participants to examine how people's lives, their choices, and their emotional landscapes and wellbeing have changed from the 1970s to the present day. The questions also offered opportunities to reflect on how people might deal with similar problems in the present. I ran the activity at several events, tailoring it to diverse audiences, but the first iteration of the activity was developed for school students aged fourteen to fifteen years as part of the University of Essex's Digital Arts Festival in April 2019.

The Digital Arts Festival creates an opportunity for young people at secondary schools in Essex to visit campus and attend workshops by academics and local arts practitioners on different topics and technologies. The theme of the 2019 festival was '#ChallengeYour-Reality', and I wanted to address young people's experiences with digital environments as well as to include a digital element. Young people on school visits to the festival were obliged to be there by their teachers – a captive audience – but even so I wanted the activities to speak to their interests. I designed a workshop called 'Am I normal? Body image from agony aunts to Instagram', which included four short interactive activities: the 'Could you be an agony

202   *Sites and spaces*

aunt?' pairing exercise in worksheet form, a group discussion about the internet and body image, a task involving designing a body-positive Instagram post, and an online quiz version of the 'Could you be an agony aunt?' activity conducted in competing teams. Due to issues of safeguarding and accessibility I did not want the young people involved to use their own Instagram accounts and devices to design an Instagram post, so I turned that task into a drawing activity. I created the online quiz to include a 'digital' element rather than asking the young people involved to reflect solely on their digital lives. Constrained by budget and time, I made the quiz using the free online quizzing website Sporcle.[13]

While the workshop was certainly less flashy than some of the other activities on offer at the Digital Arts Festival, I was concerned with ensuring that the activities spoke to themes in young people's lives. I selected problem/answer pairs representing areas including body image, confidence, and relationships. My research was on women's magazines and at that stage in the project I was still methodically working through mainstream monthly magazines including *She*, *Cosmopolitan*, and *Nova* and had not yet begun looking at magazines aimed at lesbian and bisexual women (*Arena Three*, *Sappho*) or those aimed at Black and South Asian women (*Chic*, *Black Beauty and Hair*, and *Mukti*). Most of the problem pages I had access to were created with white, cisgender, heterosexual, adult women in mind. My colleague Hannah Froom shared problem pages she had examined during her PhD research into *Jackie* magazine – a magazine aimed at teenagers – including questions sent to the Beauty Editor asking advice about cosmetics and hair.[14] From the problems Hannah shared with me, I selected letters which would hold participants' attention. As Suzie Hayman, former agony aunt for *Woman's Own*, explains: 'As an agony aunt, I think I owe my readers professionalism and empathy and knowledge and understanding [...] But I also owe them entertainment, because they're not gonna read if it's just a professional screed.'[15] I tried to choose shorter pairings and ones that were possible to match without being too obvious. I also made sure that questions about body image did not include specific advice about weight loss and dieting, as that could be potentially harmful. The advice on offer needed to be sensitive and sensible, even accounting for changing attitudes over time. Finally, it was important that some of the humour in the activity could be found by attempting to match wildly incorrect responses.

I could select only a handful of pairings for the worksheet and those I did not use I made into the online quiz. This included pairings from gay or bisexual young people. I included these on the online version rather than the worksheet because at that point I did not feel equipped to have conversations about queer topics with young people whom I was meeting for the first time that day. The year before, some of the young people who had attended the Digital Arts Festival had been a bit disruptive and the workshop length of forty-five minutes was not long enough to build the level of rapport necessary for me to feel comfortable navigating potentially homophobic responses. At the time there were frequent news stories about protests against LGBTQ+ inclusive education in schools in Birmingham.[16] As a queer person and one who had lived in Birmingham, those news stories affected me. I felt like I did not have the capacity to have those conversations. Including questions about queer experiences where the advice given was kind and encouraging felt like a compromise. It was there in the activity for those it would resonate with, but the quiz activity was fast-paced enough that we would not linger on it. Together the interactive activities provoked some interesting discussions around body image, but the girls in the groups were much more engaged than the boys, some of whom were visibly bored. The competitive element of the Sporcle quiz reinvigorated the group and the session ended on a high note despite the earlier dip in enthusiasm. On reflection, I had tried to fit too much into a forty-five minute session to overcompensate for a lack of exciting technology that I knew other workshops were using, but in essence the 'Could you be an agony aunt?' activity was born.

Adapting the activity for LGBTQ+ and sixteen+ audiences

In November 2019, I was awarded funding through the Being Human Small Award scheme to put on a weekend of events for the Being Human Festival themed around health and beauty. Being Human is the UK's national festival of the humanities, encouraging humanities researchers to produce enjoyable events for public audiences to attend at their leisure. Two of the three events we ran were

204 *Sites and spaces*

drop-in events and we wanted to include a variety of activities for visitors to engage with. I turned 'Could you be an agony aunt?' into the tabletop matching game that I described above, using all the problem pairs I had and some new ones. The first event of the weekend, 'Beauty school drop in', was about exploring what beauty means/meant to people in the past and in the present and examining how that has changed over time culturally and for individuals. Traditional beauty spaces can be alienating, especially for queer and gender non-conforming people. To address this and make the event as inclusive as possible, whilst at the same time adding to the beauty salon feel, we booked transgender activist Charlie Craggs to do manicures. Craggs's 'fabulous activism' includes her project 'Nail Transphobia', where she invites members of the public to ask her questions about trans lives whilst she paints their nails.[17] 'Nail Transphobia' aims to break down stereotypes and create allies, and for Craggs sharing in the self-care element of having your nails done is an important part of her work: 'The act of looking after yourself is an act of love, and learning to love myself saved my life.'[18] We aimed to make 'Beauty school drop in' a space where beauty could be explored in an open and inclusive way and I wanted to build this message into all the interactive activities we were running, including 'Could you be an agony aunt?'.

At this point in my research schedule, I had started to scope out more queer magazines, including magazines for lesbian and bisexual women like *Arena Three* in the 1960s and *Sappho* in the 1970s. Whilst letters pages were integral to building community in these publications, they offered a more discursive space for readers to respond to articles and each other rather than emulating the problem pages of mainstream women's magazines.[19] The *Beaumont Magazine* – a magazine from the 1990s for transfeminine 'transsexuals' and 'cross-dressers' – had what I was looking for: a problem-page column for crowd-sourced beauty tips called the 'Poser Page'.[20] With the problems and the advice both coming from readers, the 'Poser Page' functioned as a community-building space whilst also more closely emulating the problem-page dynamic that I needed for 'Could you be an agony aunt?': 'You ask the questions [...] we give you an answer and invite you, the READER, to give us your wisdom. Send your solutions to us!'[21] Questions such as this one from 1993 – 'I always take care with my eye make-up. Then I ruin it by mis-managing my mascara brushes. Any pointers?' – fit well with the beauty questions already in the activity, as did the answer which encouraged the use of 'false eyelashes, readily available from Boots, department stores etc [...] select the finer styles, not the thick ones'.[22] During the activity at 'Beauty school drop in' I explained to participants that the pairings on the table were from a variety of magazines: teenage magazines, mainstream women's magazines, and the *Beaumont Magazine* which transgender women read in the 1990s. Unfortunately, Charlie Craggs had to pull out of the event at the last moment, but through the activity I was able to have conversations with people about LGBTQ+ history and experiences with beauty and self-expression.

At the time I was pleased with how seamlessly the *Beaumont Magazine*'s beauty questions fit into 'Could you be an agony aunt?' However, I soon realised that they fit so well as to be invisible among the mainstream women's magazine questions. The activity was queer, but only if you knew it. Like subtext or coded language, a queer reading was available to those who recognised it, but it was not obvious. In December 2019 this was brought home to me when I took the activity to the annual LGBTQ+ History and Archives Conference at the London Metropolitan Archives. Our main aim in attending this event was to recruit older lesbian and bisexual women for our oral history research. We attended with a large stack of flyers and laid out the agony aunt game to draw people into discussion. Surrounded by co-produced projects that centred LGBTQ+ voices, I realised that this activity was not transparently queer and it did not garner the same interest from passers-by as it had from visitors to 'Beauty school drop in' – who, although it was a 'drop-in' event, tended to stay for a couple of hours. A number of people approached our stand to ask about the game, but when I explained that it was about agony aunts their response was often muted. Met with their lack of enthusiasm, I'd switch to talking about the oral history project and try to get them to take a flyer to pass on to any women aged between fifty and eighty. I found that younger people were more inclined to have a go at the game, but the experience left me feeling drained. I felt like the activity was not 'queer enough' for the event, and that perhaps, by extension, neither was I. In

206   *Sites and spaces*

January 2020 I took the same activity to the Goldsmiths Queer History Fair without having time to remake it, and received a similar response.

The new year brought one last in-person public engagement opportunity before the COVID-19 pandemic and national lockdown. In February 2020, the Body, Self and Family team were invited to have a stand at Valentine's Day Late event at the Royal College of Nursing organised by the University of Roehampton's 'Surgery and Emotion' project. The Late was aimed at adults interested in the history of medicine, including medical professionals. Museum and library 'lates' are usually evening events promoted to younger adult audiences as an opportunity to view exhibitions outside normal opening hours in a friendly, social space. They often incorporate interactive activities and food and drink, including alcohol. After confirming with the organisers that this was a sixteen+ event, I decided to adapt 'Could you be an agony aunt?' further.

By this point I had completed my research on *She* magazine. A monthly magazine, *She* was created in 1955 for the women its founder saw around him; women who were 'funny, vulgar, and tough'.[23] *She* spoke to women whose interests did not centre on being a housewife, although the women who read it most likely were housewives, or expected to be once they married. Amassing a regular circulation of more than 300,000 in the 1960s, '*She* blazed a lone trail of outspokenness [...] showing a healthy disregard for customary "unmentionables"'. *Cosmopolitan*'s launch onto the UK market in 1972 with a male nude centrefold threatened *She*'s place.[24] To compete with *Cosmopolitan*'s frank attitude to sex, *She* reintroduced a doctor's column in 1973. Written by Dr David Delvin, it focused exclusively on answering readers' questions about sex and reproductive health, whilst seasoned agony aunt Denise Robins continued to tackle readers' emotional problems in a separate column. Delvin's column was informative. He answered quite basic questions about the risk of pregnancy when having sex standing up, often countering erroneous information given to women by their male lovers.[25] He also answered more complex questions about types of contraceptive pill and their side effects.[26] But Delvin's column was humorous too. Striking a brasher, sillier note than Robins's more serious advice column, it followed publishing trends which saw some newspapers and magazines present problem pages 'more overtly as entertainment' by the 1970s.[27] In response to one letter writer who asked whether Delvin approved of her husband's preference for pouring 'half a glass of 1968 Burgundy' on her 'most intimate area' before oral sex, Delvin wrote, 'No, I don't … The correct year would be … (dare I say it) a '69'.[28] I thought problem/answer pairs from Delvin's column would make a nice addition to 'Could you be an agony aunt?' for a Valentine's Day-themed event aimed an adult audience in the 'Late' space.

This version of 'Could you be an agony aunt?' was a success. Having run versions of the game multiple times by this point, I was very familiar with it and with talking to visitors about our project. I knew each pairing off by heart and could answer at ease any questions about the historical context. People approached the activity with a real sense of fun, curiosity, and engagement. A group of young women were slightly scandalised by some of the questions, while some older women there with friends reminisced about teenage magazines. An older man read through some of the problems with a wry smile and then suddenly stopped. He picked up a problem from a teenage boy writing into *Woman* magazine with confusing feelings about a male friend:

> I'm 16, still at school and a pretty normal guy – or at least I was. I still date girls, but for the past six months I've been strongly attracted to another guy. He's very good looking and is looked up to by most people. But it's more than admiration in my case. We've only got a few weeks left at school and I'm desperate at the thought of never seeing him again.[29]

I helped him find the response and he was surprised and touched by how sympathetic it was (see Figure 8.1). The agony aunt, Anna Raeburn, reassured the boy that there were 'many kinds of affection' but that he was understandably 'frightened of a kind of human behaviour which, sadly, has been made into a bogey'.[30] The man told me that when he was growing up in the 1970s and realising that he was gay he would have found a response like this in his mother's magazine comforting.

Jennifer Crane, in her work on the 'Cultural History of the National Health Service (NHS)' project, writes about 'the challenge of how – and whether – to position ourselves, our own memories and beliefs' within interactions with the public. Crane found that being open

208   *Sites and spaces*

about her own life and experience with the NHS improved conversations she had with the public: 'Bringing my own NHS glasses, for example, which I wore as a child, encouraged members of the public to tell me their own childhood stories.'[31] The challenge of how to position ourselves and where to draw boundaries around our personal life in these kinds of interactions is something we each have to consider on a case-by-case basis, although there is a clear difference between telling a member of public about your glasses and talking about your sexuality.

Eli Burke explains that, 'To be visible as a queer person is to be vulnerable', but 'to be vulnerable is to develop strength and resilience. It is to reclaim your narrative in a world that wishes you erased. It is an act of resistance.' Working with intergenerational LGBTQIA+ communities as a queer/trans museum educator, Burke found that 'vulnerability is a powerful teaching tool, especially when working with a population that must grapple with it for survival'.[32] By sharing his experiences and allowing himself to be vulnerable over a ten-week-long, weekly arts programme, Burke made powerful connections and gained a deeper emotional understanding of his participants' experiences:

> Their lives and struggles made my freedom to live openly possible. I knew this intellectually, but the connections I made through our reciprocal moments of vulnerability during this program made me feel this in my body. It became an organic, breathing new truth that I could not put on a shelf.[33]

Burke reframes vulnerability 'as a form of power.'[34] Talking with this older man at the Valentine's Day Late event I felt a glimmer of this power. As he shared his experiences of the 1970s with me, I felt comfortable opening up in turn about my experiences as a queer but closeted teenager in the 2000s. We talked about the differences as well as the similarities, and of what we saw of young people today and their experiences. It was a meaningful interaction for me, and I think for him as well. He was by no means the only queer person that I had a long conversation with that evening. A bisexual woman around my age participated in the activity, and after she responded similarly to the queer voices in the agony aunt game we talked about the impact Section 28 had had on our younger selves.[35]

Understanding different responses to 'Could you be an agony aunt?'

In trying to understand why people responded so differently to 'Could you be an agony aunt?' at the Valentine's Day Late, as compared with the LGBTQ+ history fairs, I turned to museum studies literature on visitor experience. Exploring the role identity plays in visitor experience, Falk writes that 'the long-term meanings created by visitors from their time in the museum are largely shaped by short-term personal, identity-related needs and interests rather than by the goals and intentions of the museum's staff'. These 'identity-related visit motivations' are 'the series of specific reasons that visitors use to justify as well as organise their visit, and ultimately use in order to make sense of their museum experience'. These can be as varied as looking for queer connection or just having an hour to kill before catching a train. Both can exist at once and can be 'fluid and changing' to the extent that 'the same individual can engage with the same exhibitions and content in fundamentally different ways depending upon their current identity-related visit motivations'.[36]

Visiting a museum or exhibition can be a frustrating experience for queer people seeking queer representation, recognition, and connection. Margaret Middleton explains how attempting to find LGBTQ+ representation in museum settings can feel like work:

> As queer people, we are used to approaching museum visits as if we are archaeologists seeking long lost traces of our ancestors. My all-too-often accurate assumption that queerness will be missing from the interpretation means that the feeling underlying my experience in museums is one of scrutiny and scepticism. The few queer-positive museum experiences I have had are markedly more relaxing because they are not so much work.[37]

The absence of queer stories in museums can not only be tiring but also alienating. Middleton writes of the 'relief it would be to visit any museum and be met with exhibition text, tours, and other methods of engagement that demonstrate the interpretation team has noticed queer connections, deemed them worthy of mention, and imagined a potential queer visitor'.[38] While this hypothetical situation sparks relief, Burke explores the harm inherent to most learning environments

210   *Sites and spaces*

in which 'heteronormativity is pervasive [...] We are often caught in the loop of considering our identities and aware that we are not part of the accepted majority before learning can even begin.'[39] People attend LGBTQ+ history fairs expecting queer content. An LGBTQ+ history fair should be a relaxing space for a queer person where they should feel assured that LGBTQ+ identities have been considered and will be represented. Coming across an activity that hides queer experiences among heterosexual and cis-normative ones and considers queerness through the heteronormative lens of the 1970s agony aunt could be jarring in this environment, leading a participant to feel that the activity is too much work to engage with.

The same visitor approaching the same activity in a different event with a different context may well experience the activity more positively. Sean Curran, writing about the process of situating LGBTQ+ voices in National Trust historic houses, frames the feeling of searching for and finding traces of queer experiences in a more positive light. Curran deploys cruising as a metaphor to explore the feeling of encountering fleeting moments of queer recognition in historical spaces. Drawing on Mark Turner's work, Curran explains that cruising 'is not just about looking for nameless and faceless sex, but rather about forging brief and fleeting connections through "backward glances", which constitute "an act of mutual recognition amid the otherwise alienating effects of the anonymous crowd"'.[40] Viewing cruising as a still-popular and 'inherently queer way of experiencing place, and of community building', Curran nevertheless acknowledges that 'queer people are rightly no longer content with this stealth-like appropriation of spaces', with many preferring to use apps like Grindr or Hinge to insert themselves into mainstream hook-up or dating culture.[41] For many, faced with an LGBTQ+ event that is full of queer stories and queer voices, there would be no great desire to sift through a mostly straight collection of agony aunt problems to find glimmers of queer recognition.

At an event where that is not the case, however, like the Valentine's Day Late, these brief moments of queer recognition and connection can still hold their power. As Burke notes, queer people 'often come to know themselves as LGBTQIA+ in isolation. It often happens in private moments of awareness around other bodies or in familial settings where what is modelled does not "feel" right for us.'[42] Seeing glimmers of queerness and recognition in a source as domestic, heteronormative, and everyday as mainstream women's magazines is powerful. Often queer people, especially queer young people, have had to look for queer community outside the home. For a queer person to recognise and imagine the experience of a queer person in the past finding comfort from an object inside the home (in this case a queer teenage boy and his mother's magazine), and with that recognition find themselves transported back to their own past self, is a significant moment. I know from my own experience that finding glimmers of queerness amongst pages of heteronormative content is exciting, and to share that experience with another queer person is joyful. It feels good to be in the know. For the right person in the right context, then, experiencing flashes of queer recognition in unexpected places can be exhilarating rather than exhausting.

If I had the opportunity to run the 'Could you be an agony aunt?' activity at an LGBTQ+ event again, or even for a general audience, I would change it to foreground the queer experiences by dramatically reducing the number of problem/answer pairs from mainstream women's magazines and by writing the name of the publication on the pairings to make it clearer if the examples came from LGBTQ+ publications like the *Beaumont Bulletin*. I have since researched magazines aimed at Black women in Britain such as *Chic* magazine, which from 1984 closely emulated mainstream magazines, covering lifestyle, relationships, careers, and beauty from the perspective of Black British women, and its successor *Candice*, which from the late 1980s claimed a readership of 25,000.[43] I would incorporate problem/answer pairs from these publications too, prioritising discussions of LGBTQ+ themes. Although labelling the problem/answer pairs with their publication sources would make the matching component easier, successful matching would still require paying attention to the text and would allow for queer recognition without participants having to work so hard for it. Furthermore, it would counter the invisibility of Black and trans women in the activity, who, when writing in to publications aimed at themselves, did not tend to describe themselves as 'Black' or 'trans' unless it was relevant, such as with one 'dark skinned black girl' who wrote to *Chic* for make-up advice. The diversity of these women's experiences might otherwise be lost between the problems of the readers of mainstream magazines aimed at white, cis, heterosexual women where the readers writing in were assumed white unless otherwise stated.[44]

212   *Sites and spaces*

Conclusion: the 'Bodies, hearts, and minds' toolkit

'Could you be an agony aunt?' was originally designed as an activity for adolescents at the Digital Arts Festival with the eventual aim of including it in a toolkit engaging young people with histories of women's 'everyday health' and encouraging them to take control of their own wellbeing. As a project, one of the aspects we found most challenging in building the toolkit was representation. From 1960 to 1990, the period examined by the 'Body, Self, and Family' project, mass-market cultural products like women's magazines either exoticised or rendered invisible women of colour and LGBTQ+ women. The activities in our toolkit needed to portray how racism and heterosexism structured the 'everyday health' experiences of these women, through unthinking exclusion as well as documentable oppression. But we struggled with how to represent and historically contextualise invisibility in short activities and avoid reducing these women's multifaceted lives to oppression and victimhood. As we have explained elsewhere, we were

> particularly keen not to represent BAME [Black, Asian and Minority Ethnic] and LGBTQ+ women's experiences in primarily negative terms to adolescents. As they struggle with racism and heterosexism in their own lives, they need opportunities to empathise with the successes, pleasures and mundanities of the lives of past women with whom they share aspects of identity – the opportunities that white, heterosexual girls and women can take for granted.[45]

We were keenly aware of these issues as we designed activities, and were grateful for the feedback we received from the activists, educators, and community groups who helped us to shape the 'Bodies, hearts, and minds: using the past to empower the future' toolkit.[46]

In the much-simplified version of 'Could you be an agony aunt?' included in the toolkit, we included the question from the teenage boy who was 'strongly attracted' to another male friend as one of just three problem/answer pairings (Figure 8.1). In other activities throughout the toolkit, we used extracts from oral history interviews and autobiographies to include diverse experiences, and we incorporated images from the fashion pages of Black women's magazines alongside images from mainstream women's magazines in collage materials.[47] Trialling the toolkit with Healthwatch Essex Young

Queering the agony aunt 213

Dear Agony Aunt...

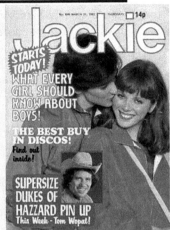

In the 1970s and 1980s, young people wrote into magazines with their problems. Although some read the problem pages and had a laugh about them with their friends, others read them carefully, seeking answers and advice. For the most part, agony aunts took questions seriously and offered suggestions meant to help.

One of these magazines was *Jackie*, which ran from 1964 until 1993. It published a mix of fashion and beauty tips, gossip, short stories and comic strips.

The centre pages of the magazine usually contained a pull-out poster of a popular band or film star, and it printed funny interviews with pop stars.

In the 1970s, it was Britain's best-selling teenage magazine, with sales figures of 600,000 copies per week.

The following examples are all copied from *Jackie*. Could you be an agony aunt? Match the questions with the answers.

Q1: I'm 16, still at school and a pretty normal guy – or at least I was. I still date girls, but for the past six months I've been strongly attracted to another guy. We've only got a few weeks left at school and I'm desperate at the thought of never seeing him again.

Q2: I need to lose weight – lots of it – and last week I finally started on a diet, but I'm cheating already! Any tips for someone with no willpower?

Q3: I am 13 and have just started to mature physically. The trouble is that at the moment I want to be with my parents more than I used to. Whenever a friend asks me to go out, I want to burst out crying. What is happening to me?

A1: It is only natural that you are conscious of this change in yourself physically and this makes you self-conscious and unsure of yourself... Invite your friends round. In the security of your own home, you will be able to establish relationships with others.

A2: You can argue that there are many kinds of affection and involvement which aren't necessarily sexual; or you can say that all relationships have sexual components... To appreciate another man's looks, charm and ability isn't necessarily evidence of homosexuality. And why should you never see him again?... You're frightened of a kind of human behaviour which, sadly, has been made into a bogey.

A3: You've got reasons for wanting to be slim so make a list of them and pin them up where they can't be missed. Set a goal – decide how many pounds you'd like to lose, but give yourself time: don't be too impatient. It's not easy but think how pleased you'll be when your friends notice how slim you're getting.

9

Figure 8.1 'Dear agony aunt' activity from the 'Bodies, hearts, and minds: using the past to empower the future' toolkit. Courtesy of Tracey Loughran, Kate Mahoney, and Daisy Payling. All rights reserved and permission to use the figure must be obtained from the copyright holder.

214 *Sites and spaces*

Mental Health Ambassadors – a group of local adolescents interested in mental health – we received feedback that we needed to incorporate more male experiences. We commissioned additional activities from historians of masculinity Mark Anderson, Richard Hall, and Katherine Jones, but also took the opportunity to be more gender inclusive. We reached out to photographer Julia Comita and make-up artist Brenna Drury, the artists behind 'Prim 'n Poppin" – a project which recreates vintage make-up advertisements to make them more inclusive – to ask if we could incorporate their project into an activity.[48] With the models' permission, they graciously allowed us to use the adverts they created starring non-binary models Cory and Kaguya as a discussion starter about what – and who – is often missing in media depictions of beauty and fashion.[49]

The conversations I had with LGBTQ+ participants playing 'Could you be an agony aunt?' encouraged me to put some of my own experiences into the 'Bodies, hearts, and minds' toolkit. In an activity called 'Sex education then and now: putting yourself in the picture', we included quotes about people's experiences of sex education in the 1960s, 1970s, 1980s, 1990s, 2000s, and 2010s, leaving a space for young people to include their experiences of sex and relationships education in the 2020s. Most of the quotes come from oral history interviews and Mass Observation responses, but, as material from those sources stopped in the 1990s, we had to look elsewhere for examples for the 2000s and 2010s. For the 2000s, we included my memories of growing up under Section 28, attributed to a character called Chris:

> We had a term of specific PSHE [Personal, Social, Health, and Economic education] teaching which looked at sex and relationships but also taught us about drugs and other things. These lessons were in the music block and taught by one of our music teachers. I vividly remember the teacher saying that homosexual relationships were valid but that she wasn't allowed to tell us that.[50]

Eli Burke writes that, as queer people, 'our intuition, vulnerabilities, personal narratives, and experiences are the most powerful places from which we can gain understanding, make more sense of things in the world, and connect with others'.[51] Playing 'Could you be an agony aunt?' with other LGBTQ+ people and sharing something of my experiences helped me better understand my queer self and trust

Queering the agony aunt 215

that I knew when and how much of it to share. The 'Bodies, hearts, and minds' toolkit reflects a diversity of experiences including my own. As LGBTQ+ inclusive sex and relationships education continues to weather attacks in 2023, I hope our toolkit can act as an inclusive resource for young people to connect with others' experiences, better understand and trust themselves, and take control of their 'everyday health'.[52]

Acknowledgements

The research on which this chapter is based was conducted as part of the Wellcome Trust Investigator Award in the Humanities and Social Sciences, 'Body, Self and Family: Women's Psychological, Emotional and Bodily Health in Britain, c. 1960–1990', WT 208080/Z/17/Z.

Notes

1 National Co-ordinating Centre for Public Engagement (NCCPE), 'Target your audience': https://www.publicengagement.ac.uk/do-engagement/understanding-audiences/target-your-audience (accessed 5 February 2023).
2 NCCPE, 'About quality engagement': https://www.publicengagement.ac.uk/do-engagement/quality-engagement/about-quality-engagement (accessed 5 February 2023).
3 Body, Self and Family, 'The project': https://bodyselffamily.org/ (accessed 5 February 2023).
4 Tracey Loughran, Kate Mahoney, and Daisy Payling, 'Reflections on remote interviewing in a pandemic: negotiating participant and researcher emotions', *Oral History*, 50:1 (2022), 38.
5 'Bodies, hearts, and minds: using the past to empower the future', https://bodyselffamily.org/blog/?page_id=137 (accessed 5 February 2023).
6 Laurel Forster, *Magazine Movements: Women's Culture, Feminisms and Media Form* (New York and London: Bloomsbury, 2015), p. 158; Tracey Loughran, 'Sex, relationships and "everyday psychology" on British magazine problem pages, c. 1960–1990', *Medical Humanities*, 49:2 (2023), 204.
7 Ros Ballaster et al., *Women's Worlds: Ideology, Femininity and the Woman's Magazine* (New York: New York University Press, 1991), p. 111.

216 *Sites and spaces*

8 Fiona Hackney, 'Getting a living, getting a life: Leonora Eyles, employment and agony, 1925–1930', in Rachel Ritchie, Sue Hawkins, Nicola Phillips, and S. Jay Kleinberg (eds), *Women in Magazines: Research, Representation, Production and Consumption* (New York and London: Routledge, 2016), p. 108.

9 Penny Morris, 'From private to public: Alba de Céspedes' agony column in 1950s Italy', *Modern Italy*, 9:1 (2004), 12; Loughran, 'Sex, relationships and "everyday psychology"', 204.

10 Claire Langhamer, 'Everyday advice on everyday love: romantic expertise in mid-twentieth century Britain', *L'Homme: Zeitschrift für Feministische Geschichtswissenschaft*, 1 (2013), 43.

11 Elizabeth Wilson, *Mirror Writing: An Autobiography* (London: Virago, 1982), p. 16; Ana Cristina Ostermann and Deborah Keller-Cohen (1998), 'Good girls go to heaven; bad girls ... learn to be good: quizzes in American and Brazilian teenage girls' magazines', *Discourse & Society*, 9:4 (1998), 534.

12 Mitchel Resnick and Ken Robinson, *Lifelong Kindergarten: Cultivating Creativity through Projects, Passion, Peers, and Play* (Cambridge, MA: MIT Press, 2017).

13 For more on converting the activity into its digital form see Tracey Loughran, Kate Mahoney and Daisy Payling, 'Women's voices, emotion and empathy: engaging different publics with "everyday" health histories.' *Medical Humanities*, 48:4 (2022). You can play 'Could you be a 1970s agony aunt?' here: https://www.sporcle.com/games/BSF/could-you-be-a-1970s-agony-aunt-2 (accessed 30 April 2021).

14 Hannah Froom, 'Menstruation, Subjectivity and Constructions of Girlhood in Britain, 1960–1980' (PhD thesis, University of Essex, 2022).

15 Suzie Hayman, interviewed by Tracey Loughran, 7 January 2019.

16 'Birmingham teaching row: how did it unfold?', *BBC News* (22 May 2019): https://www.bbc.co.uk/news/uk-england-48351401 (accessed 3 March 2023).

17 'Charlie Craggs: trans activist', V&A (Victoria and Albert Museum): https://www.vam.ac.uk/articles/charlie-craggs (accessed 4 March 2023).

18 'How Charlie Craggs is fighting transphobia one manicure at a time', *The Fader*: https://www.thefader.com/2016/07/01/charlie-craggs-nail-transphobia (accessed 4 March 2023).

19 Rebecca Jennings, *Tomboys and Bachelor Girls: A Lesbian History of Post-war Britain, 1945–71* (Manchester and New York: Manchester University Press, 2007), p. 155.

20 The *Beaumont Magazine* was published by the Beaumont Society, one of the first groups in Britain established specifically to provide support to trans people. Fleur MacInnes writes about the Beaumont Society

and its earlier publication, the *Beaumont Bulletin*, in chapter 8 in this collection.

21 *Beaumont Magazine*, 1:4 (1993).

22 *Beaumont Magazine*, 1:4 (1993).

23 Cynthia White, *Women's Magazines, 1693–1968* (London: Michael Joseph, 1968), p. 166.

24 Janice Winship, *Inside Women's Magazines* (London: Pandora Books, 1987), pp. 45, 106, 166–8.

25 *She*, April 1973.

26 *She*, July 1975.

27 Adrian Bingham, 'Newspaper problem pages and British sexual culture since 1918', *Media History*, 18:1 (2012), 54.

28 *She*, January 1976.

29 *Woman*, 2 July 1977.

30 *Woman*, 2 July 1977.

31 Jennifer Crane, '"The NHS ... should not be condemned to the history books": public engagement as a method in social histories of medicine', *Social History of Medicine*, 34:3 (2021), 1020.

32 Eli Burke, 'Intuition and vulnerability: a queer approach to museum education', *Journal of Museum Education*, 45:4 (2020), 404.

33 Burke, 'Intuition and vulnerability', 406.

34 Burke, 'Intuition and vulnerability', 403.

35 Section 28, known as Clause 2a in Scotland, was legislation introduced in 1988. It prohibited 'the promotion of homosexuality by local authorities'. In practice, this meant that local authorities could not provide books, plays, leaflets, or films that depicted LGBTQ+ relationships positively. Teachers who taught about same-sex relationships could face disciplinary action. The law was stopped in Scotland in 2000 and in the rest of the United Kingdom in 2003.

36 John H. Falk, *Identity and the Museum Visitor Experience* (Walnut Creek, CA: Left Coast Press, 2009), pp. 35–6.

37 Margaret Middleton, 'Queer possibility', *Journal of Museum Education*, 45:4 (2020), 426.

38 Middleton, 'Queer possibility', 427.

39 Burke, 'Intuition and vulnerability', 409.

40 Sean Curran, 'Queer Activism Begins at Home: Situating LGBTQ Voices in National Trust Historic Houses' (PhD thesis, University College London, 2019), p. 27, quotations from Mark W. Turner, *Backward Glances: Cruising the Queer Streets of New York and London* (London: Reaktion, 2003), p. 9.

41 Curran, 'Queer Activism Begins at Home', p. 27.

42 Burke, 'Intuition and vulnerability', 409.

218   *Sites and spaces*

43 Yinka Sunmonu, 'Chic', in Alison Donnell (ed.), *Companion to Black British Culture*, (Routledge: London, New York, 2002), p. 73; Kadija Sesay, 'Publishing, newspapers and magazines', in Donnell (ed.), *Companion to Contemporary Black British Culture*, p. 251.

44 *Chic*, July 1985. A further alternative could be to keep the pairings unlabelled but include an information sheet showing covers of each magazine featured with a sentence explaining its audience and reach. Whilst this would retain the mystery element of the activity, it would create an additional step in an activity that already requires quite a lot of reading.

45 Loughran, Mahoney, and Payling, 'Women's voices, emotion and empathy', 400.

46 'Bodies, hearts, and minds: using the past to empower the future', toolkit, p. 47, downloadable: https://bodyselffamily.org/blog/?page_id=137 (accessed 5 February 2023).

47 'Bodies, hearts, and minds', toolkit, pp. 9, 21, 28–9.

48 Prim 'n Poppin', 'About': https://www.prim-poppin.com/about (accessed 20 March 2023).

49 'Bodies, hearts, and minds', toolkit, p. 23.

50 'Bodies, hearts, and minds', toolkit, p. 34.

51 Burke, 'Intuition and vulnerability', 411.

52 Sophie Perry, 'Petition to ban "LGBT content" from UK schools crashes, burns and fails at the first hurdle', *Pink News* (31 January 2023): https://www.thepinknews.com/2023/01/31/lgbt-content-uk-schools-curriculum-petition/ (accessed 20 March 2023).

Part III

Mass media and networks of communication

Part III: Introduction

Daisy Payling and Tracey Loughran

In early 2020 Chrissie (b. 1953) spoke to us about her experiences of 'everyday health'. More than twenty-five years earlier, in her early forties, living in South Wales and not yet out as a lesbian, Chrissie found an advert in the back of *Diva* magazine for a nearby women's group and met up with them. In its early days of publication *Diva* was not yet on sale where she lived; she used to drive to London just to buy the magazine and was relieved after a few years when it started to be sold in Bristol. As a means of connecting with other women and with lesbian culture in general, the magazine meant a lot to Chrissie: 'thank God for *Diva*', she told us. At around the same time, the television soap *Brookside* featured the first pre-watershed same-sex kiss between women. This was a 'profound' moment for Chrissie, who had grown up 'glued' to television programmes featuring women she had 'crushes' on. She described the representation of gay lives on television as having 'a more profound effect than any politician or any campaign for homosexual equality'. These were not the only times mass cultural forms played an important part in Chrissie's life. As a child, she was sexually assaulted. In her late teens she read a piece in *Jackie* magazine about sexual assault. She remembered, 'they said, "It's not your fault", and that's the first time I'd ever seen that [...] it changed, it did change my life'. The article 'lifted a weight off my shoulders' and she 'blossomed'. Chrissie described *Jackie* as the 'social media of its day' and drew parallels between it and the contemporary #MeToo campaign that saw 'very strong women standing up and saying similar things today'.[1]

222   *Mass media and networks of communication*

The effects of mass media on 'everyday health' threaded through the life stories of other women interviewed for the same project. Laura remembered religiously using the calorie-counter booklet issued by a mass-market magazine to lose 'puppy fat', while as a nervous first-time mother Teri looked to mother and baby magazines for reassurance. Marie sent off for early lesbian publication *Sappho*; 'all hell broke loose' when her mother discovered the 'stash of magazines'. In the 1980s, Anna was haunted by television dramas about nuclear war, the literal 'stuff of nightmares', while Kate remembered a TV health education advert about AIDS more distinctly than her school sex education lessons. In trying to explain the sexist culture in her workplace in the early 1980s, Diana described it as like *Ashes to Ashes*, the time-travelling police drama broadcast in the 2000s. In more recent years, many women had started to rely on the internet for information about health. Karen said that she might visit her doctor about back problems she had started to experience, 'but probably before I go I'll look online and see how serious it is'. Nadine, plagued by hot flushes and night sweats, had done her own internet research on the menopause to supplement the guidance of her family doctor. Meanwhile Connie, who described herself as 'introverted', found that nowadays 'much of my social life takes place online through various forms of social media'.

The experiences of these women who came to adulthood in the second half of the twentieth century reflect the diversification and rise and fall of specific forms of mass media across this period. In 1950, magazines, cinema, and film were established forms of mass communication; television ownership was beyond the dreams of most households; and Tim Berners-Lee, inventor of the World Wide Web, was not yet born.[2] Today, headlines (read online) regularly herald the death of radio, cinema, and print media, but in the UK more than 99 per cent of households own a television and more than 96 per cent have access to the internet, while there are more than fifty-seven million active social media users, representing nearly 85 per cent of the population.[3] Whatever the precise form, from the postwar decades until the present day, across large parts of the western world mass media has been inescapable.[4] As it came to shape everyday life, so too mass media has shaped how people understand their bodies and selves, how they learn about health, and their capacities to actively seek and exchange information about

Part III: Introduction 223

their wellbeing. Part III brings together chapters exploring different networks of mass communication about 'everyday health': radical newsletters, magazines, television talk shows, and social media. It considers the positioning of differently gendered, abled, and classed bodies within networks of communication, and how different networks offer individuals and groups possibilities for exploitation, affirmation, and resistance to particular positionings of their bodies and selfhood – often at the same time. In doing so, it demonstrates the influence of different forms of media in shaping selfhood and shows how historians can use different media sources to reconstruct histories of 'everyday health'.

Whitney Wood (chapter 9) examines the publicisation of theories of natural childbirth in Canadian popular women's magazines in the postwar decades. Such magazines included health-related content in multiple formats: editorials, articles, 'expert' columns, reader letters, and advertorial content. In analysing these magazines, Wood reveals not only their importance in publicising ideas about natural childbirth but their potential as a resource for learning about many different aspects of women's 'everyday health'. Wood further considers how such features shaped the ideas and experiences of Canadian women who wrote to British obstetrician Grantly Dick-Read, in this way (partially) closing the gap in our understanding of what happens on the page and how readers responded to it – a notoriously difficult act, and one possible in this instance only because letters to Dick-Read are preserved in his archives. Wood's chapter also illuminates how mass media outlets facilitated transnational networks of communication. Dick-Read's popular texts were published in Canada, but reached many more women through mass-market magazines, as did the natural childbirth theories of Russian psychotherapist I.Z. Vel'vovskii and French obstetrician Fernand Lamaze. These magazines were a crucial medium for the international circulation of information to 'ordinary' women and influenced their day-to-day health practices.

The newsletter of Gemma, a radical group for disabled lesbians founded in 1976, was definitely not a form of mass media. At its height, the newsletter reached at most a few hundred readers. But, as Beckie Rutherford (chapter 10) shows, Gemma was a crucial network of communication for those readers because it represented disabled lesbians' lives in their fullest dimensions, at a time when the mainstream media either ignored, pathologised, or desexualised

224   *Mass media and networks of communication*

disabled people, and other radical groups often made little effort to integrate them. Gemma did what no other media outlet tried to do. Within itself, the newsletter constituted a print community that reached beyond the UK, with members in Europe, North America, and the Middle East. Out of its pages also arose face-to-face connections that almost certainly would not have happened without it: meetings at community centres, socials, picnics, wheelchair-friendly discos, meet-ups at Pride, and International Women's Day celebrations. Gemma carved out for itself a unique space within radical politics, making links with other gay and lesbian, disabled, and feminist groups. Out of its existence at the intersections of these alliances, Gemma created a distinct identity revealed through its many publications – not just the newsletters, but also a cookbook, gay guide, access guides, and prose and poetry anthologies. As the world slowly started to catch up with Gemma, members also took opportunities to make themselves visible in the mainstream media, for example through appearing on Channel 4's *Out on Tuesday*, the world's first nationally networked television series aimed at a gay and lesbian audience. Gemma enabled its members to become more fully themselves in connection with each other, and to celebrate their lives and identities in different arenas, including prising open spaces in the mainstream.

Out on Tuesday, first transmitted in 1989, sought to represent diverse queer sexualities and to include voices not usually represented on television.[5] It can be seen as one manifestation of the trend towards more outwardly democratic and participatory formats on television in this era, most visible in the rise of the talk show. A format first popularised in the USA in the 1950s, by the late 1980s the talk show had spread to most parts of the world and its set-up had mutated into less overtly hierarchical forms. These included shows hosted by women, featuring 'ordinary' people or experts by experience (in this way dovetailing with the new prestige of experiential expertise outlined in Part I), and inviting greater levels of audience participation. As Fabiola Creed (chapter 11) explores in her discussion of talk show coverage of 'tanorexia', the woman-centred, emotion-directed, and participatory self-presentation of these shows was no more than a superficial veneer. Celebrity hosts perpetuated conservative social attitudes, expertly directing studio audiences towards the 'right' responses to guests, resulting in the

Part III: Introduction   225

condemnation of those who did not fit the desired mould. In the case of 'tanorexia', this meant young, working-class women whose attempts to meet idealised feminine beauty standards led to their condemnation as irresponsible mothers. Creed reveals how the double standards and hypocrisy of the mass media fuelled contradictory pressures on women in the 1990s – a process that the next chapter shows is ongoing today, its tentacles spread throughout new forms of communication.

Louise Morgan (chapter 12) brings the section to a close, and its focus on mass media bang up to date, with an exploration of social media influencers' manipulation of 'ordinariness' in their narratives of clean eating. In the 2010s, many entrepreneurial young women exploited social media to promote 'healthy' lifestyles based on the rejection of hyper-processed foods and embrace of more apparently 'natural' ways of eating. Some aspects of this trend were new: social media, open to anyone who can sign up for an account, has more genuinely democratic potential than other forms of mass communication; unbound by the materiality of print or the limits of broadcast transmission (admittedly less of an issue in the digital age), it can reach more people, in more places, at any given point in time – partly because, unlike these other media, it is a continuous rather than episodic form; and clean eating, with its self-conscious rejection of the 'diet' label, is certainly at least a newish spin on the policing of bodies. At the same time, so many elements are depressingly familiar: these social influencers are from privileged backgrounds, lending both their condemnation of affordable foods and their denial of political stances a nasty edge; their narratives of miracle cures echo those promoted in tabloid newspapers, women's magazines, and popular television shows in earlier decades; and are their claims of achievability and relatability really so different from the long-standing magazine trope of models insisting that, like the reader, they really just love eating burgers?[6] The means of communication is new, but the structures of power are old, and as we move from the hope of the Arab Spring to major social media companies' complicity in spreading misinformation about elections, they sometimes seem as impenetrable as ever.[7]

What Morgan's chapter underlines is the importance of mass media forms for understanding approaches to 'everyday health' today and in past decades, especially when we are dealing with producers,

226 *Mass media and networks of communication*

consumers, and/or content that is likely to be dismissed as frivolous or trivial. Clean eating might or might not turn out to be a blip in the longer-term history of diet and health, but Ella Mills's *Deliciously Ella*, published in 2015, remains the fastest-selling debut cookbook of all time in the UK – a success built off the back of her hugely successful blog. For future historians, trying to understand people's relationships to their bodies, their sense of self, and their experiences of health will be impossible without recourse to social media.[8] As we peel back different forms of mass media in this section, we see that it is equally impossible to understand the broader landscape of ideas about health in the 1950s without looking at newspapers and magazines, or in the 1980s and 1990s without consulting television programmes. Creed's chapter, which makes an explicit plea for the potential of television as a resource for historians of 'everyday health' and provides a 'how-to' guide on how to use it, is especially important in showing how the stigmatisation of groups that held less power was not only perpetuated in some mass cultural forms but has also permeated the attitudes of historians who have not seen these as 'respectable' sources. Magazines, television, and social media: all propose to speak to 'everyday' lives and concerns, and therefore feature content on diverse aspects of health and wellbeing, but remain largely untapped.

Mass media therefore offers enormous potential for understanding how 'everyday health' operates through networks of communication from the local to the global level. As ever, we know more about representation than reception – what appeared on the page or screen does not tell us about audience response to it and cannot be taken as a straightforward guide to the experiences of those it represents.[9] And, as Rutherford's exploration of Gemma shows, twentieth-century mass media for the most part did not even try to represent everyone – a problem that might seem less pressing in the present age of social media, but that would be to ignore opinion amplification, biased algorithms, and problematic moderation practices.[10] But even if its promise of democracy and community is illusory, mass media still offers a way into histories of health that are less top-down than the traditional focus on science and medicine. Moreover, to a degree often unrealised, user engagement with social media offers possibilities for interaction and pushback. The women who read *Chatelaine* could also write in to the magazine and to Dick-Read; the participants on *Esther* did not have equal access to the microphone, but they

Part III: Introduction 227

could still speak on national television; Ella Mills's Instagram account has comments turned on.

These formats do not have the capacity for resistance of a genuinely ground-up enterprise like Gemma, but, perversely, mass-market forms are always potentially radical in that capitalism demands customer satisfaction. If there is any choice, unhappy consumers will turn elsewhere. As forms with broad reach that attempt to represent, even in sanitised or distorted ways, the lives of millions of people, mass media tells us something about what people *chose* to read and watch, and therefore something about what they enjoyed, loved, or at least did not hate enough to put down and switch off. As we delve into what mass media told its consumers about 'everyday health', we also delve into what aspects of their bodies, selves, and health millions of people tried to understand. This way of thinking about representation requires a move away from narratives of passivity and medicalisation. It does not mean ignoring the flaws of mass media or not critiquing its multiple exclusions. But it does mean opening out a space for agency, without ignoring the shaping role of power structures, by taking seriously the reading and viewing habits, and therefore the thoughts, feelings, and lives, of the mass of people, past and present.

Notes

1 Interviews with Chrissie and the other women discussed in this introduction were part of the project 'Body, Self, and Family: Women's Psychological, Emotional, and Bodily Health in Britain, c. 1960–1990'. These interviews will be archived at the British Library in 2024–25. Names given here are pseudonyms.

2 Ross McKibbin, *Classes and Cultures: England, 1918–1951* (Oxford: Oxford University Press, 1998), pp. 419–76; Jeffrey Richards, *Cinema and Radio in Britain and America* (Manchester: Manchester University Press, 2010); Ros Ballaster, Margaret Beetham, Elizabeth Frazer, and Sandra Hebron, *Women's Worlds: Ideology, Femininity and the Woman's Magazine* (Basingstoke: Macmillan, 1991).

3 'Home Internet and Social Media Usage', Office for National Statistics www.ons.gov.uk/peoplepopulationandcommunity/householdcharacteristics/homeinternetandsocialmediausage (accessed 22 June 2023); 'Television in the United Kingdom', Wikipedia: https://en.wikipedia.org/wiki/Television_in_the_United_Kingdom#History (accessed 22 June 2023);

228   *Mass media and networks of communication*

'Total Number of TV Households in the United Kingdom from 2013 to 2021', Statista: www.statista.com/statistics/269969/number-of-tv-households-in-the-uk/ (accessed 22 June 2023); 'Active Social Media Audience in the United Kingdom (UK) in January 2023: www.statista.com/statistics/507405/uk-active-social-media-and-mobile-social-media-users/ (accessed 22 June 2023).

4 Overviews of the history of mass media and mass communication in the UK include James Curran, 'Media and the making of British society c. 1700–2000', *Media History*, 8:2 (2000); James Curran and Jean Seaton, *Power without Responsibility: The Press, Broadcasting, and the Internet in Britain* (London: Routledge, 2009); John Corner, *Popular Television in Britain* (London: BFI Publishing, 1991); Laurel Forster and Joanne Hollows (eds), *Women's Periodicals and Print Culture in Britain, 1940s–2000s* (Edinburgh: Edinburgh University Press, 2020); Adrian Bingham and Martin Conway, *Tabloid Century: The Popular Press in Britain, 1896 to the Present* (Oxford: Peter Lang, 2015).

5 'Remembering Channel 4's Out on Tuesday', BIMI (Birkbeck Institute for the Moving Image) Blog: http://blogs.bbk.ac.uk/bimi/remembering-channel-4s-out-on-tuesday/ (accessed 22 June 2023); Caroline Spry and Rebecca Dobbs, 'The Channel 4 years: working with Stuart Marshall, a conversation between Rebecca Dobbs and Caroline Spry', *Critical Studies in Television: The International Journal of Television Studies*, 14:4 (2019).

6 '21 Models and actresses enjoying burgers', *Elle*, 10 June 2016: www.elle.com/culture/celebrities/g28360/models-eating-burgers/ (accessed 22 June 2023).

7 Nezar AlSayyad, Muna Guvenc, Anant Maringanti, Eric Sheppard, Ananya Roy, Vinay Gidwani, Michael Goldman, and Helga Leitner, 'Virtual uprisings: on the interaction of new social media, traditional media coverage and urban space during the "Arab Spring"', *Urban Studies*, 52:11 (2015); Jens David Ohlin and Duncan B. Hollis (eds), *Defending Democracies: Combating Foreign Election Interference in a Digital Age* (Oxford: Oxford University Press, 2021).

8 For some initial research in this field see Julia Coffey, *Everyday Embodiment: Rethinking Youth Body Image* (Basingstoke: Palgrave Macmillan, 2021); Wasim Ahmed and Josep Vidal-Alaball (eds), *Social Media and Public Health: Opportunities and Challenges* (Basel: MDPI, 2021); Yvonne Kelly, Afshin Zilanawala, Cara Booker, and Amanda Sacker, 'Social media use and adolescent mental health: findings from the UK Millennium Cohort Study', *EClinicalMedicine*, 6 (2018).

9 On issues around audiences/viewers/readers and reception, see Ballaster et al., *Women's Worlds*, pp. 8–42; Margaret Beetham, *A Magazine*

Part III: Introduction

of Her Own? Domesticity and Desire in the Woman's Magazine, 1800–1914 (London: Routledge, 1996), pp. 157–73; Laura Mulvey, 'Visual pleasure and narrative cinema', *Screen*, 16 (1975); Edward Snow, 'Theorizing the male gaze: some problems', *Representations*, 25 (1989); Caroline Evans and Lorraine Gamman, 'The gaze revisited, or reviewing queer viewing', in Paul Burston and Colin Richardson (eds), *A Queer Romance: Lesbians, Gay Men and Popular Culture* (London: New York and Routledge, 1995); Daisy Payling and Tracey Loughran, 'Nude bodies in British women's magazines at the turn of the 1970s: agency, spectatorship, and the sexual revolution', *Social History of Medicine*, 35:4 (November 2022).

10 Merylna Lim and Ghadah Alrasheed, 'Beyond a technical bug: biased algorithms and moderation are censoring activists on social media', *The Conversation*, 16 May 2021: https://theconversation.com/beyond-a-technical-bug-biased-algorithms-and-moderation-are-censoring-activists-on-social-media-160669 (accessed 22 June 2023); Soo Ling Lim and Peter J. Bentley, 'Opinion amplification causes extreme polarization in social networks', *Scientific Reports*, 12 (2022): https://www.nature.com/articles/s41598-022-22856-z (accessed 22 June 2023).

9

'Thirty years behind England'? Framing 'natural' childbirth in postwar Canada

Whitney Wood

Introduction

Following the North American publication of British obstetrician Grantly Dick-Read's *Childbirth without Fear* in 1944, natural childbirth theories reached new audiences, including Canadians who were interested in what they perceived as a 'new' way to give birth. 'Natural' birth, in both its Dick-Read and Lamaze-inspired forms, attracted growing coverage in the Canadian press from the mid-1940s onwards, with sustained attention throughout the immediate postwar decades. In popular magazines and newspapers, as well as letters to Dick-Read, Canadian women and experts alike discussed their perceptions of and engagement with natural childbirth ideas. In so doing, they articulated a range of attitudes surrounding women's bodies, pregnancy and childbirth, and postwar gender roles.

This chapter draws on popular magazines, newspapers, and a selection of letters from Canadians to Grantly Dick-Read to explore the ways in which Canadian women experienced and perceived reproductive health in the immediate postwar decades, with particular attention to how women framed their health before, during, and after giving birth. 'Natural childbirth' emerged as a malleable concept, and medical experts, the popular press, and parents-to-be continued to use the term in flexible ways throughout the postwar decades. While some continued to pathologise both pregnancy and childbirth and emphasise the need for continuous medical surveillance, others, in growing numbers, sought to position these reproductive health events and life stages as ordinary, everyday, and routine, requiring

'Thirty years behind England'? 231

little in the way of medical intervention. Canadian women, like their global counterparts, conceptualised their pregnancies and childbirths in various ways, demonstrating myriad understandings of what exactly constituted a 'natural' birth. Many women, however, drew on international comparisons to describe their experiences of giving birth in postwar Canada, situating these as 'antiquated' or 'modern' in the context of a transnational natural childbirth movement.

Grantly Dick-Read and 'natural' childbirth

Grantly Dick-Read was born in Beccles, Suffolk in 1890. He received medical training at the London Hospital, qualified as a physician in 1914, and went on to serve with the Royal Army Medical Corps during the First World War. By the close of the decade, Dick-Read had observed what he considered to be quintessential 'natural' births, including the relatively pain-free deliveries of a Whitechapel mother, and of a Belgian 'peasant woman' he saw deliver a child in a field.[1] These cases formed the basis of Dick-Read's theories, which centred on the idea that fear of childbirth caused muscular tension, contributing to heightened cervical contractility and spasms, resulting in increased pain. Dick-Read argued that extensive prenatal education and training in relaxation were the keys to overcoming pain during delivery and envisioned the ideal birth involving the expectant mother as an active and awake participant,[2] in contrast to the standard practice of anaesthetising mothers – most often to the point of full unconsciousness, or 'the surgical degree' – at the moment of delivery.[3]

Grantly Dick-Read's first book, *Natural Childbirth*, which popularised the term, was published in the United Kingdom in 1933.[4] His second book, *Revelation of Childbirth* (1942), was republished for North American audiences as *Childbirth without Fear* in 1944.[5] This book introduced a new audience of Canadian parents to the principles of 'natural childbirth' – an ideology that represented some of the first significant and organised opposition to the medicalisation of birth that had been ongoing since the nineteenth century.

Dick-Read's 'new' approach to childbirth, however, was markedly conservative in a number of ways. He drew heavily on

232   *Mass media and networks of communication*

nineteenth-century medical folklore that emphasised the relatively pain-free deliveries of so-called 'primitive' women – a group including both members of the working and 'peasant' classes,[6] and those who represented racial 'others', namely African women whose births he observed on travels through central Africa alongside his practice in Johannesburg in the postwar years. Dick-Read's emphasis on how the 'ideal' mother should conduct herself during labour – as conscious, composed, and silent – imposed an additional set of expectations on women, while simultaneously upholding and reinforcing physician authority. Dick-Read's approach to natural childbirth left little space for deviation from traditional gender roles, and he framed motherhood as 'the greatest conscious achievement of a woman', noting that 'she was built for that purpose'.[7] Still, his ideas enjoyed increasing popularity amongst North American audiences from the late 1940s onwards, peaking in the 1950s before his death in 1959, after which they were largely replaced by a more Lamaze-inspired (and breathing focused) form of psychoprophylaxis or pain relief during childbirth.

In Canada, natural childbirth enjoyed increasing coverage in the popular press from the late 1940s onwards. Dick-Read's Childbirth without Fear (CWF) methods (and later, the psychoprophylactic theories of Russian psychotherapist I.Z. Vel'vovskii[8] and French obstetrician Fernand Lamaze) were the subject of a number of articles in newspapers and women's magazines, including Canada's leading title, *Chatelaine*. At the close of the 1950s, *Chatelaine* had a circulation of nearly one million copies per month (in a country with a total population of approximately seventeen million).[9] While contemporary analyses failed to identify a diverse readership in terms of race and ethnicity, the magazine was widely read by both working-class and middle-class Canadians from both rural and urban areas.[10] White, married, and middle-class women, however, were the most likely to see themselves and their maternal identities readily reflected in the pages of the magazine. Until the late 1950s, these Canadian audiences regularly received the message that Dick-Read's CWF principles were synonymous with 'natural childbirth'. Accordingly, a growing number of Canadians, both parents-to-be and practitioners, wrote to Dick-Read as the method gained public attention. Canadian letter-writers generally requested more information on the method, referrals to physicians amenable to natural childbirth techniques,

'Thirty years behind England'?   233

and overwhelmingly expressed their appreciation to this British doctor. This chapter includes analysis of letters sent by over sixty women from all regions of Canada between 1946 and his death in 1959, included among hundreds of letters from expectant mothers located throughout the UK, the United States, the British Commonwealth, and globally, in the Dick-Read papers housed at the Wellcome Library for the History of Medicine. In accordance with archival restrictions, all lay letter-writer names are pseudonyms.

Remarkable for the frank discussions of individual pregnancy and birth experiences they contain, letters to Dick-Read, and to Canadian magazines and newspapers, offer a valuable window into how these women framed their health before, during, and after giving birth. These personal narratives reveal how women made sense of competing medical and cultural messages in framing their individual and subjective reproductive health experiences. Alongside popular women's magazines that published a range of health-related editorials, articles, 'expert' columns, reader letters, and advertorial content in the postwar decades, these sources allow historians to begin to 'chart those ideas about health and illness that framed the backdrop of "ordinary" life (itself a concept that gained increasing cultural and political purchase in the postwar period'.[11] In unpacking the embodied and subjective history of 'natural' birth in postwar Canada, three key themes emerge: the malleability and slipperiness of 'the natural' when it came to how individual mothers conceptualised their own delivery experiences; the ways in which Canadians – as cultural commentators, medical experts, and parents-to-be – sought to reframe pregnancy and birth as healthy, normal, and routine life events; and, in the context of an increasingly global natural childbirth movement, the ways in which women turned to transnational comparisons to temporally situate their experiences of giving birth in postwar Canada.

Defining 'natural' birth

Historian Jessica Martucci, writing on the history of natural motherhood and breastfeeding in twentieth-century America, argues that though the term 'natural' figures prominently – and holds considerable power – in a range of health-related discussions it remains 'slippery',

234   *Mass media and networks of communication*

its meaning varying according to context, time, and place.[12] This is absolutely true when it comes to historical discussions of so-called 'natural' birth. In mid-century descriptions a variety of terms were used, including Childbirth without Fear, 'prepared childbirth', and 'educated childbirth', but, echoing Dick-Read's 1933 UK title, 'natural childbirth' quickly came to predominate. This trend can be contextualised by attention to older, early twentieth-century debates on whether pregnancy and childbirth existed as physiological (more natural) or pathological (more disease-like) bodily states, discussions that were recurring and commonplace amongst North American medical experts.[13] Over time, increasing pathologisation and medicalisation played an integral role in fuelling the shift from home to hospital for birth.[14] At the same time, however, there was growing medical and cultural emphasis on the value of a return to nature as an antidote to the damaging effects of 'overcivilisation' and modern life.[15] While some aspects of the birth experience – including Caesarean sections – were consistently recognised as unnatural (though allowing for the display of medical authority, knowledge, and expertise), there was a great deal of wiggle room in terms of what fell under the umbrella of 'natural' birth. This flexibility is reflected in how experts discussed natural childbirth, how popular magazines and newspapers represented the method, and how women described and reflected on their own birth experiences.

By the mid-twentieth century, the popular press offered consistent messages on the value of medical science in promising 'a happier future for women'. Writing in 1943, *Chatelaine* columnist Adele Saunders stressed the need for continued medical supervision and intervention when it came to women's health. Though 'pioneer women' and women 'through the ages' faced a range of 'physiological handicaps' and 'minor ailments' inescapably connected with 'menstruation, child-bearing, and menopause', scientific advancements made 'the future of being a woman ... brighter now than ever before. In other words,' *Chatelaine* readers learned, 'your daughter and the little girl next door are growing up at a time when science is planning to make life healthier and therefore happier for women.'[16] Articles and advertisements further underscored the authority of the trained physician in all health matters, and particularly reproductive ones, as 'intelligent women' were advised to rely on their doctors from the moment they discovered they were pregnant.[17]

'Thirty years behind England'?   235

In their examination of natural childbirth in the 1970s, Flannery Burke and Jennifer Seltz identify 'the tension between natural-as-wild and natural-as-practised' as a persistent characteristic of natural childbirth training programmes. Though medical experts and supporters of natural birth 'had complicated and sometimes conflicting visions of nature [...] they all tended to locate the keys to natural birth in the mind–body connection'.[18] Nature, however, was often framed as requiring modern medical management and control. As emerging experts, including Dick-Read, sought to win public support for their theories, they described their methods in ways that reflected these tensions and ambiguities: while underscoring the value of nature and the natural, they were also careful to recognise the authority of the medical establishment, and accordingly to emphasise the value of medical science in the 'practice' or mastery of natural childbirth techniques.

Answering reader questions in a January 1958 *Chatelaine* feature article, Dick-Read was, unsurprisingly, asked first and foremost to provide a definition of 'natural childbirth'. Responding to this question in conversation with *Chatelaine* home-planning editor Evelyn Hamilton, Dick-Read asserted that natural childbirth

> means that a woman has her baby using the machinery and equipment that nature has provided for her to bear a child. Like any other natural process it does not ask for or necessitate interference. But since this simple concept was lost to sight through centuries of ignorance, superstition, and the dangers that used to surround childbirth, civilized woman was almost deprived of the ability to give birth naturally.[19]

This response from the leading figure in the mid-century natural childbirth movement understandably reflected dominant interpretations of the method. But, when later asked if the method would 'allow anesthesia and surgical help when necessary', Dick-Read responded:

> Certainly. The fallacy that natural childbirth means using no anesthetics is grossly untrue and unfair, and has deterred many women from using this method. I have said repeatedly that no woman should be allowed to suffer more pain or discomfort than she is willing to bear. She should not be allowed to be gallant, either, out of conviction or loyalty to her doctor. The needless suffering of pain in childbirth is a very dangerous thing. I would rather see the scar of a Caesarean

236   *Mass media and networks of communication*

operation than the lasting scars left on a woman's mind by severe and prolonged pain.[20]

Here, then, we can see Dick-Read's emphasis on the malleability of his CWF methods as an attempt to assuage the concerns both of *Chatelaine*'s women readers as well as of physicians, the majority of whom remained sceptical of natural childbirth techniques throughout the postwar decades. Nevertheless, despite Dick-Read's flexible framing of a 'successful' natural birth, a clear hierarchy of birth experiences was established that held 'natural' births, variously defined, above their medicalised counterparts.[21]

Canadian physicians sympathetic to natural childbirth methods adopted similar approaches, underscoring the value of exercises to attain physical relaxation in birth, but offering flexible – and perhaps more realistic – definitions of natural childbirth. In a November 1960 *Chatelaine* article, Dr H.B. Atlee, Emeritus Chief of the Department of Obstetrics and Gynecology at Dalhousie University in Halifax, Nova Scotia, emphasised that he used the term 'natural childbirth [...] in its widest definition'. Atlee continued, 'What is natural childbirth? In the narrow sense of making the actual process of labor more bearable, it means to some a method of attaining physical relaxation through exercises, and to others a routine of reassurance that drives out fears.'[22] Rigid definitions, Atlee continued, had the potential to negatively affect both expectant and new mothers, and the reputation of the method. 'Because in ten percent of cases no pain seems to be felt,' Atlee noted, 'natural childbirth was first looked to as a painless method. But used in that hope it can only result in disillusionment. While it undoubtedly helps in bearing pain, it does not in the large majority of cases remove it entirely, nor does it preserve the woman entirely from the ravages of fear.' Despite these caveats, Atlee concluded, 'there is a difference between feeling and bearing pain', and training in natural childbirth allowed women to develop stoicism, remove fear associated with the birth experience (thereby lessening pain), and channel their energies during delivery 'into useful effort rather than emotional protest'.[23]

This emphasis on the flexibility and malleability of 'natural childbirth' continued into the 1960s as new techniques and methods appeared, and Dick-Read's ideas were supplanted by Lamaze-inspired methods which gradually came to be synonymous with 'natural

'Thirty years behind England'? 237

childbirth' for many North American audiences. A 1964 *Chatelaine* article on 'Childbirth with hypnosis', for example, noted that 'twenty to thirty techniques' that aimed 'to free childbirth from severe pain: "childbirth without fear", "painless childbirth", "natural childbirth", "psychophysical preparation for childbirth"', were unified by their emphasis on 'a degree of mental serenity and a calm relaxed approach to childbirth which few women are able to retain throughout their labor'.[24]

Echoing these flexible definitions, Canadian women framed their 'natural' birth experiences in a number of ways, some of which included considerable medical interventions. Writing to Grantly Dick-Read in 1955, Laurel Rice of Toronto described taking a sedative upon her arrival at the hospital and the administration of ether at the moment of birth, without her consent and despite her explicitly stated desire for a so-called 'natural birth'. Nevertheless, she reported that she was 'very happy that the delivery was so easy', and gave 'all the credit' to Dick-Read.[25] In 1958, another Toronto mother, Fay Grabowski, reported to Dick-Read that she had 'just produced a 10lb 2½oz boy by Natural Childbirth', but included the note that the administration of Demerol – a pain-relieving opioid – during the transition stage of labour 'took the sharp edge off the pain' and 'helped tremendously'.[26]

Eight years later, in the May 1966 issue of *Chatelaine*, Canadian mother Patricia Land recounted her experience giving birth via the Lamaze method in England in a piece entitled 'What the Russians can teach us about painless childbirth'. Offering an analysis of 'natural birth' that demonstrated that Lamaze-inspired methods had largely displaced Dick-Read's initial ideas, Land reported that after labouring for several hours following psychoprophylactic principles: 'the examination showed that my cervix was only very slightly open. The midwife was afraid that if I stayed awake throughout the first stage, which promised to be long, I would be too tired to cope correctly with the second (pushing) stage. I was given sedation.'[27] Land framed the use of sedative drugs during the first stage of labour as a valuable tool that allowed the expectant mother to rest and conserve her strength for the pushing work that followed. Individual narratives, then, complicate historical and present understandings of the 'natural', a term that was and continues to be used to describe a range of birth experiences.[28]

238   *Mass media and networks of communication*

Positioning pregnancy and childbirth as 'everyday' health events

Throughout the immediate postwar decades, expectant mothers who sought a 'new' way to birth, as well as medical experts who promoted alternative birth methods, made space – to varying degrees – for certain medical interventions, including the use of drugs and anaesthesia, in the delivery room. Those who advocated for natural childbirth and birth reform, however, may have been more unified in a fundamental desire to bring pregnancy and childbirth – life events that most mainstream North American practitioners in the mid-twentieth century pathologised and positioned as moments requiring acute and significant medical care – into the realm of the 'everyday'. Loughran, Mahoney, and Payling define 'everyday health' as 'the emotional, psychological, and bodily state-of-being in individuals' day-to-day lives, and the strategies they pursue (or do not) to maintain equilibrium in this state-of-being'.[29] Birth reformers sought to bring childbirth into the realm of the 'ordinary' and 'everyday', and, as Burke and Seltz argue, 'postwar women's ordinary experience and environmental imaginaries frequently included birth'; on a basic level, 'postwar women experienced the nature of their own birthing bodies […] amid contradictory and contested representations of women's bodies, women's labor, and motherhood as natural'.[30]

Relying on bottom-up sources including women's own letters to popular publications and leading figures in the natural childbirth movement provides a valuable window into women's 'everyday' experiences of and thoughts on their own bodies, reproduction, pregnancy, and childbirth. Within these sources, individual women and mothers-to-be responded to and negotiated often competing articulations of medical and cultural expertise and authority. Demonstrating the deep entanglement of body, mind, and emotion in natural childbirth discourses, the reframing of pregnancy and birth as 'everyday' health events entailed two distinct steps: first, removing the stigma, ignorance, and fear that surrounded childbirth; and second, repositioning birth as a 'normal' and 'happy' part of making a family in the mid-twentieth century.

Writing to Dick-Read in October 1948, Karen Birch of rural Alberta captured the enduring stigma and pathologisation that surrounded pregnancy and childbirth in the first half of the twentieth

'Thirty years behind England'? 239

century. Birch recounted her first introduction to the mechanics of giving birth when, at the age of thirteen in the mid-1930s, she had the chance to look at the textbook of a family friend enrolled in a correspondence nursing course:

> I picked up her book and turned to – 'Home delivery of a Baby.' Mother snatched it from me, flipped over the pages, and handing it back, said, 'There ... read how to lay out the dead – that's more suitable.' In an aside to her friend, Mother commented, 'It's disgusting the way children take such an interest in these unnatural things.' !!! That episode speaks for itself and is quoted verbatim. I never forgot it.[31]

Historically rooted taboos surrounding open discussions of the female body and women's sexuality contributed, for many Canadian women, to lack of knowledge surrounding reproductive health events, including pregnancy and birth, well into the twentieth century.[32]

In the postwar period, Canadian medical experts recognised the lingering and still damaging effects of this maternal ignorance, particularly when these gaps in knowledge were filled by 'old wives' tales' and horror stories. Dr Marion Hilliard, head of the Department of Obstetrics and Gynaecology at Women's College Hospital in Toronto, described such stories as 'fears passed down lovingly from mother to daughter like family heirlooms'. The fear of giving birth, Hilliard suggested, was a familiar and recurring source of anxiety for many Canadian women, easily passed between generations, 'providing the mother mentions often enough how agonizing the process is, and remembers to pity, aloud, every woman in the neighbourhood who becomes pregnant. Her daughter will be terrified during her pregnancy, if she has one.'[33] Hilliard, widely recognised as Canada's leading woman doctor in the postwar decades, and a regular columnist in *Chatelaine*, described a familiar encounter with a patient: 'Late one afternoon a few weeks ago a patient sat on the edge of a chair in my office, gripping her purse tightly and looking everywhere but at my face. "Doctor," she began in a taut voice, "I'm afraid I'm pregnant."' Hilliard recognised that 'some women are ill at ease with their bodies and those changes which nature causes within them. They distrust and fear the processes of female evolution.' She suggested that most women's fear of giving birth was not fear of pain – as others, including Dick-Read, had argued – but instead fear rooted in not knowing 'what to expect'.

240   *Mass media and networks of communication*

These uncertainties, Hilliard argued, made the whole of pregnancy, for many women, a 'Nine-Month Case of Jitters'.[34]

Those women who took the time to write to Dick-Read had, since the late 1940s, articulated a different view of childbirth. Darlene Bell of Vancouver, British Columbia, wrote to Dick-Read in November 1951 for his advice on how to counter her own physician's arguments against CWF: upon hearing her requests for a drug-free birth, he 'put it to me that I might just as well contemplate having my appendix out without an anaesthetic'. Bell stated her own view of birth in reporting how she responded to her doctor's argument: 'My reaction: I feel it is a function – not a disease, and this argument has no parallel.'[35] Laurel Rice, who reported her experience of anaesthetisation without consent, wrote a letter of complaint to her doctor following her 1955 birth, in which she positioned childbirth as 'a perfectly natural function', and stated that the doctor's role was 'to assist and aid [...] and not interfere'.[36] Writing three years later, Moira Kaufman of Winnipeg, Manitoba, described her 1957 pregnancy as 'extremely healthy and active', and her labour and delivery, conducted according to Dick-Read's teachings, as an 'amazing' and 'thrilling' experience that was a 'mutual delight' for both her and her husband.[37]

Medical and lay supporters of natural childbirth suggested that education and training in the method improved individual birth experiences but also removed much of the ignorance and fear that continued to surround pregnancy and birth. The demystification of childbirth and the imperative to cultivate a healthy and prepared mindset in the expectant mother was framed as an important undertaking. Canada's leading medical experts emphasised the 'everyday' and 'normal' nature of pregnancy and birth. A January 1955 *Chatelaine* article entitled 'It's fun raising a family!' asked current or future mothers to carefully consider their attitudes toward pregnancy:

> The trickiest point in any pregnancy is your own personal point of view. If you look on childbearing as an abnormal act of courage on your part or carry in your heart a sense of grievance against your own husband, your whole pregnancy will be colored by this attitude. If on the other hand you look on it as one of the happy periods in your life, if you think of the birth of your child as a normal act, then your nine months' period of waiting will mean a fuller life for both you and your husband.[38]

'*Thirty years behind England*'? 241

Still, this normalisation of childbirth was not without its limits; this particular article juxtaposed discussions of the routine nature of childbirth with lengthy discussions of the many 'bodily discomforts' associated with pregnancy.[39] In a 1960 article arguing that 'Childbirth should be easier', H.B. Atlee conceded, 'I doubt it will ever be possible to have a baby without some stress and discomfort. One twentieth of a living organism cannot be torn from an organism without a sense of cataclysm and anguish.' Atlee went on, however, to write, 'Let us instead ask ourselves if it is not possible to change pregnancy and childbirth into a process so satisfactory that stress and anguish lose their terrifying power.'[40] The time had come, Atlee suggested, for a shift in societal attitudes towards pregnancy and birth, and, more broadly, 'toward the whole status of the modern married woman'.[41]

Through the 1960s, Canadian women learned through the popular press that new natural childbirth techniques, including hypnosis, could render childbirth 'A NORMAL HAPPY EVENT'.[42] Part of this transformation entailed broadening the range of 'normal' birth experiences, and letting mothers-to-be know what they could expect during birth, through extensive prenatal education and dedicated training in natural childbirth. Canadian mother Patricia Land, giving birth in England in 1965, described her prenatal classes: 'As delivery approached, we were told about the possible variations of labor, and what would be done about each by the medical staff. As almost no labor follows in every detail the "normal" pattern, this was enormously reassuring.'[43] Though childbirth education could, in this sense, 'de-pathologise' or normalise the delivery experience, repositioning birth as a more 'ordinary' health event, Canadians like Land remarked that some countries were further 'ahead' than others in the pursuit of birth reform, and looked to transnational comparisons to make sense of their own natural childbirth experiences.

Situating Canadian birth cultures in transnational context

Individual women who embraced and promoted natural childbirth regularly relied on international comparisons to frame their birth experiences, often positioning these as 'antiquated' or 'backwards' – and, at times, echoing established and explicitly racialised juxtapositions, as 'primitive' – in contrast to what they saw as the

242   *Mass media and networks of communication*

more 'enlightened' obstetric practices of other countries. Individual comments that focused explicitly on the embrace or rejection of natural childbirth principles were often contextualised by broader comparisons. Women who wrote to Dick-Read in the early 1950s pointed out to the British doctor that midwives were not permitted to practise in Canada and suggested that this negatively impacted on their birth experiences. Hattie Jones, for example, reported to Dick-Read in 1951 that the lack of midwives in the Canadian context led to harmful practices, including holding the baby back during delivery, to ensure the doctor was present.[44] Anne Weston, who had recently emigrated to British Columbia from Germany, wrote in 1953 that she found the Canadian 'set-up appalling – no midwives and the only place to have your baby is the hospital', and contrasted her recent childbirth with her two previous deliveries, completed with the assistance of a German midwife, both babies 'born peacefully at home'.[45]

In April 1958 a *Chatelaine* piece weighing the potential benefits – and drawbacks – of midwives in the Canadian system made similar transnational comparisons. Considering the question 'Do we need midwives in Canada?' the article in question showcased two opposing viewpoints. Mrs Anna Davies, a housewife and mother of three, argued in favour of the introduction of midwifery, while Dr Elizabeth Wiley, 'one of Canada's busiest obstetricians', suggested that the Canadian system would not benefit from the introduction of midwives, and that 'the majority of Canadian doctors' were 'strongly' opposed to such a shift. Davies, espousing the pro-midwifery viewpoint, held up the British system where, readers were told, 'midwives deliver eighty percent of all babies – and infant mortality is far below Canada's' as an ideal model. The piece continued to position Canadian obstetric care in a particularly damning light:

> Canada has the second highest standard of living in the world, but it ranks thirteenth among the nations in infant survival. We are well behind such countries as Sweden, Denmark, New Zealand, Switzerland, and Britain [...] In Canada, the word 'midwife' still evokes memories of a superstition-ridden old woman ignorant of all modern technique, spiteful toward doctors and casual toward patients. In other parts of the world, most notably Britain, 'midwife' means the opposite: a smooth, efficient, well-trained obstetrical nurse who plays an indispensable role in the community.[46]

'Thirty years behind England'?   243

The dominant Canadian view of midwives as 'superstition-ridden', 'ignorant' practitioners divorced from the latest medical science, expertise, and technique was markedly contrasted with the more modern and enlightened British perspective. Davies went on to suggest that the growing use of midwives in Canada could play an important role in reducing widespread maternal ignorance and fears surrounding childbirth, thereby contributing to the de-pathologisation or 'normalisation' of the birth experience, helping to reposition childbirth alongside a broader range of reproductive health events experienced by many Canadian women over the course of their lives.[47]

In response to this article, *Chatelaine* received a number of letters from readers located across the country, publishing a selection of these in the June 1958 issue. Doris M. Wilson of Duncan, British Columbia, wrote to express her disbelief in Dr Wiley's assertion that the introduction of trained midwives was 'going backward', and reported favourably on her experience giving birth in India, expressing hope that Canada would soon start a training school for midwives.[48] Mary C. Ellison of Ottawa, Ontario wrote that while Dr Wiley's support for existing status quo in Canadian obstetric practice 'may have been able to fool you Canadians', as a newcomer to Canada she saw the fault in the obstetrician's arguments: 'I'm English and disgusted with your dollar-grabbing doctors and medical services over here. Any country without a state welfare scheme is poor indeed.'[49] Here, the progressivism embodied in England's National Health Service, contrasted with the embryonic state of universal health insurance in the Canadian context, functioned as another marker of modern and enlightened maternity care.[50]

Speaking with *Chatelaine* in the same year, Dick-Read touched more explicitly on the status of natural childbirth both in Canada and internationally. In response to the interviewer's suggestion that 'few Canadian doctors follow[ed] [his] methods', Dick-Read countered, 'I find many Canadian doctors are following natural childbirth procedures with increasing satisfaction', but also commented, 'In Canada, there seems to be a tendency in some places to order the women what to do, and things still occur which in most primitive native tribes would be considered an offence against decency – for instance, a woman may be strapped down and given an anaesthetic against her will.'[51] Dick-Read suggested, additionally, that a generational divide among health practitioners shaped how they received the

244 *Mass media and networks of communication*

new method, noting that many physicians 'cannot be persuaded to try anything new to them, even if medical literature commends its advantages to mother and baby'.[52] Finally, he noted that even those Canadian physicians who did embrace the method did so in an 'out of date' way, following the older recommendations for prenatal instruction that included greater reliance on physiotherapy-inspired gymnastic exercises than Dick-Read found either 'desirable or helpful'.[53]

Readers echoed Dick-Read's assessment. Sheila Thompson of Hamilton, Ontario, for example, wrote in to congratulate the magazine on its interview, and reported:

> I have had three children by this 'natural' method [...] I was shocked and dismayed on my arrival in Canada [from England] two years ago, to find that many doctors appeared to be using methods of delivery which were in current use in the late 1920s in England. Friends of mine who have had babies in both England and Canada agree. Surely the choice of natural childbirth is every mother's right, and not the doctor's prerogative?[54]

Chatelaine editorialised, posing the question: was Canada 'thirty years behind England' when it came to obstetric care?

These types of global comparisons continued, and perhaps became more explicit, over the following decade. Reporting on the Second International Congress of Obstetrics and Gynecology held in Montreal in the summer of 1958, Joan Morris assessed 'the current status of natural childbirth' in transnational perspective, highlighting the progress other countries, including Italy, China, Poland, Australia, India, Sweden, and the United States, had made in implementing natural childbirth methods. In contrast, in Canada there were only small pockets of support in cities including Halifax, Hamilton, Toronto, Ottawa, and Montreal.[55] As Lamaze-inspired approaches came to reflect perceptions of 'natural birth' in the 1960s, popular representations of alternative birth practices continued to situate Canadian birth practices as antiquated and behind the times. Canadian mothers and experts alike, including Hamilton obstetrician Dr Murray Enkin, positioned psychoprophylaxis as a 'well-accepted obstetrical approach', but noted that, despite its 'spread to 46 countries', psychoprophylaxis was 'still largely ignored' and 'not too widely accepted' by the Canadian medical establishment.[56]

'Thirty years behind England'? 245

Conclusion

A note in the November 1960 issue of *Chatelaine* asked readers:

> From your personal experience, how would *you* improve maternity care and delivery for Canadian mothers? Whether you have a small but useful suggestion to make, or a major change, tell us about it. *Chatelaine* will pay $50 for the best letter – and publish it wholly, or excerpted, in a future issue.[57]

In response, Diana Bacon of Ottawa, Ontario, suggested that women 'be quietly persistent' in advocating for the type of care they sought from hospital staff, and their desired type of birth experience. Bacon included the note: 'The nurses are much more likely to treat you as an intelligent, self-controlled woman, if you act like one.'[58]

Women were concerned with their comportment in the birthing room, but perceptions of their behaviour by both medical experts and expectant mothers alike were inextricably shaped by gender, race, class, and age. Writing to Dick-Read, Karen Birch, for example, described a previous experience during which she, in her words, 'witnessed [...] a natural childbirth, and didn't realize it', as 'a Cree Indian woman from a reserve' near her rural Alberta town, who was in a neighbouring bed in the maternity ward, experienced a fifteen-hour labour:

> During that time, she lay quietly, her arms down by her sides, her eyes closed. The sheet over her rose and fell with the contractions. I was in a welter of pity for her ... I said, 'Aren't you in pain? Shall I call the nurse?' She opened her black eyes, and a sweet smile lighted up her bronze face. She said in a most maternal manner, 'No-no, little girl, do not mak' the fuss. I lak' having baby.' And closed her eyes and went on with her business. After she left to have her baby, we modern young mothers bleated derisively, 'Like having a baby!' We concluded that she was just a dumb Indian and didn't know any better.[59]

Gender, race, class, and age intersected to shape how this mother's conduct was positioned as 'antiquated' in comparison to that of 'modern' mothers. These intersecting factors, alongside others, continue to fuel historically rooted medical sexism and racism that shapes individual encounters with Canadian healthcare systems.

246   *Mass media and networks of communication*

'Natural' childbirth held multiple and shifting meanings in the immediate postwar decades, with many Canadian practitioners and parents-to-be finding the concept flexible enough to include considerable medical intervention. Despite these ambiguities, as Burke and Seltz argue, 'the desire and consumer demand for the natural [...] has been a constant'.[60] The fixation on the term and the need to distinguish 'natural' births from their 'non-natural' counterparts indicates the continuing power of 'nature' in shaping perceptions of 'good' birth experiences. Individual experiences, and access to less-medicalised or alternative birth options, were and continue to be mediated by geographic location, class, and race, with a variety of structural factors shaping women's abilities to make demands of their doctors. That said, those who sought natural childbirth and promoted birth reform in the immediate postwar decades were often unified in their desire to reject the pathologisation of pregnancy and birth and bring these life events into the realm of 'everyday health', turning to transnational comparisons to situate and contextualise their own birth experiences, and effectively make the case that the time had come for Canadian birth reform.

Notes

1 Wellcome Library (hereafter WL), Dick-Read, Grantly, Autobiography (?Draft of articles published in *Woman*), PP/GDR/A.92, Grantly Dick-Read, Autobiography – Unpublished Manuscript, Instalment Two, 22–4; Instalment Three, 7.

2 WL, Dick-Read, Grantly, Publishing, Press, Films, Lectures, etc., Lectures and Courses, PP/GDR/C.71, Lecture on 'Pains of Labour,' delivered at Norwich, 17 October 1933.

3 Writing in *Chatelaine* in 1957, Dr Marion Hilliard recorded the status quo in mid-century Canadian obstetric practice: 'The good obstetrician a few years ago was the doctor who put his patient under heavy sedation the moment she arrived in hospital and kept her totally unconscious throughout the entire process. The mothers wakened the next morning with no recollection at all of participating in a birth.' Marion Hilliard, 'Your first baby', *Chatelaine* (January 1957), 46.

4 Grantly Dick-Read, *Natural Childbirth* (London: William Heinemann, 1933).

'Thirty years behind England'? 247

5 Grantly Dick-Read, *Revelation of Childbirth: The Principles and Practice of Natural Childbirth* (London: William Heinemann, 1942); Grantly Dick-Read, *Childbirth without Fear* (New York: Harper and Brothers, 1944).

6 See, for example, George J. Engelmann, *Labor among Primitive Peoples: Showing the Development of the Obstetric Science of To-day, from the Natural and Instinctive Customs of All Races, Civilized and Savage, Past and Present* (St Louis, MO: J.H. Chambers & Co., 1883).

7 Evelyn Hamilton, 'Dr. Grantly Dick-Read answers your questions on NATURAL CHILDBIRTH', *Chatelaine* (January 1958), 17.

8 Paula Michaels, *Lamaze: An International History* (Oxford: Oxford University Press, 2014), pp. 93–113.

9 Valerie Korinek, *Roughing It in the Suburbs: Reading* Chatelaine *Magazine in the Fifties and Sixties* (Toronto, ON: University of Toronto Press, 2000), p. 35.

10 Korinek, *Roughing It in the Suburbs*, pp. 24, 66–8.

11 Tracey Loughran, Kate Mahoney, and Daisy Payling, 'Women's voices, emotion, and empathy: engaging different publics with "everyday" health histories', *Medical Humanities*, 48:4 (2022), 395. Loughran, Mahoney, and Payling additionally note that 'reader content was carefully selected and heavily edited, and while it is the best available evidence of what certain readers thought and felt, it requires delicate handling'.

12 Jessica Martucci, 'Beyond the nature/medicine divide in maternity care', *AMA Journal of Ethics* 20:12 (December 2018); Jessica Martucci, *Back to the Breast: Natural Motherhood and Breastfeeding in America* (Chicago, IL: University of Chicago Press, 2015).

13 Wendy Mitchinson, *Giving Birth in Canada, 1900–1950* (Toronto, ON: University of Toronto Press, 2002); Whitney Wood, '"Bound to be a troublesome time": Canadian perceptions of pregnancy, parturition, and pain, c. 1867–1930', in Jennifer Evans and Ciara Meehan (eds), *Perceptions of Pregnancy from the Seventeenth to the Twentieth Century* (Basingstoke: Palgrave Macmillan, 2017).

14 In Canada, this shift was ongoing into the mid-twentieth century. Mitchinson, *Giving Birth in Canada*, pp. 158–89.

15 Whitney Wood, '"The luxurious daughters of artificial life": female "delicacy" and pain in late-Victorian advice literature', *Canadian Bulletin of Medical History*, 31:2 (2014).

16 Adele Saunders, 'The future of being a woman', *Chatelaine* (November 1943), 13.

17 Kate Aitken, 'For *Chatelaine*'s young parents: it's fun raising a family!' *Chatelaine* (January 1955), 48.

248   *Mass media and networks of communication*

18 Flannery Burke and Jennifer Seltz, 'Mothers' nature: feminisms, environmentalism, and childbirth in the 1970s', *Journal of Women's History*, 30:2 (2018), 64.

19 Hamilton, 'Dr. Grantly Dick-Read answers your questions', 17.

20 Hamilton, 'Dr. Grantly Dick-Read answers your questions', 27.

21 Dick-Read, for example, continued his commentary on the role of anaesthesia in 'natural' birth by stating: 'Critics have said that it is bad for a woman psychologically if she fails to achieve a natural birth when she has trained for it. If my method is properly used, she will know that she has a 96 percent chance of success. This teaching takes care of disappointment and success so that neither of these normal emotions will be exaggerated.' For more on medical and personal attitudes towards 'success' and 'failure' in natural birth, see Whitney Wood, 'Pride, shame, and anger: women's struggles to "achieve" natural childbirth in postwar Canada', in Lara Campbell, Michael Dawson, and Catherine Gidney (eds), *Feeling Feminism: Activism, Affect, and Canada's Second Wave* (Vancouver, BC: University of British Columbia Press, 2022).

22 H.B. Atlee 'Childbirth should be easier', *Chatelaine* (November 1960), 54.

23 Atlee 'Childbirth should be easier', 54.

24 Anne Barrie, 'Childbirth with hypnosis', *Chatelaine* (May 1964), 42.

25 WL, Dick-Read, Grantly, Natural Childbirth Correspondence: Mothers, PP/GDR/D.92, Laurel Rice to Grantly Dick-Read, 24 May 1955.

26 WL, Dick-Read, Grantly, Natural Childbirth Correspondence: Mothers, PP/GDR/D.95, Fay Grabowski to Grantly Dick-Read, 24 August 1958.

27 Patricia Land, 'What the Russians can teach us about painless childbirth', *Chatelaine* (May 1966), 60.

28 Margaret Macdonald, 'Gender expectations: natural bodies and natural births in the new midwifery in Canada', *Medical Anthropology Quarterly*, 20:2 (June 2006).

29 Loughran et al., 'Women's voices, emotion, and empathy', 394.

30 Burke and Seltz, 'Mothers' nature', 67.

31 WL, Dick-Read, Grantly, Natural Childbirth Correspondence: Mothers, PP/GDR/D.90, Karen Birch to Grantly Dick-Read, 12 October 1948.

32 See Katharine Arnup, *Education for Motherhood: Advice for Mothers in Twentieth-Century Canada* (Toronto, ON: University of Toronto Press, 1994).

33 Marion Hilliard, 'The four fears that prey on women', *Chatelaine* (July 1955), 42.

34 Hilliard, 'The four fears that prey on women', 33, 40.

35 WL, Dick-Read, Grantly, Natural Childbirth Correspondence: Mothers, PP/GDR/D.90, Darlene Bell to Grantly Dick-Read, 16 November 1951.

'*Thirty years behind England*'? 249

36 WL, Dick-Read, Grantly, Natural Childbirth Correspondence: Mothers, PP/GDR/D.92, Laurel Rice to Grantly Dick-Read, 24 May 1955.
37 WL, Dick-Read, Grantly, Natural Childbirth Correspondence: Mothers, PP/GDR/D.92, Moira Kaufman to Grantly Dick-Read, 1 February 1958.
38 Aitken, 'For *Chatelaine*'s young parents', 48.
39 Aitken, 'For *Chatelaine*'s young parents', 51.
40 Atlee, 'Childbirth should be easier', 33.
41 Atlee, 'Childbirth should be easier, 58.
42 Barrie, 'Childbirth with hypnosis', 63 (capitalisation in the original).
43 Land, 'What the Russians can teach us about painless childbirth', 58. Land allowed for variations in birth experiences and continued on the following page, 'The process of normal labor, handled according to psychoprophylactic principles, is roughly as follows. Let me emphasize that a labor can, like mine, deviate in many ways from this pattern and still be perfectly normal.'
44 Jones wrote, 'Because there are no midwives here it is thought to be a crime of the worst sort to allow a baby to be born without a doctor.' WL, Dick-Read, Grantly, Natural Childbirth Correspondence: Mothers, PP/GDR/D.91, Hattie Jones to Grantly Dick-Read, 12 January 1951.
45 WL, Dick-Read, Grantly, Natural Childbirth Correspondence: Mothers, PP/GDR/D.93, Anne Weston to Grantly Dick-Read, 8 April 1953.
46 'Do we need midwives in Canada?', *Chatelaine* (April 1958), 17.
47 'Do we need midwives in Canada?', 85.
48 Doris M. Wilson, 'Canadian midwives? YES', *Chatelaine* (June 1958), 6.
49 Mary C. Ellison, 'Canadian midwives? YES', *Chatelaine* (June 1958), 6.
50 Many Canadian provinces would have hospital insurance schemes in place by the close of the 1950s, with 'universal' Medicare emerging during the decade that followed. At the time this letter was written, however, the contrast between the English and Canadian healthcare systems was clear. For more on this see Whitney Wood, 'Medicare and maternity: historicizing inequities in women's health', in Esyllt W. Jones, James Hanley, and Delia Gavrus (eds), *Medicare's Histories: Origins, Omissions, and Opportunities in Canada* (Winnipeg, MB: University of Manitoba Press, 2022).
51 Hamilton, 'Dr. Grantly Dick-Read answers your questions', 27. On the following page, he commented, 'Some hospitals in Canada appear to be far behind the rest of the civilized world in the standard of care of mothers when their babies are born.'
52 Hamilton, 'Dr. Grantly Dick-Read answers your questions', 28.
53 Hamilton, 'Dr. Grantly Dick-Read answers your questions', 28.

250   *Mass media and networks of communication*

54 'Readers take over – childbirth: thirty years behind England?', *Chatelaine* (March 1958), 6.
55 Joan Morris, 'Special *Chatelaine* report on the latest news about having your baby', *Chatelaine* (November 1958), 21, 73–4, 78.
56 Land, 'What the Russians can teach us about painless childbirth', 25.
57 'How would YOU improve maternity care?', *Chatelaine* (November 1960), 56.
58 Diana Bacon, 'How *you* would improve maternity care: a *Chatelaine* report', *Chatelaine* (August 1961), 18.
59 WL, Dick-Read, Grantly, Natural Childbirth Correspondence: Mothers, PP/GDR/D.90, Karen Birch to Grantly Dick-Read, 12 October 1948.
60 Burke and Seltz, 'Mothers' nature', 81.

10

'I started a new life when I joined Gemma': disability, community, and sexuality in Gemma newsletters, 1978–2000

Beckie Rutherford

Introduction

'I started a new life when I joined Gemma – I'd like everyone to have this chance.'[1] When this comment was made in 1991, Gemma had been organising for fifteen years and had grown to several hundred members. Gemma was a support group and friendship network for disabled lesbians, and its name was inspired by the Latin meaning for 'bud' or 'shoot' to capture the idea of something small with the potential to grow.[2] The growth and longevity of the group testifies to its ongoing success at building a community to challenge the isolation of disabled lesbians. Gemma is still organising and circulating newsletters to this day and the eighty-nine newsletters produced between 1978 and 2000 offer intimate insight into the everyday lives of disabled women in late twentieth-century Britain.

Gemma was formed within the distinct culture of consciousness-raising fostered by the Women's Liberation Movement (WLM) and adopted similar approaches to empower and politicise its members.[3] Although Gemma did not promote itself as a political group, its history exhibits the growing politicisation of disabled women throughout this period. Gemma became increasingly well known to other groups associated with the WLM, the Disabled People's Movement and the Gay Liberation Movement (GLM), and established frequent connections and collaborations as a result. The demographic of Gemma embraced all three of these movements and its members were often encouraged to contribute to projects and publications

252 *Mass media and networks of communication*

about disabled women's experiences of healthcare, sexuality, and various other topics.[4] Essentially, Gemma was actively engaged in generating and disseminating knowledge about disabled womanhood – specifically that of disabled lesbians – just as the subject was beginning to be recognised as valuable and of interest.

In spite of its unique location in relation to multiple liberation movements, historical recognition of Gemma remains negligible.[5] The longevity of Gemma's existence is unmatched by any other disabled women's group of this period. The consistency of its newsletter production (four per year for at least three decades) is remarkable, considering the threat that funding cuts and widening social inequality posed to grassroots organising during the 1980s and 1990s.[6] Other disabled women's groups – for example the Liberation Network of People with Disabilities (founded 1979) and Sisters Against Disablement (founded 1981) – capture a snapshot of disabled women's organising during this period.[7] However, Gemma's history is key to documenting change over time in terms of how disabled women developed and articulated understandings of themselves and their bodies. This has a significant bearing on writing the history of disabled women's everyday lives and experiences of health in late twentieth-century Britain.

Gemma's fundamental contribution to the task of locating and historicising everyday health in postwar Britain is to centre disabled women's agency and the richness of their everyday lives. Tropes of passivity and victimhood are widespread in both popular and academic narratives, and disabled people are rarely positioned as historical agents except directly in relation to disability. Disabled people constitute the largest minority group in Britain, encompassing differences of gender, race, class, sexuality, and age.[8] Yet their voices, stories, and experiences are all too often absent from broader histories of modern Britain. To date, historians of disability have focused mainly on the medicalisation and pathologisation of disabled bodies.[9] Illuminating this as a history of oppression was an essential undertaking, but this approach has failed to fully remove the ongoing, tacit association between disability and medicalisation.[10] Recent scholarship has broadened the field of modern British disability history by centring the social and working lives of disabled people and by engaging only minimally with their construction as medical subjects.[11] However, there is still little historical research on disabled women's experiences and the negotiation of gender, sex, and sexuality within their everyday lives.

Disabled women remain almost entirely absent from both feminist and lesbian histories. They are rarely mentioned within scholarly literature on the WLM, and any popular references to their growing visibility within feminist or lesbian organising during the 1980s and 1990s are brief and generalised.[12] The predominance of non-disabled socialist feminist perspectives within WLM historiography obscures the voices of disabled women captured in contemporary feminist texts, such as Elsa Beckett's recollection of the foundation and purpose of Gemma, or Kirsten Hearn's reflection on her politicisation as a blind lesbian.[13] These stories are essential to shaping the histories of feminist and lesbian organising in Britain, and their underuse reproduces the very exclusion that inspired Gemma's foundation.

Gemma's history contributes to the task of historicising everyday life and health within postwar Britain in three primary ways. First, the newsletters indicate the radical shift that took place within disabled communities in late twentieth-century Britain towards theorising disability as a collective experience of social oppression, rather than a medical identity rooted in individually impaired bodies. This disrupted the principle at the heart of the medical model of disability, which defines disability as personal deficit (a fault or weakness located within an individual body) and has historically been used to control and oppress disabled people. This shift directly informed how the women in Gemma thought of themselves and their right to inclusion in the growing women's and gay liberation movements. Second, the sheer wealth of activity documented in the Gemma newsletters showcases the vibrancy of disabled women's social and political lives and the diversity of interests and identities nurtured within the group. The newsletters reveal Gemma's powerful sense of internal community as well as myriad connections to other groups organising in relation to gay, lesbian, and disability politics. Third, Gemma's existence illustrates disabled women's growing sexual agency and its connections to emotional wellbeing. Within Gemma, disabled lesbians could explore and embrace sexuality on their own terms, and in doing so reject ableist paradigms that granted them little sexual agency.[14] These three avenues of inquiry – redefining disability, building community, and embracing sexuality – are essential to progressing the writing of disabled women's history because they

254   *Mass media and networks of communication*

look beyond the medicalisation of disability and centre disabled women as historical agents.

The history of Gemma

Gemma was established in 1976 by two disabled lesbians, Elsa Beckett and Frances Bernard. Beckett responded to Bernard's penfriend advert in the lesbian magazine *Sappho*, as both shared a desire to 'try to find other women like ourselves'.[15] Gemma's primary aim was to lessen disabled lesbians' sense of isolation and to facilitate their access to the growing number of lesbian groups and publications flourishing within the fervour of the WLM. Gemma was determined to raise awareness of the access needs of disabled women and therefore opened its membership to non-disabled lesbians. Beckett recalled, 'Some of us would have able-bodied lovers and friends who would want to be in the group and whom we would want to be there; we didn't want to repeat discrimination.'[16] She further explained that initially Gemma aimed to inspire other feminist and lesbian groups to become more inclusive. However, at that time 'we were perhaps not confident enough to persist as an effective pressure group [...] we thought our own integrated group might act as a model.'[17] With this in mind, a handful of women began meeting in members' homes in June 1976, and in February 1978 Gemma printed its first newsletter. From then on Gemma printed four newsletters a year and meetings were moved to community centres and women's centres in London – the Camden Lesbian Centre was a popular choice until its funding was withdrawn in 1996.

In the summer of 1980, London-based Gemma events were fixed to the second Sunday of each month, with the aim to alternate between group meetings and more sociable get-togethers. Gradually, the frequency of both meetings and socials increased and the 'Gemma Diary' printed on every newsletter's front page became increasingly long and varied. Social activities included picnics, play readings, swimming sessions, wheelchair-friendly discos, film screenings, and museum visits. Members also engaged in several ongoing creative projects such as 'Gemma's Gay Little Cook Book', a recipe book compiled from members' suggestions and sold during Gay Pride Week in 1981. One member's short play, *What's the Use in Her*

'I started a new life when I joined Gemma' 255

Coming? She Can't Dance, drew its inspiration from the response of a non-disabled organiser when asked to make a lesbian disco physically accessible.[18] As well as compiling an increasingly long quarterly newsletter, Gemma also published anthologies of members' poetry, prose, and creative writing. These coincided with anniversaries and milestones in Gemma's history and aimed to celebrate and reflect on the group's achievements.[19] By 1986 Gemma had also produced three access guides, two of which had a national focus and provided a wealth of information on the accessibility of lesbian and gay venues across Britain. The third was a detailed 'gay guide' specifically for disabled Londoners and supported by funding from the Greater London Council.

Gemma attracted women of all ages ('from teens to 80 plus') and its steadily increasing membership consisted of roughly half disabled and half non-disabled women.[20] The latter included the friends and partners of disabled members, but non-disabled lesbians with no prior connection to the group were also drawn to Gemma's community. In 1986, Beckett expressed disappointment that '[f]ew ethnic minority women have joined us thus far'.[21] It is unclear why Gemma remained predominantly white, but photographs in one of its later anthologies reveal that at least one woman of colour regularly attended socials and Gay Pride events.[22] The November 1984 newsletter acknowledged the need to translate the Gemma information leaflet into 'Punjabi, Urdu, Gujerati and other languages of ethnic minority women' in an attempt to reach non-native English speakers, although it is unclear if this ever came to fruition.[23] Gemma did take great pride in its small number of international members, based as widely as Sweden, Germany, Israel, and North America. In early 1991 it was reported that 'a new member in America is taking on the work of being the distributer for the newsletters tapes there'.[24]

All Gemma's meetings and most social events took place in central London, and the lack of momentum to organise elsewhere was a consistent frustration for the group's founders. Nevertheless, for members unable to leave their homes or travel, the Gemma penfriends list was vital for connecting and communicating with other disabled lesbians. The list was embedded within the newsletter until early 1984, when it became too lengthy. From then on it was printed separately and available on request. Reflecting on the intimacy of letter writing, Elsa Beckett explained, 'While there is a privacy in

256   *Mass media and networks of communication*

the support we give each other the effect is one of a network of solidarity', adding that '[l]etters are a great force in feminist solidarity'.[25] As Gemma expanded and the number of visually impaired members increased, correspondence via tape recordings or braille became more common and Beckett advocated the need for all members to extend their range of communicative techniques to avoid perpetuating exclusion. Many of the friendships forged within Gemma were lifelong and it was not uncommon for members to form romantic relationships and choose to spend their lives together.[26]

Redefining disability

The Gemma newsletters demonstrate how, from the mid-1970s onwards, disabled people began framing disability as a form of social oppression rather than a medical identity. Throughout the 1980s and 1990s the experience of disability was increasingly redefined, as the direct result of inaccessible environments and prejudiced attitudes rather than impaired bodies.[27] The backdrop to this understanding was the development of the social model of disability. In 1975 the Union of Physically Impaired Against Segregation declared that 'disability is a situation, caused by social conditions', and in 1983 the term 'social model' was coined by sociologist Mike Oliver.[28] Since then, it has become a cornerstone of both disability studies and disability rights activism in Britain. The social model pinpoints physical barriers and social prejudice as fundamental sources of disability, arguing that the problem lies with built environments and societies that fail to understand and adapt to the needs of people with impairments. It rejects the notion of disability as an individual problem located within impaired bodies, and reorientates the discussion towards resolvable issues of physical access and social attitudes.[29]

The knowledge and attitudes present within Gemma reflect this understanding of the causal relationship between society and disability. Campaigning for better access clearly aligned with a social-model understanding of disability, and Gemma members consistently foregrounded poor access as a key factor preventing their engagement with the WLM and GLM. They were confident in identifying physical barriers as the source of their exclusion and refused to conceal their

'*I started a new life when I joined Gemma*' 257

growing frustration. In February 1982 one member declared, 'And how about a barrier-free lesbian community in Britain? [...] At present many women's groups behave as if their access info might be useful to the KGB.'[30] A few months later, another member referred to visually impaired women's ability to access feminist and lesbian literature as 'an absolute and fundamental human right', indicating that normalising braille and tape-recorded books should not be a matter for debate.[31] Towards the end of the 1980s, as discussions about access slowly became more widespread, Gemma increasingly promoted its expectation that non-disabled lesbian communities should be more adaptable. One example of this was a May 1989 advert for a vacancy in a lesbian housing co-op in Twickenham which explained that, 'Interested disabled women would need to join this co-op and make their suggestions re the design and layout of their accommodation before the conversion takes place so that their individual needs can be catered for.'[32] This clearly reflects the belief that disabled and non-disabled lesbians were equally entitled to join this community and that adapting the physical environment to make this possible was entirely feasible.

As well as highlighting the hostile effects of physical barriers, Gemma members spoke openly about how discriminatory attitudes fundamentally excluded them from lesbian society. In August 1986 one member shared her experience of answering a lesbian penfriend advert in *Time Out* magazine: 'To my amazement I had a reply saying she did not wish to write to anyone with a disability [...] This made me think, are we less of a human being or are they afraid of something they don't understand.' In spite of the setback, she vowed, 'I for one do not intend to hide under a rock or give up the fight [...] Being disabled does not mean we are incapable of love, understanding or sex.'[33] This indicates a growing understanding within Gemma that disabled women's ostracisation was a form of social injustice, not an inevitable or justifiable outcome of impairment. Another member expressed a similar sentiment in August 1992: 'The group has freed so much of my energy – partly by allowing me to express my anger at the exclusion of lesbians with illness/disability and showing me it is not my personal problem.'[34] The Gemma community was clearly a vital space in which disabled lesbians could express their frustration at the discriminatory attitudes prevalent within feminist and lesbian groups. Its newsletters provide

258   *Mass media and networks of communication*

crucial insight into the more widespread shift whereby disabled people began to attribute the 'problem' of disability to social attitudes rather than the alleged failings of individual bodies.

Since the early 1990s there has been growing criticism, particularly from disabled women, of the way in which the social model determines physical and social barriers as the sole causes of disability. Disabled feminists such as Liz Crow and Jenny Morris have argued that while the social model is an essential tool for the empowerment and liberation of disabled people, it is often applied in a way that fails to acknowledge the centrality of impairment within disabled people's lives. Crow wrote:

> As individuals, most of us simply cannot pretend with any conviction that our impairments are irrelevant because they influence so much of our lives. External disabling barriers may create social and economic disadvantage but our subjective experience of our bodies is also an integral part of our everyday reality.[35]

The everyday experience documented in the Gemma newsletters powerfully testifies to this critique. Gemma members confidently identified inaccessible environments and prejudiced attitudes as sources of their oppression, but also spoke candidly about the pain and inconveniences caused by their impairments. Gemma is therefore an apt case study for tracing how disabled people politicised and radically redefined disability on their own terms in late twentieth-century Britain. Gemma proves that it was possible to acknowledge the challenging reality of an impaired body whilst supporting the principle of disability as social oppression and, crucially, that impairment did not prevent these women from going about their everyday lives.

Building community

Gemma demonstrates the myriad ways that disabled women socialised, parented, involved themselves in politics, pursued careers and creative projects, and much more. Both the newsletters and penfriend network provided means of organising and sharing news, and the newsletters give insight into the development of Gemma's activities over time. In 1987, Elsa Beckett wrote:

'I started a new life when I joined Gemma'   259

What do we write about? The minutiae of our lives, how we manage with money, wrangles with Social Security and hospitals, relatives, hopes and disappointments, joyful news of lovers, children, a new baby, homophobia, politics, books, television, radio programmes, our companion animals. Women abroad write about their lives, lesbian groups (or lack of them), and feminism there.[36]

The question 'What do we write about?' gestures to the non-disabled world's doubt that disabled women could have very much to write about. However, Gemma testifies to the richness of disabled women's social and political lives throughout the 1980s and 1990s, and their connections to the broader landscape of liberation politics. As well as nurturing its internal community through the shared interests and concerns described above, Gemma was also committed to developing its identity as 'part of a vast grassroots network' of gay, lesbian, and disabled people's groups.[37]

The Gemma community created great opportunities for socialising, and members were free to partake as much or as little as they liked. As well as picnics, parties, and museum visits, the group organised celebrations of events such as International Women's Day. To mark this occasion in 1989, the group hosted feminist women's choir the Pre-Madonnas and secured funding from the Camden Women's Unit 'for our transport, creche, publicity and entertainment'.[38] Two years later it was reported that 'We had a lovely afternoon celebrating International Women's Week at the Camden Lesbian Centre. About fifty women and some very well behaved children enjoyed a buffet provided by Gemma, singing by The Tokens, poetry and fun.'[39] These reports indicate that members balanced socialising with childcare and that children were welcome at Gemma events. This insight into the everyday life of Gemma members helps to overturn the long-standing prejudices which deem disabled women incapable of either socialising or being mothers.[40] Occasionally fluctuations in health affected Gemma members' ability to attend social events but the group's general outlook was optimistic, trusting that women would get involved whenever and in whatever capacity suited them. The August 1985 newsletter mentioned a Gemma lunch ('with marvellous food') recently held in one member's garden, reporting that: 'These lunches are our favourite Gemma events, we are sorry that more of you couldn't come along but sadly with a group like ours illness so often intervenes. Never mind – next time!'[41] Such cheerful pragmatism

260   *Mass media and networks of communication*

in response to a disappointing turn-out no doubt aided the steady growth and longevity of Gemma's community.

From the outset, Gemma was supported by and connected to a number of other lesbian and gay groups. Frances Bernard was also involved with lesbian magazine *Sappho* (1972–81) and the two groups fostered a close relationship during Gemma's early years.[42] *Sappho* regularly listed Gemma to help increase its visibility, whilst Gemma donated money to *Sappho* to try to save it from financial collapse in 1979.[43] When *Sappho* did fold, towards the end of 1981, the Gemma newsletter reported with sadness: 'So much grew from Sappho – and without it Gemma would not have come into being [...] a mainstay has been lost.'[44] Other early supporters included *Sequel* (a short-lived feminist magazine for isolated lesbians) which featured Gemma on the front cover of its third issue, and KENRIC, which was already established as the longest-running UK lesbian organisation by the late 1970s.[45] A donation from KENRIC to Gemma in early 1980 inspired its first group anthology, and six years later joint social events with KENRIC were still regularly reported in the Gemma newsletter.[46]

As well as building relationships with non-disabled lesbian groups, Gemma also developed close connections with groups run by disabled gay men such as Gaycare and the Gay Men's Disabled Group. Gaycare was founded in the same year as Gemma and aimed to bridge the gap between disability services and lesbian and gay aid initiatives.[47] The two fledgling groups organised several joint social events, and in 1979 Gemma's newsletter editors suggested an official affiliation with Gaycare.[48] In 1982, Elsa Beckett encouraged two gay men, Julian Salmon and Glen McKee (both wheelchair users) to set up a male equivalent to Gemma, and the Gay Men's Disabled Group (GMDG) was launched. These examples illustrate Gemma's close connection to some of Britain's earliest lesbian groups, as well as its pivotal role instigating the organisation and visibility of the gay disabled community more broadly.[49]

From the mid-1980s, Gemma newsletters included updates on members' involvement with the organised large-scale gay rights protests proliferating in and around London. The August 1985 newsletter contained a lengthy, enthusiastic report on the 'Pride 85 Carnival Parade' (Figure 10.1), during which one Gemma member commented, 'It is wonderful to have lived to see this day.'[50] A few

'I started a new life when I joined Gemma' 261

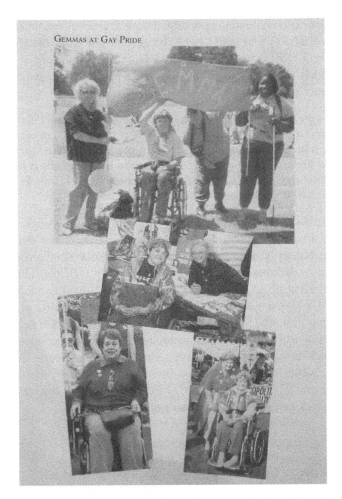

Figure 10.1 'Gemmas at Gay Pride', in Gemma anthology, *Silver Leaves* (June 2001). Courtesy of Special Collections and Archives, Bishopsgate Institute. All rights reserved and permission to use the figure must be obtained from the copyright holder.

years later, several Gemma members took part in the 'Stop the Clause March' in central London, protesting the proposal of Section 28.[51] For Gemma members unable to take to the streets, there were other opportunities to engage in the ongoing resistance against Section 28. The November 1988 newsletter invited Gemma members to

262 *Mass media and networks of communication*

complete an anonymous Lesbian Custody Project questionnaire – a political action that could easily be carried out from the comfort and security of home.[52] Disabled Gemma members were quick to highlight the unique threat that Section 28 posed to the gay disabled community:

> the general attack on the lesbian/gay community will hit those of us with disabilities particularly hard: we will not be allowed to use any accessible council-funded property, our information will be banned from libraries and reference books, we could not have stalls at fund-raising events in halls, public parks etc. If lesbian/gay centres are forced to close our hopes of integration will be gone.[53]

This bleak picture indicates two important aspects of Gemma's position within the broader lesbian and gay community ten years into its history. First, it was now a firmly established and recognised presence – information about Gemma was widely available in libraries and reference books; its members regularly ran stalls at gay fundraising events; and the group used lesbian and gay centres to organise meetings and other events. Second, by 1988 Gemma was secure in its identity as an integrated group aiming to inspire further integration and inclusion, despite significant setbacks such as Section 28. The future wellbeing of Gemma's community was tied to that of the lesbian and gay community as a whole, and Gemma saw its personal difficulties as part of a wider struggle.

Embracing sexuality

Gemma provided a trusted space where disabled women could form friendships on the basis of lesbian identity, and sexuality was therefore fundamental to the group's existence. Members were well aware of the stigma attached to both lesbianism and disability and clearly valued the Gemma community all the more because of this. In September 1994 one member wrote, 'We know that to some able-bodied hets, who think that while lesbians must be sex fiends, disabled women must be asexual, we're a contradiction in terms, but in Gemma, we can be OURSEVLES [sic].'[54] The Gemma newsletters demonstrate that sex was an important part of members' everyday lives, and that during the late 1980s and 1990s disabled lesbians

'I started a new life when I joined Gemma' 263

increasingly explored and celebrated their sexuality in diverse ways. Therefore, one of the crucial contributions Gemma makes to the broad history of disabled people's experiences of sex and sexuality is to demonstrate that disabled lesbians' sex lives flourished, in contradiction to the widespread stigma designating disabled people as either uninterested in or incapable of being sexual.[55]

The Gemma community demonstrates the varying ways that disabled women chose to explore and embrace their sexuality, making it clear that there was no archetypal way to be a disabled lesbian. Gemma encompassed a vast age range, and from its inception the group was firmly inclusive of women who identified as bisexual, despite widespread ambivalence and hostility towards bisexuality at this time.[56] Consequently, there was wide variation in how different members chose to express their sexuality. Within the Gemma newsletters, members were free to enthusiastically endorse pornography ('Keep it coming, girls, and plenty of it!')[57] and share news of gatherings dedicated to discussing sex and relationships ('We found that one day was not nearly enough for all we wanted to say').[58] In line with the growing visibility and celebration of lesbian culture, some members were comfortable embracing their lesbian identity in the public eye. This included, 'the FIVE Gemmas who took part in the OUT ON TUESDAY lesbian/gay TV programme' in 1990. Feedback for this programme from the wider lesbian and gay community was favourable, and another Gemma member described it as 'one of the most interesting lesbian documentaries I've ever seen'.[59] Similarly, several Gemma members were involved in a grassroots project to compile a 'lesbian millennium calendar', which suggests eagerness to represent Gemma within broader lesbian culture. A photo of some Gemma members featured in the calendar and the September 1999 newsletter reported that 'Profits will go to aid the work of Gemma and we're delighted and proud to be associated with it.'[60]

It is equally important to recognise Gemma members who preferred to be discreet about their sexuality. The newsletter's letter pages reveal that many did not feel comfortable being 'out' to their family, friends, or carers. Gemma's founders were keenly aware of this and navigated the issue sensitively, for example by posting newsletters in plain, unidentifiable envelopes and offering advice on how to initiate phone calls that might be answered by a carer or family

264   *Mass media and networks of communication*

member. Furthermore, not all Gemma members welcomed the sexually graphic creative writing that occasionally featured in Gemma's anthologies. In June 1994 one member declared, 'I have just read "Facets" and was very taken aback by the contents. I think the sex scene was too explicit, and moreover contained the word C – T, which I am sure many women found offensive'.[61] Many, often older, members were also frank about their decisions to be celibate, but they still sought friendship and connection with other lesbians via Gemma's network.[62]

The newsletters offer insight into an ongoing debate within the Gemma community about whether it was appropriate to use the penfriends list to find sexual partners. Gemma's official stance was that it was 'NOT a date-line or dating agency', but over time it did acknowledge its role as a 'friendship network from which everlasting relationships have sometimes developed'.[63] One example of these 'everlasting relationships' indicates that disabled lesbians ignored the assumption that they would form romantic or sexual partnerships only with other disabled women:

> A few weeks ago I met a Gemma who is severely disabled. In a very short time we found love in one another's company and it has achieved great results in her – all her nurses and care attendants have remarked on the improvement in her health, and we are determined to keep this up [...] We both feel we owe our new-found happiness to Gemma without which we would never have met, so a very big 'thank you'. Also I am sure you will be pleased to know a real relationship has been formed between a disabled member and an able-bodied one.[64]

Tom Shakespeare, Kath Gillespie Sells, and Dominic Davies highlight the ableist assumption that disabled people will 'stick with their own kind'.[65] However, this anecdote demonstrates that attraction and desire could exist between disabled and non-disabled women. Furthermore, it proves that exploring such a connection could be beneficial to both women's physical and emotional wellbeing. The author of this letter (a non-disabled woman called 'Steve') was evidently aware of Gemma's aim to normalise friendships and relationships between disabled and non-disabled women. It is worth noting that throughout and beyond the period covered by this chapter Gemma was coordinated for the most part by a lesbian couple, one

'*I started a new life when I joined Gemma*' 265

of whom was non-disabled. Elsa Beckett was a wheelchair user but her partner, Kathryn Bell, did not identify as disabled.[66] Both women dedicated an extraordinary amount of time and labour to Gemma (many of the early Gemma socials were held in their home) and their 'integrated' partnership was deeply admired within the group.[67]

Not only did Gemma defy the stereotypes of disabled women's asexuality, but the group was frequently involved in grassroots knowledge production about lesbian sexuality. Adverts and notices in Gemma newsletters reflect the wealth of books, pamphlets, and magazines on women's sexuality generated throughout the 1980s and 1990s. Other groups often approached Gemma to contribute information from a disabled lesbian perspective. For example, the November 1984 newsletter contained an advert for 'a book planned on the politics of LESBIAN SEX & SEXUALITY' and a request for members to 'please contribute even if you don't think it's word-perfect'.[68] There was a growing sense within the Gemma community that disabled women were entitled to inclusion and representation within conversations about sexuality. The November 1990 newsletter also contained the following call to arms:

> SHEBA FEMINIST PUBLISHERS are seeking short stories for their forthcoming anthology EXCITEMENT – stories about sex in the 90s by women [...] A Gemma comments on this: 'I will be surprised if there is anything reflecting disabled lesbians in it. Do you think there is any possibility we could ask for anonymous contributions from Gemmas, that we could compile into a contribution? I'm interested in challenging the able-bodied assumptions and stereotypes about sex, and also just to be there, to be part of it, not quietly lying under the carpet, unspeakable'.[69]

It is unclear if Gemma did end up contributing to this project. However, this member's desire to challenge 'able-bodied assumptions and stereotypes about sex' exemplifies the confidence and sexual agency fostered within Gemma. Although the wellbeing and privacy of its members was of paramount importance (hence 'anonymous contributions'), Gemma also inspired pride and an outward-looking spirit when it came to celebrating and educating people about lesbian sexuality. Gemma's history makes it clear that disabled women were

266   *Mass media and networks of communication*

consistently 'there' and 'part of it' in many spaces where they were not expected to be.

Conclusion

Illuminating Gemma's story provides more than just a compensatory history and achieves more than simply adding disabled women into existing narratives of gender and sexuality. Gemma was uniquely situated in relation to feminist, disability, and gay liberation politics. Its engagement with all three is integral to historicising the full complexity of these movements and their role within everyday life in late twentieth-century Britain. Gemma newsletters showcase the shift that took place as disabled communities began to radically redefine disability according to the social model. Informed by this new thinking, Gemma consistently challenged the curators of non-disabled lesbian spaces by foregrounding poor access and attitudes as the problem, not their individual bodies. Acknowledging this perspective is critical because it refuses the narrative of medicalisation and invites us to reflect on disabled women's lives in terms of agency rather than oppression.

The newsletters further reveal the vibrancy of Gemma as a social and political community, and its wide-reaching connections to other grassroots liberation groups. Given persistent, harmful assumptions about the lack of value in disabled people's everyday lives, and the continuing tendency to homogenise disabled people, recognising the diversity fostered within communities like Gemma is even more urgent. The newsletters' insight into disabled women's navigation of sex and sexuality further exhibits not only disabled women's agency but also important variations in how they chose to exercise it. As one member jubilantly pointed out: 'in Gemma, we can be OURSEVLES [sic]'.[70] These selves included women of all ages, who identified as lesbian, bisexual, disabled, non-disabled, single, married, sexually active, or celibate; a strikingly diverse community united by its founding aim to be inclusive and not 'repeat discrimination'. The three avenues of inquiry pursued in this chapter – redefining disability, building community, and embracing sexuality – carry enormous potential to rethink and subsequently develop a broader history of disabled people's everyday lives in late twentieth-century

'I started a new life when I joined Gemma'   267

Britain. Gemma's story is a small but essential contribution to this task.

Notes

1 *Gemma*, 57 (November 1991), 7. All Gemma newsletters mentioned in this chapter were consulted at the Feminist Archive South, University of Bristol Special Collections.
2 Elsa Beckett, 'Women like us: the history of Gemma', in *Silver Leaves* (self-published *Gemma* anthology, June 2001), p. 2.
3 Sue Bruley, 'Consciousness-raising in Clapham: women's liberation as "lived experience" in South London in the 1970s', *Women's History Review*, 22:5 (2013); Sarah Crook, 'The women's liberation movement, activism and therapy at the grassroots, 1968–1985', *Women's History Review*, 27:7 (2018).
4 For example, in 1983 the women's peace magazine *Lysistrata* wrote to Gemma requesting 'the experiences, feelings and opinions of women with disabilities about the women's peace movement', *Gemma*, 23 (May 1983), 6. In 1990 Gemma invited members to put their names on file for when Gemma was approached for interviews or television programmes: *Gemma*, 52 (August 1990), 2–3.
5 The only historical analysis of Gemma I have located is an unpublished MA thesis: Noah Littel, '"Minority Consciousness Gone Mad?" Exclusion, Inclusion and Self Organisation of Disabled LGBTI People in the Dutch and British LGBT+ and Disability Movements, in the Late Twentieth Century' (MA thesis, Leiden University, 2019).
6 The abolition of the Greater London Council in 1986 removed a key source of funding for London-based projects aiming to foster equality, diversity, and inclusion. See Peter Dorey, 'A farewell to alms: Thatcherism's legacy of inequality', *British Politics*, 10:1 (2015); Lucy Delap, 'Feminist bookshops, reading cultures and the Women's Liberation Movement in Great Britain, c. 1974–2000', *History Workshop Journal*, 81:1 (2016).
7 See Beckie Rutherford, 'Disabled Women Organising: Rethinking the Political within British Liberation Movements, 1976–1998' (PhD thesis, University of Warwick, 2023).
8 There are approximately thirteen million disabled people living in Britain. Equality and Human Rights Commission report, 'Being disabled in Britain: a journey less equal' (2017), p. 5: www.equalityhumanrights.com/sites/default/files/being-disabled-in-britain.pdf (accessed 1 November 2022).

268 *Mass media and networks of communication*

9 Sharon L. Snyder and David T. Mitchell, *Cultural Locations of Disability* (Chicago, IL and London: University of Chicago Press, 2006); Coreen McGuire, *Measuring Difference, Numbering Normal: Setting the Standards for Disability in the Interwar Period* (Manchester: Manchester University Press, 2020); Patrick McDonagh, C.F. Goodey, and Timothy Stainton (eds), *Intellectual Disability: A Conceptual History, 1200–1900* (Manchester: Manchester University Press, 2018).

10 The same criticism applies to Anne Borsay's seminal *Disability and Social Policy in Britain since 1750: A History of Exclusion* (Basingstoke and New York: Palgrave Macmillan, 2005), which focuses primarily on the social marginalisation of disabled people due to their perceived physical and mental deficiencies.

11 Martin Atherton, *Deafness, Community and Culture in Britain: Leisure and Cohesion, 1945–95* (Manchester: Manchester University Press, 2018); David M. Turner and Daniel Blackie, *Disability in the Industrial Revolution: Physical Impairment in British Coalmining, 1780–1880* (Manchester: Manchester University Press, 2018); Lucy Delap, 'Slow workers: labelling and labouring in Britain, c. 1909–1955', *Social History of Medicine*, First Published Online, 14 July 2023: https://doi.org/10.1093/shm/hkad043 (2023).

12 For example, in her article for the British Library website, Louise Kimpton Nye briefly mentions disabled women alongside working-class, Black, Jewish, and lesbian women, but does not discuss their experiences in detail: '*Spare Rib*: changing perspectives and new ideologies': www.bl.uk/spare-rib/articles/changing-perspectives-and-new-ideologies (accessed 1 November 2022).

13 Natalie Thomlinson, *Race, Ethnicity and the Women's Movement in England, 1968–1993* (Basingstoke and New York: Palgrave Macmillan, 2016), p. 8; Elsa Beckett, 'Women like us', in Gail Chester and Sigrid Nielsen (eds), *In Other Words: Writing as A Feminist* (Abingdon and New York: Routledge, 1987); Kirsten Hearn, 'Oi! What about us?', in Bob Cant and Susan Hemmings (eds), *Radical Records: Thirty Years of Lesbian and Gay History, 1957–1987* (Abingdon and New York: Routledge, 1988).

14 For definitions of 'ableism' and 'disablism' see www.scope.org.uk/about-us/disablism/ (accessed 1 November 2022). The terms can be used interchangeably, but here I refer to 'ableist paradigms' to emphasise the assumption that matters of sex and sexuality apply only to non-disabled people.

15 Beckett, 'Women like us' [1987], p. 203.

16 Beckett, 'Women like us' [1987], p. 203. Within the disabled community there is ongoing variation in favouring the terms 'disabled people' and 'non-disabled people' (identity-first language) or 'people with disabilities'

'I started a new life when I joined Gemma'   269

and 'people without disabilities' (people-first language). 'Able-bodied' and 'abled' are also used to describe non-disabled people. In line with the British tradition that advocates disability as an experience of social and political oppression, I advocate identity-first language and use the terms 'disabled people' and 'non-disabled people' throughout this chapter. See Colin Cameron, 'Why we are disabled people, not people with disabilities', *Disability Arts Online* (2 July 2015), https://disabilityarts.online/magazine/opinion/disabled-people-not-people-disabilities/ (accessed 1 November 2022).

17 Elsa Beckett, 'Gemma: breaking barriers', in 'Women and Disability', *GLC Women's Committee Bulletin*, 26 (January 1986), 52.

18 Beckett, 'Women like us: the history of Gemma', p. 4.

19 By 2000 Gemma had produced four anthologies: *Findings* (1980), *Sparkles* (1989), *Facets* (1991) and *Amethyst* (1998).

20 Beckett, 'Women like us: the history of Gemma', p. 2.

21 Beckett, 'Gemma: breaking barriers', p. 52.

22 Beckett, 'Women like us: the history of Gemma', pp. 6–7. The women in the photographs are not named, so I am unable to identify this woman.

23 This newsletter also reported that 'The Gemma leaflet is now available in Welsh, Hebrew, Hindi, French, Dutch and Frisian': *Gemma*, 29 (November 1984), 3.

24 *Gemma*, 54 (January/February 1991), p. 2.

25 Beckett, 'Women like us' [1987], pp. 205, 208.

26 Beckett, 'Gemma: breaking barriers', p. 53; *Gemma*, 29 (November 1984), 3; *Gemma*, 30 (February 1985), 6.

27 The Disability Studies Department at the University of Leeds defines impairment as 'an injury, illness, or congenital condition that causes or is likely to cause a loss or difference of physiological or psychological function' and disability as 'the loss or limitation of opportunities to take part in society on an equal level with others due to social and environmental barriers'. See https://disability-studies.leeds.ac.uk/wp-content/uploads/sites/40/library/Northern-Officers-Group-defining-impairment-and-disability.pdf (accessed 1 November 2022).

28 *The Union of the Physically Impaired Against Segregation and The Disability Alliance discuss Fundamental Principles of Disability* (Leeds: The Disability Archive, 1997 [1976]), p. 4: https://disability-studies.leeds.ac.uk/wp-content/uploads/sites/40/library/UPIAS-fundamental-principles.pdf (accessed 1 November 2022); Mike Oliver, *Social Work with Disabled People* (London: Red Globe Press, 1983).

29 Tom Shakespeare, 'The social model of disability', in Lennard J. Davis (ed), *The Disability Studies Reader*, 4th edn (London and New York: Routledge, 2013).

270 *Mass media and networks of communication*

30 *Gemma*, 17 (February 1982), 5.

31 *Gemma*, 20 (November 1982), 7.

32 *Gemma*, 47 (May 1989), 5.

33 *Gemma*, 36 (August 1986), 3.

34 *Gemma*, 60 (August 1992), 3.

35 Liz Crow, 'Including all of our lives: renewing the social model of disability', in Jenny Morris (ed), *Encounters with Strangers: Feminism and Disability* (London: The Women's Press, 1996), p. 210. See also Jenny Morris, *Pride against Prejudice: Transforming Attitudes to Disability. A Personal Politics of Disability* (London: The Women's Press, 1991), p. 10.

36 Beckett, 'Women like us' [1987], p. 204.

37 *Gemma*, 87 (June 1999), quotation from 'Gemma Annual Report 1998' enclosed at the back of this newsletter.

38 *Gemma*, 47 (May 1989), 3.

39 *Gemma*, 55 (May 1991), 1.

40 For Gemma members, the attitudinal barrier to motherhood was twofold, encompassing prejudice against the right of both lesbians and disabled women to have children. On the former see Rebecca Jennings, 'Lesbian motherhood and the artificial insemination by donor scandal of 1978', *Twentieth Century British History*, 28:4 (2017). On the latter, see Kath Gillespie Sells, Mildrette Hill, and Bree Robbins, *She Dances to Different Drums: Research into Disabled Women's Sexuality* (London: King's Fund, 1998).

41 *Gemma*, 32 (August 1985), 3.

42 Frances died just two years after Gemma was established but continued to influence remaining members: *Gemma*, 4 (November 1978), 1. In 2001 co-founder Elsa Beckett wrote, 'I have missed her inspiration and humour very much': 'Women like us: the history of Gemma', p. 5.

43 *Gemma*, 7 (August 1979), 2.

44 *Gemma*, 16 (November 1981), 2.

45 *Sequel* seems to have ceased publication in 1984 or 1985. KENRIC (founded 1965) is still running today. See 'History: through the decades': https://kenriclesbians.org.uk/about-kenric/kenric-history/ (accessed 1 November 2022).

46 *Gemma*, 9 (January 1980), 4; *Gemma*, 35 (May 1986), 1–2.

47 See Littel, 'Minority Consciousness Gone Mad?'

48 *Gemma*, 5 (February 1979), 2.

49 GMDG ceased to organise in 1988. See Littel, 'Minority Consciousness Gone Mad?'

50 *Gemma*, 32 (August 1985), 3.

'*I started a new life when I joined Gemma*' 271

51 Section 28, known as Clause 2a in Scotland. This legislation prohibited 'the promotion of homosexuality by local authorities'. In practice, this meant that local authorities could not provide books, plays, leaflets, or films that depicted LGBTQ+ relationships positively.

52 *Gemma*, 45 (November 1988), 3.

53 *Gemma*, 42 (February 1988), 6.

54 *Gemma*, 68 (September 1994), 6.

55 Tropes about disabled lesbians' lack of sexual agency are rooted in the historic infantilisation and pathologisation of disabled people of all genders and sexualities. A groundbreaking disabled-led study identified many of these tropes in 1996: see Tom Shakespeare, Kath Gillespie Sells, and Dominic Davies, *The Sexual Politics of Disability: Untold Desires* (London: Cassell, 1996). For a pioneering analysis of disabled lesbians' sexual oppression see Gillespie Sells, Hill, and Robbins, *She Dances to Different Drums*, pp. 38–64. Disabled journalist and author, Frances Ryan, regularly comments on the persistence of regressive, ableist attitudes in the present day: Frances Ryan, *Crippled: Austerity and the Demonization of Disabled People* (London: Verso, 2019).

56 Martha Robinson Rhodes, 'Bisexuality and Multiple-Gender Attraction in Britain, 1970–1990: A Queer Oral History' (PhD thesis, University of Birmingham, 2020).

57 *Gemma*, 49 (November 1989), 4.

58 *Gemma*, 38 (February 1987), 4.

59 *Gemma*, 51 (May 1990), 2.

60 *Gemma*, 88 (September 1999), 5.

61 *Gemma*, 67 (June 1994), 4.

62 *Gemma*, 20 (November 1982), 3.

63 *Gemma*, 59 (May 1992), 1.

64 *Gemma*, 37 (November 1986), 4.

65 Shakespeare, Gillespie Sells and Davies, *Sexual Politics*, p. 92.

66 In February 2020, Kathryn was still the main coordinator for Gemma, having taken up the role after Elsa's death.

67 *Gemma*, 114 (March 2006), 1.

68 *Gemma*, 29 (November 1984), 7.

69 *Gemma*, 53 (November 1990), 4.

70 *Gemma*, 68 (September 1994), 6.

11

Talk shows and 'tanorexia': motherhood and 'sunbed addiction' on British television in the 1990s

Fabiola Creed

Introduction

'I think you're being really selfish to your children. Cause like you're risking your own life and everything' – Studio audience member to 'sunbed addicted' mother Dawn Harley.
  ('Tanorexia', *Esther*, BBC2, 4.55pm, 18 June 1997).

This stern declaration, shouted by the last audience member to speak, summarised the overriding sentiment towards all 'sunbed addicted' mothers on the 'tanorexia' episode of *Esther*, Esther Rantzen's talk show. The response of the studio audience, most of whom were women (many accompanied by their daughters), further intensified this powerful condemnation; most stood up and passionately clapped in agreement. The camera then zoomed onto Dawn Harley's two sons who were a part of the trial-like spectacle. The oldest, aged eleven, immediately smiled and clapped. The youngest, aged seven, first looked around in confusion. He then clapped himself, feeling the communal pressure from the audience members. Harley, both her autonomy and parental authority undermined, looked at her children with distress and agitation. The audience member continued by asking, 'What's more important, a tan or your life?' Trying to regain authority in front of her children, Harley asserted 'a tan'. The host, Esther Rantzen, concluded: 'and there [...] *we* have defined [sunbed] addiction'.

This public trial of a 'sunbed addicted' or 'tanorexic' mother demonstrates the problematic undertones of the women-centred talk

Talk shows and 'tanorexia' 273

show genre which became popular on British television in the 1990s, and provides a snapshot of the paradoxes of third wave feminism within popular culture. Using 'tanorexia' as a case study, this chapter shows how the very platforms designed to give women new agency in public spaces sometimes disempowered and discriminated against them. In historicising the intersection of public health concerns around skin cancer and 'sunbed addition' with the popularity of 1990s women-centred talk shows, this chapter shows how talk shows are valuable sources for the history of women's 'everyday health' and wellbeing. An in-depth analysis of *Esther*'s 'tanorexia' episode, including how its prominent themes related to discussions of 'sunbed addiction' on other British talk shows, reveals that expectations of 'selfless' motherhood were central to the show. As such, 'tanorexic' mothers were stigmatised more than their male counterparts. This stigmatisation affected *all* women, not only those who were mothers; even in late twentieth-century Britain, most women could not avoid discussions on prospective motherhood as part of their 'female' identity.[1] The ideal of motherhood, implied or portrayed, therefore had the potential to exert monumental pressures on *all* women participating in or watching these talk shows.

Women's health and wellbeing in the media, c. 1945–90s

After the Second World War, the huge expansion of mass media platforms and genres slowly moved many private discussions on everyday health and social issues into more public spaces.[2] From the 1960s, women increasingly used the print press to publicly discuss their own wellbeing issues, creating networks that, paradoxically, could both provide support and stigmatise women's everyday lifestyle and consumption choices.[3] It took longer for 'ordinary' women to access and use television broadcasts to speak about their own everyday wellbeing.[4]

Before the 1980s, women's health concerns were mainly discussed on television through male-produced 'factual' shows such as formal news reports, public health campaigns, educational documentaries, and medical programmes, and more occasionally through fictional and therefore dramatised representations.[5] Most of this television content, however, was not produced, managed, and hosted by women.

274   *Mass media and networks of communication*

Women struggled to enter and remain in 'above the line' roles as directors and producers and were instead clustered in 'below the line' roles as hairdressers, continuity 'girls', production assistants, and negative cutters.[6] Nor were these programmes structured, as they were in the print press, as 'supportive' communal discussions between women. By the 1990s, however, the British television industry consisted of more women, which led to more female-centred television programmes, including talk shows.

The television talk show originated in 1950s America, but soon spread throughout the world.[7] From the 1960s, 'chat shows', where the host(s) interviewed celebrities, and 'talk shows', where 'ordinary' members of the public were interviewed, became popular. Some shows eventually combined elements of both formats. Several subgenres of talk show shortly emerged, but certain features remained the same. They all featured at least one host, who set the show's tone and managed the discussion on one preselected topic by interviewing either one or multiple guests with relatable first-hand experience, and also audience members (either the studio audience or members of the public who called in) and/or a panel of 'experts'. The most common types of 'expert' were spokespersons from industry, government, education, criminal justice, public health, medicine, charity, or religious groups. Shows also featured 'experts by experience': consumers, patients, victims, sufferers, survivors, affected family or friends, or simply someone providing a perspective from a different culture or country. The predictable structures and relatable themes of the talk show allowed viewers to follow individual episodes, even if they had never seen any of the others.

Before the 1980s, not one woman had been a sole host for a talk show in the USA or UK, and very few women even co-hosted with men. In the USA, this was rectified in the mid-1980s as a wave of solo female-fronted talk shows emerged, including *The Sally Jessy Raphael Show* (1983–2002), *The Oprah Winfrey Show* (1986–2011) and *The Late Show with Joan Rivers* (1986–88).[8] A similar wave of British talk shows hosted by and named after women emerged only in the 1990s. The four most popular women-centred British talk shows starting in this decade were *The Chrystal Rose Show* (1993–95), *Esther* (1994–2002), *The Vanessa Show* (*Vanessa*) (1994–98) and *Trisha* (1998–2010). As the studio and television audiences for daytime shows were mostly women, topics centred on 'ordinary' women's issues and mostly featured women as 'experts by experience'.[9] At the same time, more and more women became a part of the production team (from the executive producers to the series content creators) for these new women-centred talk shows in Britain.[10]

Motherhood and women-centred talk shows

These British television programmes encouraged an 'American-style' public confession culture. On American talk shows, both guests and studio audiences talked willingly about private health, emotional, and familial issues. At first, this openness did not resonate with British sociocultural expectations of reticence.[11] The British public struggled to speak candidly on television, even though it was now more acceptable for women to voice their everyday issues through the print press.[12] The team on *The Chrystal Rose Show* struggled to find topics that the British would comfortably discuss, finding that most audience members wanted to simply listen rather than participate, unless the issue directly applied to them.[13] However, when topics addressed a wellbeing issue related to motherhood, audience members enthusiastically, even aggressively, voiced their own opinions – suggesting widespread belief that women's actual and assumed reproductive roles were always open to debate.[14] Any discussion topic even loosely related to motherhood therefore became a double-edged sword for the women involved; as talk show guests, mothers simultaneously received both 'support' and intense scrutiny from the public.

The producers and hosts of talk shows asserted that their programmes provided mini-therapy sessions for the guest(s) and 'public therapy' for viewers. They specified that the British public needed confession-style psychotherapy to help them 'loosen up' on commonplace issues that caused emotional distress.[15] These assertions did not go unchallenged. In the print press, critics publicised concerns about the ethics behind *Esther*'s staged 'therapy sessions' or, as they termed it, 'victim television'. Rantzen responded by sharing stories to show how *Esther* had, in some cases, saved the lives of its participants and viewers.[16] Nonetheless, it is difficult to avoid viewing 'morality tales' as the central component of talk shows.[17]

276   *Mass media and networks of communication*

Jane Shattuc argues that the talk show genre is 'structured around the moral authority and educated knowledge of a host and/or an expert who mediates between guests and audience'. To captivate the viewing public, talk shows had to both focus on the emotional and social 'human-interest story' of prominent new stories, and enact cultural conflict, crisis, and resolution through the on-stage drama.[18] As such, emotionally provocative topics were often deliberately oversimplified to invite public reactions of condemnation. As boundaries 'between normal and deviant, public and private, real and fictional' were blurred, an artificial community could respond more harshly towards individual guests because the 'drama' felt detached from real life.[19] Andrew Tolson similarly suggests that by focusing on the psychological and the personal, rather than external factors such as the environment, poverty, or commercial pressures, hosts intensified negative judgements of guests' attitudes, lifestyles, and behaviours.[20] Although the new talk shows were 'women-centred', it is therefore not surprising that their attitudes towards female guests were deeply problematic.

On the surface, these new women-centred talk shows could be perceived as a positive result of third wave feminism. This genre gave some women a space to therapeutically share their private issues with other women, amplifying their everyday concerns to the viewing public, forming a new community in the process, and potentially inciting collective action.[21] Moreover, some television scholars have argued that talk shows undermined the traditional view that only medical or official experts offered reliable and valuable knowledge, in contrast to knowledge based on everyday life experience.[22] Talk shows could therefore be seen as creating new opportunities for female empowerment, especially as the voices of 'ordinary' women rarely dominated previous television shows. At the same time, the stigma related to women's 'addictions' – particularly those relating to aesthetics and/or affecting mothers – still reflected traditional expectations, and therefore public judgement.[23] Ultimately, these platforms permitted greater scrutiny of women's lifestyle, wellbeing, and consumption choices. Moreover, the 'support' offered by female talk show hosts consisted of pressuring women (mainly mothers) to change their everyday habits, arguing that this would 'improve' both their own and their children's lives. Mother-related issues attracted most attention and the harshest responses, as it was assumed mothers should 'know better'.[24] In reality, this 'public therapy' often provoked a backlash towards women's autonomy – especially when they exercised liberal attitudes towards 'beautifying' their bodies in public spaces.

Skin cancer and 'sunbed addiction' as public health concerns

This stigmatisation of some women's choices is evident in talk show coverage of 'sunbed addiction'. During the mid-1990s, increased melanoma incidence and mortality rates sparked a 'global' panic on skin cancer – mainly in Europe, America, and Australia. In Britain, sunbeds became the prime target of campaigns because they were highly visible and quantifiable, whereas everyday sun exposure could not be controlled. As medical authorities assumed that removing sunbeds would be an easy way to prevent skin cancer, the media attacked Britain's sunbed industry.[25] Dermatologists pressured providers to either instigate tighter restrictions or remove sunbeds entirely, claiming that providers were exploitative, profit-focused, 'pernicious', and unconcerned about their consumers' health.[26] However, lack of consensus within the medical profession and contradictions within anti-sunbed warnings undermined most attempts to weaken the sunbed industry's commercial power.[27] Next, new groups, including Cancer Research UK, ultraviolet (UV)-free tanning industries, and some legal authorities, attempted to weaken the sunbed industry. Yet only the legal authorities were somewhat successful by reducing the overseas expansion of the industry.[28] Moreover, UV-free tanning endorsement actually revived 'natural' UV-tanning culture, including sunbed use. Sunbed providers fought back through the media, arguing that their machines provided a vital source of vitamin D, and cured many mental and physical health issues and skin conditions. Although sunbed advertising within the mainstream media did somewhat decline,[29] these companies continued to advertise directly to consumers, using the same 'health' and 'safety' claims.[30]

Clearly, the commercial power of the sunbed industry was not deteriorating quickly enough for concerned medical experts or media producers. They therefore intensified their focus on forcefully discouraging people from using sunbeds, first through the print press and later through television. Newspaper journalists, dermatologists,

278   *Mass media and networks of communication*

psychologists, cancer specialists, and non-governmental organisations confirmed that 'sunbed addiction' or 'tanorexia' was spreading through Britain. Reports of 'sunbed addiction' first appeared in the *Guardian* and *Daily Mail*, and then in popular women's magazines.[31] *Cosmopolitan* – which had its own long history of contradictory attitudes to women's health, beauty, and bodies – described 'tanorexia' as a 'compulsion to be suntanned [through sunbeds], whatever the time of year [...] [or] cost', because 'addicts' never felt tanned enough. The article suggested that only women risked developing skin cancer through sunbed use.[32]

This moral panic around women's tanning habits was furthered by national television programmes that reached millions. In January 1996 a 'sunbed report' on BBC1's *Beauty Consumer Watchdog* featured 'sunworshippers who are as hooked on UV as others are on cigarettes'.[33] A little more than a year later, ITV's current affairs programme *3-D* included a nine-minute report 'on the health risks associated with sunbed[s]' as part of a thirty-minute episode titled 'Burning Issue – Healthy Choice?'[34] Two talk shows also showcased an episode on 'tanorexia': ITV's *The Vanessa Show* (13 October 1996), and BBC2's *Esther* (18 June 1997).[35] Talk show producers chose subjects that had opposing arguments, were socially broad enough to attract large audiences, and were popular in the print press or among viewer mail and call-ins.[36] 'Tanorexia', a public health issue that appeared to affect women, featured on both *Esther* and *The Vanessa Show*. Aired on mainstream channels to millions of people, these shows legitimated 'tanorexia' and reached much further than the print press.

Women-centred talk shows dedicated hundreds of episodes to topics around women's wellbeing, with most related to some aspect of motherhood. The two shows examined here, *Esther* and *Vanessa*, presented episodes on wide-ranging issues related to children (television, bullying, crime, gifted children), sex and relationships (teenage parenthood, contraception, abortion, 'coming out', monogamy, marital complications and abandonment, relationships with prison-bound criminals), health (AIDS, eating disorders, breast cancer, surgery), and motherhood ('natural born mothers', in vitro fertilisation, older parents, grandparents, caring for elderly parents).[37] Both shows featured episodes on 'sunbed addiction' that aimed to entertain, surprise, inform, and 'educate' a public comprised of mostly women, who formed the bulk of daytime television viewers.[38] However, these topics were tackled in quite different ways on each show.

ITV's *Vanessa* leant more towards the American-style 'public therapy' talk show genre, treating the studio audience – and, by implication, the viewers – as 'experts' and shunning formal expertise. Even when tackling serious issues, it focused on guests' personal lives, feelings, and relationships rather than other aspects of these topics.[39] It moved to BBC1 in 1999 after being 'dropped' by ITV and was then 'retired' altogether following a scandal about recruiting fake guests.[40] *Esther* was better known and more respected by the public than *Vanessa*. It ran from 1994 to 2002, aired over six hundred episodes in total, and increased from three to five episodes a week over this time, demonstrating its rising popularity. It was usually shown at 5pm and each episode was watched by roughly one to two million viewers, on average.[41] Although described by the *Radio Times* as a 'British interpretation of *The Oprah Winfrey Show*', Esther was serious in intent and often featured medical experts. The show was nominated in categories for the best/most popular chat show by the British Academy of Film and Television Arts and the National Television Awards in 1996 and 1997, and by 1999 had the highest ratings of any British-made talk show. *Esther* was one of the only talk shows not discredited on the grounds of fake stories and productions and was praised for the 'positive good' it achieved.[42] For these reasons, my discussion here mainly focuses on *Esther*.

Rantzen herself was key to perceptions of the show (Figure 11.1). She was already famous from BBC1's contemporary magazine-style consumer affairs programme *That's Life!* (1973–94), and for founding the national helpline Childline in the mid-1980s for children and young adults suffering from abuse.[43] Rantzen described herself as experienced in 'meeting people, listening to people and also working in very emotional areas', and her previous career demonstrates her investment in issues around women's and children's wellbeing.[44] As a show on the mixed-genre channel BBC2, *Esther* had to appeal to a broad adult audience. *Esther* was therefore perceived as a serious show, even if it was dramatic. Rantzen interviewed a mixture of celebrity guests and ordinary people. She sought to arouse 'disagreement and controversy' among the guests, but also wanted episodes to conclude with participants feeling glad that they had met and shared their experiences on the show.[45] Like other talk shows, *Esther*

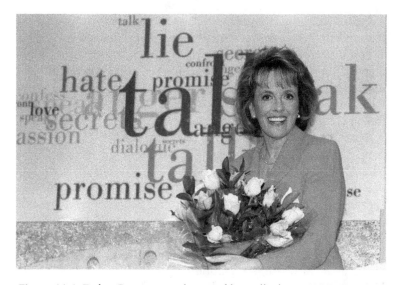

Figure 11.1 Esther Rantzen on the set of her talk show, 1998. Courtesy of Michael Stephens/Alamy Stock Photo. All rights reserved and permission to use the figure must be obtained from the copyright holder.

was supposed to present a 'balanced' and 'democratic' discussion for viewers through Rantzen's management of the conversation.[46] However, at least in the case of 'tanorexic' mothers, this 'democratic' balance was an illusion.

'Tanorexia' on *Esther*: power and control

Esther's 'tanorexia' episode featured guests representing different aspects of the issue, helping to create the impression that there would be an even-handed discussion. The three main guests were positioned centrally within the semi-circular stage and could be seen by everyone in the studio. The guests were Dawn Harley, an upper working-class mother in her thirties or forties; Diana, a red-haired, extremely fair-skinned skin cancer sufferer, two decades older than Harley; and Paul Gordon, a male sportswear model in his early twenties. In the front row of the audience sat dermatologist Dr Margaret Price, addiction psychologist Dr Mark Griffiths, a female Australian public health educator, pale model Miriam Banister and

Talk shows and 'tanorexia' 281

her boyfriend, and Kathy Banks, a representative of The Sunbed Association (TSA). The studio audience curved around the main stage, facing the guests. Asking questions and controlling the microphone, Rantzen walked around the studio. This set-up suggested a relatively balanced discussion.

In practice, however, the guests' performances of their standpoints established a biased hierarchy of respect, and further encouraged the stigmatisation of 'tanorexic' mothers. The representatives from each stakeholder group were extremely different in terms of personality and appearance; each 'character' reflected the stereotype of their faction. This made them memorable and manageable, and therefore suited to television's need for drama to entertain viewers. On *Esther*, the skin cancer 'survivor' (Diana) was much older, dressed conservatively in beige, exposing no skin, and spoke seriously. She used her horrifying experience as a sunbed user and then melanoma patient to scare Harley and the audience. The skin cancer 'survivor' on *Vanessa* was exactly the same: older, conservatively dressed and serious.[47] *Esther*'s medical experts also dressed conservatively, had upper-class accents, and spoke with authority to educate the audience. The contrast of 'respectable' melanoma survivors and medical experts with flamboyant 'tanorexics' reinforced stereotypes.

The 'tanorexic' men on *Esther* and *Vanessa* both had working-class accents and were depicted as feminised because of their attention to appearance. Nevertheless, they were not as stigmatised as Harley, who was the only female 'sunbed addict' interviewed in depth on television (*3-D*, *Vanessa* and *Esther*) in the mid-1990s. All shows presented Harley as an 'ordinary' upper working-class mother of two young boys. She was twice married, which Rantzen highlighted in a condescending tone, and had started tanning when she moved to Arizona in the 1980s. Harley always had bright blonde hair, exposed her tanned limbs through brightly coloured outfits, and wore make-up and jewellery; the *Esther* credits showed a make-up artist applying heavy bronzer on her face. With a southern English working-class accent, she spoke clearly, confidently, and passionately about why she used sunbeds. Her polite demeanour meant that hosts could easily deflect the conversation when she became agitated. Harley's comparison with conservative melanoma survivors framed her as irresponsible – a mother whose 'self-destructive' tanning habit prevented her from prioritising her children. The aggressive stance of five out of seven audience members who challenged Harley

282   *Mass media and networks of communication*

contributed to her disempowerment – and as audience members occupied the highest level in the studio, their authority was elevated as they literally spoke down to her on the main stage.

The claim of editorial balance was deceptive in other ways. Of the seventeen people including Rantzen who spoke during the episode, 17 per cent were neutral, 28 per cent were in favour of sunbeds, and 55 per cent were against them. Rantzen, who controlled the microphone, selected more anti- than pro-sunbed audience members to speak, and gave them more time collectively. Although Harley spoke for the second-longest amount of time after Rantzen, Rantzen's calculated questions framed Harley as unintelligent, vain, trivial, and reckless. The only time that Harley's 'addiction' was disputed, Rantzen interrupted and asserted that 'Dawn is an addict', and then asked Harley how many health clubs she belonged to. Throughout this discussion, the camera focused on the reactions of medical experts and outraged audience members, to encourage anti-sunbed reactions. The combined microphone time allotted to the two medical experts and the Australian public health educator, all strongly against sunbeds, accounted for roughly one third of the thirty-minute show. Rantzen invited the dermatologist Dr Price to speak on ten separate occasions, and only called twice on Banks (TSA's secretary) – both times interrupting her and withdrawing the microphone. Rantzen challenged Banks and supported the medical experts, but her back-and-forth movement between pro- and anti-sunbed speakers hid this imbalance. This presentation heightened the emotional stakes of 'sunbed addiction' and reinforced stigma against mothers who apparently consumed 'recklessly' and against the best interests of their children.

The skewing of the programme against sunbed users upheld Rantzen's opinion of her show's purpose, and her own persona as host. Rantzen saw the show as providing people with a 'positive' public service and claimed that guests wanted to appear on the show for two main reasons: to 'find a solution for themselves' and/ or to 'protect others'. These guests were 'determined to bring about change' by broadcasting their first-hand experiences to the public.[48] Rantzen was willing to defend 'ordinary' women against medical experts. She did this on an episode about myalgic encephalomyelitis, which led to *Esther* being described as 'victim television' by a columnist. Rantzen challenged this statement in a *Radio Times* interview,

Talk shows and 'tanorexia'

validating her reasons for challenging the medical expert in support of the public.[49] However, Rantzen's background, including her work with Childline, suggests that her concerns about children's wellbeing superseded that for women, especially if children were apparently under the care of 'immoral' mothers.

From the outset, Rantzen was more judgemental about 'tanorexic' mothers than the medical experts. In her mid-fifties, Rantzen performed her trademark 'host' personality as a tough-love mother figure; she was formidable, extremely articulate with an upper-class accent, and drew on a long history of media-related accomplishments. Both the media and public heralded her as the 'strong-minded, outspoken, [and] charismatic doyenne of TV'.[50] On the 'tanorexia' episode, Rantzen was dressed immaculately in a shoulder-padded power suit and expensive jewellery. Her physical presence and opinions dominated the studio space. Speaking to Harley, she used a sharp tone and dismissive body language, controlling the conversation to frame her as 'selfish' regarding her children; she interrupted, overpowered, ignored, and made stern hand gestures to quiet those who were either neutral or empathetic towards mothers who used sunbeds. This intimidating presence discouraged guests, medical experts, industry representatives, and the audience from challenging her, and the watching public likely felt the communal pressure to judge these mothers themselves.

'Tanorexia' on *Esther*: mothers and children

Rantzen managed the discussion to frame Harley as an irresponsible mother who placed both herself and her children at risk. After the opening credits, Rantzen walked onto the stage and declared:

> If you thought that a golden suntan was the sign of health, you better forget it. Because doctors now say that sunshine gives you wrinkles and skin cancer. But that won't put off the people in our studio, because we have addicts here, who are fanatical sun worshippers. They ignore all the risks because they are tan junkies or tanorexics.

Rantzen explained that the purpose of this episode was to understand 'what drives these addicts on, even though they know it can literally be fatal for them'. She started by asking Harley about her 'addiction'

284   *Mass media and networks of communication*

and the frequency of her sunbed use, before revealing that Harley had potentially already experienced skin cancer. Harley protested that it was only an abnormal mole that grew and therefore needed removal, but Rantzen suggested it was a 'warning sign' and asked Dr Price's opinion. After asserting that it was a 'free country', Dr Price explained that parents needed to be aware of the risks to protect children who could not make their own health decisions. Rantzen then asked Harley's sons, 'does she let you go out in the sun? And get sunburn? The way she does?' Harley's oldest son hesitated but eventually responded that his mother did. Rantzen sternly asked Harley if she was worried about her son's skin. Harley, leaning forwards in desperation, explained that her children 'definitely' had high-factor sun creams because she 'wouldn't put them through that'. Rantzen then asked the youngest son what he thought about his mother's sunbathing. He proudly replied that he 'really want[ed] to go on a sunbed'. Despite Harley's assertion that he was 'much too young', the studio audience gasped in horror at this apparent emulation of his mother's 'reckless' behaviour.

Rantzen then spoke to Dr Price about why people used sunbeds, and asked Diana about her tanning habits before she developed skin cancer, and her subsequent operations and chemotherapy. Diana reinforced the theme of irresponsible motherhood by telling Harley 'you're doing this to your children'. Diana also reprimanded Harley for reducing the time she spent with her children and asserted that she could prevent her children from developing skin cancer if she stopped using sunbeds herself. Rantzen, Diana, Dr Price, and the Australian public health educator (from Queensland) confirmed that UV exposure did cause 'lethal melanoma' and discussed the differences between children's anti-skin cancer campaigns in the UK and Australia. This segment placed skin cancer and children's wellbeing at the core of the episode.

The Australian public health educator tried to convince Harley to use fake tan to stop her becoming a 'brown leather bag'. Banister, the pale model, explained that she wore fake tan for modelling to avoid sunbed-induced wrinkles. Gordon, the male sportswear model, was lightly questioned about his own sunbed use, in comparison to Harley's interrogation. Finally, Griffiths, the psychologist, discussed the association of tanning with sex appeal, holidays, wealth, health, and 'feeling good'. He also explained that 'addicts' neglected 'everything'

Talk shows and 'tanorexia'

except their obsession, which contributed to the notion that Harley was neglecting her children.

Halfway through the show, Rantzen invited audience members to answer questions. These focused on exposing 'sunbed addicts' and rooting out those against sunbed use. The first woman invited to speak blamed her mother for telling her that she looked 'awful' in the winter and 'lovely' in the summer when she was younger and admitted addiction. Almost twenty minutes in, Rantzen finally asked Banks, the sunbed industry representative, a question. Banks agreed that sunbed use could be a problem, but defended sensible sunbed use and tanning itself as 'a basic mechanism to protect ourselves against UV radiation'. For the last ten minutes of the show, Rantzen spoke to other panellists and studio members, asking about other sunbed-induced health issues, including life-changing skin conditions, retina damage, melanoma, the surgical removal of tumour-embedded muscles, and the reduced life expectancy of young people. Anti-sunbed participants sharing these experiences intentionally directed their comments towards Harley rather than Gordon. A 'relapsing sunbed addict' and her extremely fair-skinned (and therefore 'very high risk') daughter were then invited to speak. The daughter immediately asserted that her mother went to great lengths to protect her from the sun as a child, and that she was now an ardent user of 'fake tan'. The disapproval of 'sunbed addicted' mothers centred on the risk it could pose to their children.

On *Esther* and *Vanessa*, 'tanorexia' was depicted as a genuine condition affecting women and men, and the pleasurable use of sunbeds was pathologised. The mere presence of an 'addiction expert' endorsed the associations between sunbed use and drug problems, while Rantzen and medical experts constantly compared sunbed use to smoking cigarettes and drinking alcohol. When Harley described herself as a nurse who paid her National Health Service taxes and did not drink, smoke, or use drugs but felt happy through sunbed use, Rantzen invited forceful audience members to pressure her to change her habits. She was called selfish, irresponsible, and vain, and accused of neglecting her duties as a mother. At the end of both shows, and in contrast to the men, Harley had been aggressively condemned.

In this way, 'tanorexia' was also implicitly framed as a women's condition, with women's 'tanorexic' tendencies portrayed as more

286   *Mass media and networks of communication*

'immoral' than those of men. Rantzen and Feltz interrogated Harley but were kinder to the men, while medical experts, 'melanoma survivor' guests, and most of the studio audience also judged her more harshly, despite Harley's perpetual politeness. On both talk shows, the male 'sunbed addicts' were reproached, but in a more light-hearted manner. On *Vanessa*, Feltz even flirted and laughed with Mike. On *Esther*, Rantzen asked Gordon only four questions, including whether photographers and clients wanted him to look suntanned. Gordon explained that male models were pressured to be tanned, especially for 'sportswear and body shots'. Satisfied with his explanations, Rantzen and the audience responded sympathetically. The pressures on women, including mothers, to look desirable were underplayed, even though many speakers (including Rantzen) affirmed the attractiveness of tanned women, and Harley admitted she used sunbeds to 'deal' with her 'weight problem'.[51] The constant but unacknowledged focus on women's appearances may have contributed to white working-class mothers being more open about their sunbed use, and therefore more easily framed as 'insecure', vain, and self-destructive. Overlooking the aesthetic pressures on mothers lent the stigmatisation of 'tanorexics' an explicitly misogynistic edge.

Conclusion

Talk shows allow historical insight into representations of 'ordinary' women and their everyday health and social concerns. The talk show genre has been heralded as an influential site supporting the lifestyle and consumption choices of 'ordinary' people. Because audience participation is central to talk shows, this genre illuminates public opinion on health and social issues at the time – even if these 'public' voices were stage-managed by the host.[52] They are therefore important sources for historians of women's everyday health, motherhood, and moral panics in late twentieth-century Britain.

Close analysis of the 'tanorexia' episode of *Esther* in this chapter illustrates the wider value of talk shows for historians of health and wellbeing. The genre provides the audio-visual representations of its subjects, including their rhetorical and emotional reactions. Visual elements are crucial; television scripts are valuable on their own, but the underlining power dynamics of talk shows are most evident when viewing the footage. The camera angles, *mise en scène*, spatial hierarchies, seating arrangements, clothing and make-up of participants, and the subtle bodily and facial reactions of everyone on set are all integral to understanding the emotions and on-stage dynamic between the host, guests, 'experts', and audience members. Analysis of individual episodes can be supplemented using the contextual information around production content and people's reception that is offered by print press coverage, and both television archives and journals, but viewing footage is still useful on its own.[53]

The insights that talk shows offer are all the more important because researchers struggle to access the histories of 'ordinary' women through television; in part because 'everyday' television for women was deemed unworthy of archiving when programmes were expensive to retain.[54] With these suggestions in mind, I argue that there is another feminist issue related to television archiving: accessing television in comparison to print press archives can be costly for scholars, and it often requires more time to locate, access, and utilise these sources. Consequently, audio-visual can prove more inaccessible for scholars with less socioeconomic resources, even though these sources would be invaluable for those invested in the history of 'everyday' women. To navigate these methodological issues, free or cheap and digitally accessible 'archives' can provide footage of 'ordinary' women (and people in general) through television.[55]

Talk shows also complicate our understandings of the relationship between public and private because they blurred the boundaries between these realms. The audience at home watched an 'ordinary' person's issues unfold, merging 'real' and 'talk show' life. Like other talk shows, *Esther* encouraged the new 'experts' of the informed public to comment, judge, and act on changing the decision making of an individual.[56] For Rantzen, 'exposing one's feelings in private' was no different from doing so 'in front of a studio audience and millions of viewers'.[57]

In relation to 'tanorexia', this approach, followed by mostly women on the show, disempowered mothers, despite the genre's potential to cooperatively promote women's agency and encourage empathy. The examples discussed here reveal instead how the media can deploy illusions of 'balance' to persuade audiences, in this instance in support of conservative and pronatalist attitudes. *Esther* and *Vanessa* consolidated public perceptions of sunbed addicts as irrational, and

288 *Mass media and networks of communication*

those who were mothers as immoral. Rantzen, the medical experts, and studio audience acted as judge, jury, and witnesses to the charge that Harley must change for the good of her children, and even society. This condemnation of her behaviour reflects historical bias towards mothers who consumed 'unhealthily' or deviated from supposedly instinctive 'selflessness'. The 'democratic' balance of the talk show was an illusion. Instead, this show reinforced sociocultural stigma against 'tanorexics', especially those who were mothers. 'Tanorexic' women on these shows were ridiculed and belittled, especially when compared to male sunbed users. There was no gender equality on these shows.

Acknowledgements

This research was supported by the Wellcome Trust, WT 203287/Z/16/Z.

Notes

1 Angela Davis, *Modern Motherhood: Women and Family in England, 1945–2000* (Manchester: Manchester University Press, 2012).

2 Virginia Berridge and Kelly Loughlin (eds), *Medicine, The Market and Mass Media: Producing Health in the Twentieth Century* (London: Routledge, 2012); Kelly Loughlin, 'Networks of mass communication: reporting science, health and medicine from the 1950s to the 1970s', in Virginia Berridge (ed), *Making Health Policy: Networks in Research and Policy after 1945* (Amsterdam: Rodopi, 2005); Alex Mold, Peder Clark, Gareth Millward, and Daisy Payling, *Placing the Public in Public Health in Post-War Britain, 1948–2012* (Basingstoke: Palgrave Macmillan, 2019).

3 Elizabeth Toon, 'The machinery of authoritarian care: dramatising breast cancer treatment in 1970s Britain', *Social History of Medicine*, 27:3, (2014), 559; Lynn Abrams, 'Heroes of their own life stories: narrating the female self in the feminist age', *Cultural and Social History*, 16:2, (2019), 205; Tracey Loughran, '"The most helpful friends in the world": letters pages, expertise and emotion in British women's magazines, c. 1960–80', in Laurel Forster and Joanne Hollows (eds), *Women's Periodicals and Print Culture in Britain, 1940s–2000s* (Edinburgh:

Edinburgh University Press, 2020); Amy Tooth Murphy, '*Arena Three* magazine and the construction of the middlebrow lesbian reader', in Forster and Hollows (eds), *Women's Periodicals and Print Culture in Britain*; Katrina Louise Moseley, 'Food, Body Weight and Everyday Life in England, c. 1954–1990' (PhD thesis, University of Cambridge, 2020).

4 Vicky Ball and Melanie Bell, 'Working women, women's work: production, history, gender', *Journal of British Cinema and Television*, 10:3 (2013).

5 Katherine Dow, 'Looking into the test tube: the birth of IVF on British television', *Medical History*, 63 (2019); Jane Hand, 'Visualising Food as a Modern Medicine: Gender, the Body and Health Education in Britain, 1940–1992' (PhD thesis, University of Warwick, 2014); Kelly Loughlin, 'The history of health and medicine in contemporary Britain: reflections on the role of audio-visual sources', *Social History of Medicine*, 13:1 (2000); Penny Tinkler, *Smoke Signals: Women, Smoking and Visual Culture* (Oxford: Berg, 2006), pp. 185–210; Jesse Olszynko-Gryn, 'Thin blue lines: product placement and the drama of pregnancy testing in British cinema and television', *British Journal for the History of Science*, 50:3 (2017).

6 Ball and Bell, 'Working women, women's work'.

7 Jane M. Shattuc, *The Talking Cure: TV Talk Shows and Women* (London: Routledge, 1997); Bernard M. Timberg and Robert J. Erler, *Television Talk: A History of the TV Talk Show* (Austin, TX: University of Texas Press, 2010); Peter Lunt, 'Television, public participation, and public service: from value consensus to the politics of identity', *Annals of the American Academy of Political and Social Science*, 625:1 (2009); Andrew Tolson (ed.), *Television Talk Shows: Discourse, Performance, Spectacle* (Mahwah, NJ: Lawrence Erlbaum, 2001); Joshua Gamson, *Freaks Talk Back: Tabloid Talk Shows and Sexual Nonconformity* (Chicago, IL: University of Chicago Press, 1998).

8 Jane M. Shattuc, 'The confessional talk shows', in Glen Creeber (ed.), *The Television Genre Book*, 3rd edn (London: British Film Institute/ Palgrave Macmillan, 2015), p. 197.

9 Andrew Tolson, 'Talking about talk: the academic debates', in Tolson (ed.) *Television Talk Shows*, p. 23; Shattuc, 'The confessional talk shows', p. 197.

10 On *Esther*, the producer, editor, and unit manager were women, as were one of the two researchers, and three of the five production team members. BFI. 'Tanorexia', *Esther*, British Film Institute, Stephen Street Archive (hereafter BFI). 'Tanorexia', *Esther*, BBC2 (aired 4.55pm, 18 June 1997).

290 *Mass media and networks of communication*

11 Sarah Lyall, 'Television: Stiff upper lips on British talk shows (lower, too)', *New York Times*, 7 May 1995, p. 33; Tolson, 'Talking about talk', p. 25.

12 Jennifer Crane, *Child Protection in England, 1960–2000: Expertise, Experience, and Emotion* (Basingstoke: Palgrave Macmillan, 2018), p. 60.

13 Lyall, 'Television', p. 33.

14 Melanie Latham, *Regulating Reproduction: A Century of Conflict in Britain and France* (Manchester: Manchester University Press, 2002); Jesse Olszynko-Gryn and Caroline Rusterholz, 'Reproductive politics in twentieth-century France and Britain', *Medical History*, 63:2 (2019).

15 Lyall, 'Television', p. 33.

16 Esther Rantzen, 'That's the accusation of her critics. As her new series begins, Esther Rantzen hits back', *Radio Times*, 292:3806, 1 January 1997, p. 27; Esther Rantzen, 'Esther takes the talk-show high ground (Letters)', *Broadcast*, 5 March 1999, p. 17.

17 Tolson, 'Talking about talk', p. 8.

18 Shattuc, 'The confessional talk shows', p. 198.

19 Tolson, 'Talking about talk', p. 9; Laura Grindstaff, *The Money Shot: Trash, Class, and the Making of TV Talk Shows* (Chicago, IL: University of Chicago Press, 2002); Vicki Abt and Mel Seesholtz, 'The shameless world of Phil, Sally and Oprah: television talk shows and the deconstructing of society', *Journal of Popular Culture*, 28 (1994).

20 Tolson, 'Talking about talk', pp. 23–4.

21 For debates on whether women-centred talk shows created an exploitative staging of personal intimacy or if they provided 'feminist therapy' and connected to public political agendas, see Helen Wood, *Talking with Television: Women, Talk Shows, and Modern Self-Reflexivity* (Champaign, IL: University of Illinois Press, 2009), p. 9.

22 Anne-Marie Simon-Vandenbergen, 'Lay and expert voices in public participation programmes: a case of generic heterogeneity', *Journal of Pragmatics*, 39:8 (2007).

23 Jahn L. Forth-Finegan, 'Sugar and spice and everything nice', *Journal of Feminist Family Therapy*, 3:3–4 (1992); Julia Skelly, *Addiction and British Visual Culture, 1751–1919: Wasted Looks* (Farnham: Ashgate, 2014); Julia Skelly, *The Uses of Excess in Visual and Material Culture, 1600–2010* (London: Routledge, 2018); Tinkler, *Smoke Signals*; James Nicholls, *The Politics of Alcohol: A History of the Drink Question in England* (Manchester: Manchester University Press, 2009).

24 BFI. 'Tanorexia', *Esther*.

25 Fabiola Creed, 'Advertising, Stereotypes and 'Addiction': Understanding Sunbed Representation in England, 1970s–1990s' (PhD thesis, University of Warwick, 2020).

26 Anon., 'Call to ban council sunbeds', *Guardian*, 11 October 1996, p. 4; Health Education Authority, 'Calls to phase out sunbeds from council premises' (London: HEA, 1996) [Press release can/96/005].

27 Jane Alexander, 'Lighten up your life with a ray of sunshine', *Daily Mail*, 25 February 1995, p. 34.

28 Anon., 'Closure hit Hawtin', *Financial Times*, 5 December 1997, p. 20.

29 Fabiola Creed, 'Sunbeds, dihydroxyacetone (DHA) fake tan and Melanotan injections: a history of "safe" tanning technologies', in Rachel Elder and Thomas Schlich (eds), *Technology and Health in the Age of Patient Consumerism* (Manchester: Manchester University Press, forthcoming).

30 Philips International Company Archive, Eindhoven, The Netherlands. 'Domestic appliances and personal care products', Philips English Catalogue, February 1997.

31 Eleanor Bailey, 'Burning ambitions: why the sun is going down on tanning', *Guardian*, 27 January 1995, p. 9; Steve Tooze, 'Tanorexia', *Daily Mail*, 16 May 1996, pp. 44–5.

32 David Machin and Joanna Thornborrow, 'Branding and discourse: the case of *Cosmopolitan*', *Discourse & Society*, 14:4 (2003), 454; Dan Glaister, 'Tanorexics', *Guardian*, 12 April 1996, 15.

33 BFI. *Beauty Consumer Watchdog* (Presenter: Alice Beer), BBC1 (Aired 7.30pm, 8 January 1996); Des Christie, 'Dial P for panic', *Guardian*, 9 May 1997, 26.

34 ITV Film Archive. *3-D, BURNING ISSUE – HEALTHY CHOICE?* (Presenter: Julia Somerville), ITV Yorkshire Television (Aired 7.00–7.25pm, 8 May 1997).

35 ITV Film Archive. 'Addicted to sunbeds', *The Vanessa Show*, ITV (Aired 2.20pm, 13 October 1996); BFI. 'Tanorexia', *Esther*.

36 Shattuc, 'The confessional talk shows', p. 197.

37 Anon., Episode Guide for *Esther* from 1994 to 2002, Internet Movie Database (IMDB): www.imdb.com/title/tt0216470/?ref_=nm_flmg_slf_114 (accessed 25 March 2021); Anon., *Esther* Episodes, BBC2: www.bbc.co.uk/programmes/p013bzvw/episodes/guide (accessed 25 March 2021); Lyall, 'Television', p. 33.

38 Timberg and Erler, *Television Talk*, pp. 7–8.

39 Lyall, 'Television', p. 33; for more on the 'evolution of talk on *Vanessa*', see Wood, *Talking with Television*, pp. 77–80.

292   *Mass media and networks of communication*

40 Sherryl Wilson, 'Real people with real problems? Public service broadcasting, commercialism and *Trisha*', in Catherine Johnson and Rob Turnock (eds), *ITV Cultures: Independent Television over Fifty Years* (Maidenhead: Open University Press, 2005), pp. 163–4; John Ellis, 'Documentary and truth on television: the crisis of 1999', in Alan Rosenthal and John Corner (eds), *New Challenges for Documentary* (Manchester: Manchester University Press, 2005), p. 353; Janine Gibson, 'Vanessa show gets the chop', *Guardian*, 10 June 1999.

41 Lyall, 'Television', p. 33; Jason Deans, 'Rantzen calls time on BBC2 talk show', *Guardian*, 23 April 2002; Anon., 'Chat's life! Rantzen and Greer return', *Radio Times*, 282:3693, 22 October 1994, pp. 6–7.

42 Anon., 'Chat's life!'; Rantzen, 'That's the accusation of her critics', p. 27; Rantzen, 'Esther takes the talk-show high ground', p. 17.

43 Crane, *Child Protection in England*, pp. 55–9.

44 Anon., 'Chat's life!'

45 Lyall, 'Television', p. 33; Deans, 'Rantzen calls time on BBC2 talk show'; Anon. 'Chat's life!'

46 Helen Wood, '"No, YOU Rioted!" The pursuit of conflict in the management of expert and lay discourses on Kilroy', in Tolson (ed.), *Television Talk Shows*.

47 ITV Film Archive, 'Addiction to sunbeds', *Vanessa*.

48 Anon., 'Chat's life!'

49 Rantzen, 'That's the accusation of her critics', p. 27.

50 Anon. 'Chat's life!'

51 BFI. 'Tanorexia', *Esther*.

52 Shattuc, 'The confessional talk shows', pp. 197–9; Wood, *Talking with Television*, p. 63.

53 Billy Smart and Amanda Wrigley, 'Television history: archives, excavation and the future. A discussion', *Critical Studies in Television*, 11:1 (2016); Brett Mills, 'Invisible television: the programmes no-one talks about even though lots of people watch them', *Critical Studies in Television*, 5:1 (2010).

54 Rachel Moseley and Helen Wheatley, 'Is archiving a feminist issue? Historical research and the past, present, and future of television studies', *Cinema Journal*, 47:3 (2008); Anon., 'BBC Archives – wiped, missing and lost', BBC Archive: www.bbc.co.uk/archive/bbc-archives–wiped-missing-and-lost/z4nkvk7 (accessed 15 July 2022).

55 These 'archives', along with commercial sites of television, film, and general audio-visual content, can be found at Manchester Metropolitan Film Archive, North West Film Archive, East Anglia Film Archive, BBC Genome, the Wellcome Trust, British Pathe, YouTube, Ebay, Amazon, Box of Broadcasts and the Internet Archive (Classic Television). If the

BFI Stephen Street and BFI Reuben Library are too costly to visit, there are also dozens of small yet free-to-access local or regional television and film archives across Britain that can be found through online searches. If contacted, some archivists and technicians will send the relevant clips digitally.

56 Wood, *Talking with television*, p. 95.

57 Anon., 'Chat's life!'

12

'Having been there ... I know how hard it is': relatability and ordinariness in twenty-first-century British clean eating

Louise Morgan

Introduction

'*The Eat-Clean Diet* was written for you, the confused but motivated reader who has struggled with weight gain and loss longer than you may want to admit.'[1] Tosca Reno's 2007 diet guide opens with this statement, immediately placing the reader at the centre of her clean eating narrative. As one of the first figures to link a wholefood diet to the phrase 'clean eating', Reno's impact on twenty-first-century food culture is hard to overstate, particularly in the United Kingdom, where clean eating experienced a sharp rise and fall in both popularity and prominence from 2014 onwards. During this time, clean eaters such as Ella Mills (née Woodward, known as 'Deliciously Ella') turned their popular blogs and Instagram accounts into lucrative media careers, with bestselling cookbooks, appearances on television and radio, and frequent mentions in the tabloid press. In Britain, the successful clean eaters were predominantly upper middle-class women, although they argued that clean eating was achievable for all genders, ages, and classes.[2] Clean eaters exploited social media to promote both their relatability and ordinariness, and clean eating as a practice, introducing these ideas to the everyday lives of large online communities. This relatability was emphasised by conversion narratives that told how clean eaters developed their way of life and helped to demonstrate the achievability of clean lifestyles – how small changes in diet would improve the everyday health of the individual.

Clean eating's popularity declined following fierce criticism from food writers, scientists, and body-positive activists. This group linked

'Having been there ... I know how hard it is'   295

clean eaters' message of individual responsibility for health to the British government's austerity measures. As the safety net of the welfare state weakened, food banks and charities stepped in to provide access to food for those who were unable to afford it. Despite clean eaters choosing not to comment on politics, against the backdrop of increasing food poverty their insistence on clean eating as an affordable lifestyle that ordinary individuals could follow left them seeming out of touch, and as unwittingly promoting neoliberal approaches to healthcare such as 'healthism' (the view of personal health as the responsibility of the individual, and ill health as a personal failing).

This chapter explores the key role of relatability in the rise of clean eating and in critical challenges to it. It uses the career of one clean eater, Ella Mills, as a case study to illustrate how clean eaters emphasised the ordinariness of diet plans and lifestyles that could nevertheless produce extraordinary bodies in optimum health. It demonstrates how developing internet cultures have changed the way people interact with mass media, becoming part of online communities following seemingly 'ordinary' influencers. As the internet continues to be a large part of our everyday lives and everyday health, historians will need to engage with these online sources to access the lived experiences of historical actors.

What is clean eating?

Clean eating is a commitment to eating mostly wholefoods – unrefined plant foods such as vegetables and wholegrains – in as close to their natural state as possible, removing any food believed to be 'processed'. 'Processed', in this context, means any food understood to have been altered to prolong its shelf life or improve flavour; for example, white flour as opposed to wholemeal, or jarred sauces rather than home-made. This nearly always includes refined sugar, chemical preservatives, often dairy and meat, and any 'unpronounceable' ingredient with a long, multisyllabic chemical name, such as tert-Butylhydroquinone, a preservative found in vegetable oils, also known as E319. However, as critics such as Anthony Warner would later point out, almost all foods have a chemical name, which could fall into this category – for example, caffeine can also be known as

296 *Mass media and networks of communication*

Methyltheobromine.[3] In making ordinary ingredients, proven fit for consumption by various international food and health agencies, extraordinary, clean eaters set out a diet which their followers believe to be a natural and pure way of eating. In removing these elements from the diet, followers of clean eating believe that they are getting the best possible nutrition in a world that encourages fast food and eating for convenience.

The ideas present in the modern-day clean eating movement combine various diets and nutritional trends from past centuries, including the low-carbohydrate, high-protein elements of the Atkins diet, and the emphasis on wholefoods and what is historically considered natural from the Paleo diet, both of which were first developed in the 1970s and rose to popularity in the early 2000s.[4] However, rather than dieting with the sole aim of slimming down, clean eaters recentre their lives and diets around the ideals of clean eating, with a broader emphasis on mental wellbeing and mindfulness, alleviation of chronic symptoms, and natural products in cosmetics and the home. Clean eating often goes hand in hand with an emphasis on physical fitness, with advocates including body builders, personal trainers, and yoga teachers. The nature of these changes is supposed to positively impact on the everyday health and behaviour of followers who make small changes to improve their overall existence.

The first use of the word 'clean' linked to this style of eating is attributed to Tosca Reno and Alejandro Junger, both based in North America. Reno and Junger independently pioneered diets and detoxes which advocated the avoidance of alcohol, sugar, and over-processed food. They also emphasised good diet as a method for achieving good health and demonstrated an interest in 'superfoods' – foods believed to have extraordinary nutritional benefits.

Junger completed medical school in his native Uruguay before moving to New York, where he worked as a cardiologist, and then to India, where he found inspiration among the 'alternative' medicine of South-East Asia. This led to his interest in toxicity, which he understood to be the build-up of chemicals not naturally found in food, and therefore toxic to humans. This build-up, Junger believed, could lead to health issues including fatigue and digestive problems. To counteract these effects, Junger developed the 'Clean Program': an intense three-week diet that eliminated entire food groups, and several meals, and replaced them with juices. It banned caffeine,

'Having been there ... I know how hard it is'   297

dairy products, eggs, red meat, alcohol, and all preservatives, stipulated fresh, organic food, and encouraged filtered water. Junger insisted 'the thinner the liquid, the more intense the detox'. Each week of the diet promised different results: 'a surge of vibrant energy and clarity of mind, as toxins are released', allowing the individual to grasp 'what hunger really is', in week one; the disappearance of 'symptoms of imbalance' such as 'skin problems, weight issues, allergies, and intestinal issues' in week two; and 'physiological balance' with the removal of all toxins, and initial reversing of processes of disease and ageing as the cleanse ended in week three. Ultimately, Junger claimed, completion of the programme felt 'like cleaning dirty spectacles: you get a fresh vision of your world'.[5] Early celebrity endorsement from actress and wellbeing fanatic Gwyneth Paltrow enabled Junger's book to become a *New York Times* bestseller. His programme became a staple in the world of detoxing and furthered the concepts of 'clean' and cleansing.[6]

Where Junger's work focused on removing the toxicity created by modern life, American health and fitness writer Tosca Reno's work instead used clean eating principles to achieve the traditional goal of diets – weight loss. A former teacher, Reno described how meeting her second husband, Robert Kennedy, 'one of the biggest and most iconic publishers of fitness, health and bodybuilding magazines in the world', changed her from 'just an ordinary housewife living an ordinary life' into a successful bodybuilder.[7] Reno documented her physical transformation in her 'Raise the Bar' column in *Oxygen* magazine, which led to book contracts. Her 2007 diet and cookbook *The Eat-Clean Diet* was the first to directly link the concept of 'clean' with weight loss, health, and beauty. It set out her rules for a clean diet, most of which are still fundamental to the wider concept of clean eating over a decade later. These included eating regular, small meals every day; drinking plenty of water; and avoiding 'unclean' foods such as 'overprocessed, refined foods, especially white flour and sugar', saturated and trans fats, colas and juices, alcohol, and 'calorie dense foods that contain little or no nutritional value'. Reno viewed herself 'as the person who created and founded the Eat Clean movement', understanding the movement as nothing short of a 'revolution'.[8] Unlike most of the later clean eaters, Reno explicitly presented clean eating as a diet. Her books featured 'before and after' photos of her clean eating progress,

298 *Mass media and networks of communication*

alongside quotes from people who had successfully followed Reno's plan to lose weight.

The second wave of clean eaters, who rose to popularity in Britain during the second decade of the twenty-first century, were much less focused on possible weight loss. Rather, they emphasised the benefits of clean eating to the internal body and everyday health. These clean eaters often described how clean eating helped alleviate and cure illnesses apparently caused by their bodies' failure to cope with an 'unclean' diet. The most striking example of this approach is found in Ella Mills' biography. After suddenly falling ill during her undergraduate degree, Mills described how: 'I literally couldn't walk down the street, I slept for sixteen hours a day, was in chronic pain, had blackouts, never-ending heart palpitations, unbearable stomach issues, constant headaches [...] I was bedridden ninety-five per cent of the time.'[9] She was eventually diagnosed with postural tachycardia syndrome (PoTS), 'an abnormality of the autonomic nervous system' that causes dizziness, fainting, palpitations, and fatigue.[10] Mills later revealed other diagnoses of Ehlers-Danlos syndrome, which affects the production of collagen, and mast cell activation disorder, which causes random allergic reactions by activating mast cells. Treatments for these ill-understood conditions currently centre on symptom relief rather than cure, while advice on advocacy websites focuses on lifestyle changes.[11]

Overnight, Mills completely changed her diet in order to control her symptoms, starting 'a wholefoods, plant-based diet' and giving up 'all meat, dairy, sugar, gluten, anything processed and all chemicals and additives'. In part, Mills's attitude stemmed from a desire to avoid medication. She explained one of the key successes of her new diet as that 'in less than two years I was off all the medication I should have been on for life'.[12] This account reinforced her dietary choices as a necessity, rather than a short-lived diet focused on weight loss and body aesthetics: 'I eat the way I do because [...] it's the only way that I'm able to manage my illness. I want to – and have to – eat nourishing food all the time.'[13] It also puts forward clean eating as a holistic lifestyle bordering on alternative healing. For Mills, this management of her everyday health provided a solution to longer-term health issues.

This alignment of illness management with dietary practice is indicative of wider cultural shifts around this time. While weight-loss

'Having been there ... I know how hard it is' 299

diets had been linked directly to medical treatment for conditions such as diabetes for several decades, the late twentieth and early twenty-first centuries saw weight-loss diets increasingly also marketed as diets for health.[14] For example, the Fast Diet, popularised by journalist Michael Mosley in 2012, prompted widespread interest in intermittent fasting – Mosley's 5:2 diet consists of eating normally for five days a week and fasting by eating only five hundred calories for the remaining two. This diet book undeniably emphasises weight loss, with its cover depicting a measuring tape functioning as a belt, but it also suggests that intermittent fasting can help manage eczema, asthma, and psoriasis.[15] This broader context of societal concerns about weight loss and health, along with the belief that it is the individual's responsibility to manage chronic conditions, allowed its advocates to offer clean eating as a solution, while also marketing the approach as a sustainable and desirable lifestyle. Importantly, however, clean eating was not presented as directly comparable to weight-loss diets, even those which emphasised health. Rather, clean eaters believed they were encouraging people to make food choices which would shape entire lifestyles.

The food choices Mills outlined in her blog and multiple bestselling cookbooks were nearly identical to those of Tosca Reno. Both advocated for vegetables, organic food, no refined sugar, and limited processed carbohydrates. However, where Reno stressed strict rules, Mills emphasised that these ideals were not restrictive, sharing recipes for 'brownies, pizza and ice cream' which followed this guidance.[16] Where Reno encouraged lean meat, fish, and limited amounts of organic dairy, Mills followed a plant-based diet, although she avoided the term 'vegan' because it was possible to be a 'very unhealthy vegan'. Her lifestyle was instead 'all about whole, natural foods that nourish your body'.[17] In emphasising individual experiences of illness and dieting, clean eaters promised a new way of living which could alleviate symptoms, free followers from calorie counting, and make individuals truly happy – as long as they avoided processed foods.[18]

Clean eating and conversion narratives

To appeal to broad audiences, clean eaters relied on appearing relatable. If clean eaters were ordinary women living ordinary lives,

300   *Mass media and networks of communication*

then readers would believe that they too could achieve extraordinary bodies. To achieve this sense of relatability, clean eaters drew on diverse methods: using lived experiences to demonstrate expertise in the subject, usually in absence of genuine nutritional qualifications; sharing intimate details of their personal lives, including symptoms and weight, in published cookbooks and social media posts; and tying these elements together in the broader narratives of their clean eating journeys. As Adrienne Rose Bitar outlines in her study of American diet literature, these stories draw on similar tropes to religious conversion narratives, following 'along the arc of the Fall of Man' to 'remember an original, innocent world and mourn the descent of the human race into modern disease'.[19]

Similarly, clean eaters' life stories simultaneously emphasised the ordinary nature and immense potential of the individual, in heroic narratives of overcoming difficulty to achieve ultimate health and happiness.[20] Theologian Bruce Hindmarsh argues that rather than 'simply reporting data', authors of written religious conversion narratives 'are telling a story'. The autobiographical nature of these narratives implies trust in the author as reliable narrator, forming 'a kind of contract with the reader that the author intends to interpret his or her own life sincerely'. This contract encourages particular responses in readers because 'as soon we identify a good, we understand ourselves with reference to this good as nearer or further from it, and this puts us in a kind of moral space and on a journey that can be narrated'.[21] In (unconsciously) mimicking the narrative structures of heroic conversion narratives, clean eating books ultimately demanded an emotional and ethical response. By identifying clean narratives as 'good', readers place themselves in relation to this 'good' and aspire to become as good as clean eaters. To make this an achievable goal and to prove their authority on the subject, clean eaters draw on three key themes in their narratives: experiential expertise, individualism, and community.

Experiential expertise

The appeal of clean eating relies on its apparent success in transforming lives. Authors shared their own experiences of changing relationships with food, along with challenging illnesses and disorders, demonstrating their ability to relate to readers experiencing similar

'Having been there ... I know how hard it is'   301

issues. Clean eaters described, in ways which encouraged readers to trust their opinions, how they developed expertise to overcome these challenges.

Each narrative began with stories of reliance on junk or 'dirty' food. Most authors described relatively healthy childhoods, with wholesome home-cooked meals, outside play, and regular exercise. They contrasted this romanticised picture of happy childhood with early adulthood at university as a time of sugary alcohol on nights out, fast food, limited exercise, and high stress. In their search for quick, easy food and energy boosts, authors turned to food and drinks high in sugar, caffeine, carbohydrates, and preservatives. They justified their need for a complete lifestyle change by building on the American myth of the 'Freshman Fifteen' to shock readers with outlandish claims.[22] Mills described herself as 'a sugar monster, and I mean a total addict', who in her first year of university 'basically lived off a delicious mixture of Ben & Jerry's Cookie Dough ice cream, mountains of chocolate (preferably filled with gooey caramel) and lots of fizzy pick 'n' mix'.[23] The intention was to offer readers a sense of relatability, not to shame them; clean eaters who now had healthy lifestyles were once stereotypical students who consumed excessive amounts of junk food and alcohol, and their stories proved that it was easy to change that lifestyle. If the sugar-addicted writer could lose weight, improve her health, and become more beautiful through drastically changing her eating habits, anyone could.

Authors enhanced this sense of relatability by next detailing the breaking point which led them to clean eating. For Mills, this was a fateful holiday that worsened her chronic symptoms. She described 'being brought home, semi-conscious, in a wheelchair'.[24] This climactic event spurred her into action; like many clean eaters suffering from health issues, Mills uncovered the world of holistic and alternative medicine. She became interested in the concept of healing and was deeply influenced by Kris Carr, an American documentary maker and writer, whose clean eating-like 'Crazy Sexy Cancer' diet apparently prolonged her life expectancy after diagnosis of stage four cancer.[25] Other clean eaters similarly insisted on health rather than weight loss, presenting clean eating as an all-encompassing lifestyle rather than a traditional diet focused on weight loss and quick results.[26] Indeed, they presented clean eating as a sustainable long-term solution

302   *Mass media and networks of communication*

to problems created by dieting, such as obsessive calorie counting and regaining lost weight.[27]

Regardless of whether clean eaters focused on internal body and illness, or appearance and mental health, the ultimate outcome was the same. Clean eating miraculously cured the medical, emotional, and physical symptoms with which the story started. They used a discourse of awakening to describe this healing. Mills exclaimed, 'I felt healed! My healthy eating adventure had really worked [...] It felt like a miracle [...] I felt free and truly like myself again.'[28] Best of all, the miracle of clean eating was not a mystical, unachievable goal. Clean eaters like Mills used their own stories as proof that even the most ordinary of people could achieve health and happiness through extraordinary transformations.

Individualism

In their miraculous revelations, clean eaters believed they had found the solution to the problems of wider society. Mills referenced wider concerns about the quality of life in the modern world, discussing rising levels of obesity, poor work–life balance, increasing reliance on screens, and 'recent studies [which] show that just 27% of the UK population get their five-a-day'.[29] Such statements and statistics, often unevidenced, justified the social and moral mission of clean eaters. They not only helped individuals lose weight and feel better but were also helping to change society. Readers could also aspire to the utopian ideals of a simpler, happier, clean life. They often depicted achieving this lifestyle as easy; a person given the choice between an apple and a chocolate bar does not need a nutritional qualification to understand that the apple is the healthier choice. Clean eating was simply a series of healthier choices, encouraging readers to enjoy the sweetness of apples rather than chocolate bars, spurred on with recipes for clean eating sweet snacks such as energy balls made of dates and almond butter or brownies made with sweet potatoes.[30]

This belief in improving society through individual actions linked clean eating to neoliberalist ideologies of individual responsibility for health. Clean eating promised to create a healthy ideal body that also met traditional western beauty standards. Departing from the ideal of late twentieth-century waif-like supermodels, this body

'Having been there ... I know how hard it is'   303

must now be fit and able as well as thin, toned, white, glossy, and flawless.[31] The renewed emphasis on ability in this ideal reflects the wider growth of 'healthism'. Initially defined by political economist Robert Crawford in 1980, 'healthism' is 'the preoccupation with personal health as a primary – often *the* primary – focus for the definition and achievement of wellbeing; a goal which is to be attained primarily through the modification of life styles'.[32] In clean eating narratives, healthism interweaved with (implicit) views of ill health and sickness as the result of individual failure. Clean eaters preferred to remain conspicuously apolitical, neither presenting illness as caused by individuals nor engaging fully with wider societal debates or campaigning for policy changes at a state level. However, they did believe that individuals were responsible for improving their own health. Mills's success as a clean eater was intertwined with her body's failure, while her reluctance to remain on prescription medication or to depend in the long-term on health systems reflects healthism. Such dependence would be antithetical to the clean eating belief in individual responsibility for health and happiness.

Clean eaters were careful to avoid dispensing specific health advice. Their cookbooks contained disclaimers reminding readers to consult medical professionals for advice regarding health and diet. Despite Mills's direct link between the alleviation of her PoTS symptoms and her new diet, it was readers' own responsibility to realise that this was not prescriptive health advice. Legally, clean eaters had to avoid even implicit claims to medical expertise. Rather, Mills promoted general 'wellness'. However, if the purpose of clean eating is to achieve a state of 'wellness', with the health and medical implications of the term, these cookbooks did make quasi-medical claims.

Community

Clean eaters accentuated organic growth, rather than claims to business acumen, in explaining their success. This emphasis on organic growth partly reflected the reality of clean eaters' rapid success. They quickly became 'microcelebrities' through encouraging readers' engagement and emotional investment by sharing their personal stories. The stress on organic growth also mirrored the importance of all things 'natural' in a clean lifestyle – likewise, clean eaters' audiences had grown sustainably, nurtured with daily contact on

Mass media and networks of communication

social media, as opposed to traditional diet literature's reliance for success on celebrity endorsement and large marketing budgets. In this sense, the weight given to organic growth in their narratives was another strategy to emphasise relatability.

Nevertheless, clean eaters' narratives followed the story-like structure of the traditional diet literature they railed against. Having suffered and found a cure, clean eaters' heroic conversion narratives conclude with the desire to share the lessons learned from their experiences. Others must learn about this miraculous cure; absolutely everyone can and should convert to their lifestyle. Authors invited readers to join them in this venture, creating online communities based around their lifestyle. Mills stated that 'Deliciously Ella [...] stopped being just about my personal journey, and instead became about a sense of community, a shared belief and ways to expand, introduce and make plant-based eating more aspirational and delicious.'[33] This community building invited readers into clean eaters' lives, with real-time updates on their diets and days, and was therefore vital to the rise of clean eating and the maintenance of its relatability, as well as its presence in the everyday life of millions.

In this respect, clean eating followed similar trends to the fashion and beauty industries. The rise of the internet and the popularity of social media enabled young women pursuing hobbies or passions to set up blogs and social media pages, in this way creating heavily invested micro-communities. In setting themselves up as 'public persona[s] to be consumed by others', using 'social media to amass enough fans to support themselves through their online creative activities while remaining unknown to most and ignored by mainstream media', influencers also became 'microcelebrities'.[34] The term 'microcelebrity' highlights the perceived 'authenticity' of the relationship between the individual who creates the content and its consumer. This authentic relationship is established through the consumer's ability to peer directly into the creator's life, unlike traditional celebrities whose relationship to fans is filtered through publicists and the media.[35] Fans could directly interact with microcelebrities (including clean eaters), sending them direct messages, receiving replies to comments, and voting in polls. As such, the influencer as microcelebrity occupies a unique space as both celebrity and consumer brand, as indicated by usernames which became brand names, such as Deliciously Ella. Fans imagined clean eaters as authentic individuals,

'Having been there ... I know how hard it is' 305

followed them as celebrities, and created aspirational communities around them.

As in religious conversion narratives, clean eaters used their autobiographies to 'cement' their relationship to their new communities, 'taking on the language and appropriating the narrative of that community'.[36] As in traditional diet literature, they encouraged readers to join 'a shared dream to remake a lost world' by adopting the language and narrative of clean eating.[37] This concept of a 'shared dream' was seen throughout clean eating books, as authors spoke directly to readers, inviting them to imitate this lifestyle and reassuring them that they could achieve this dream. Readers were expected to follow this same heroic narrative and transform their lives from ordinary to extraordinary. Furthermore, through engagement with clean eaters' social media, this 'shared dream' could become a shared life, as readers were invited to witness, 'like', and comment on meals with friends, yoga classes, dates, and weddings in clean eaters' lives, generating a tangible relationship between creator and consumer.

Readers became attached to clean eaters because they believed in the inherent goodness of their lifestyles, centred on clean food, exercise, and happiness. In becoming attached, readers wished to 'convert' or change their own lifestyles and join the heroic narrative. This narrative was not exclusively found in books, read once and then abandoned, but demonstrated across social media profiles, with new content posted daily. Readers could continue this narrative for a prolonged time, as they bore witness to the clean eater's success. This insight into and connection with the (heavily edited) ordinary lives of clean eaters further cemented readers' belief in the achievability of a lifestyle that required nothing more than dedication to a clean diet.

The backlash

This apparent achievability at first made it difficult to critique clean eating. As food writer Bee Wilson noted, 'at first, clean eating sounded modest and even homespun: rather than counting calories, you would eat as many nutritious home-cooked substances as possible'.[38] Meanwhile, chef and food scientist Anthony Warner lamented that 'its holistic approach, its lack of hard rules and its selective embracing

306 *Mass media and networks of communication*

of occasional fragments of science' made 'engaging with clean eating as hard as nailing gluten-free jelly to a wall'.[39] Nevertheless, as clean eating reached public prominence it prompted a backlash. In 2015, a group of anti-clean eaters emerged in the mainstream British media, including Wilson, Warner, chef Nigella Lawson, and food writer Ruby Tandoh. These critics shared their concerns about the trend, especially clean eating's moralistic overtones and its similarities with traditional fad diets. This backlash had thematic ties with fat activism and the body-positive movement, particularly in its critiques of a thin-obsessed society controlled by the weight-loss industry.[40]

Critics often focused on the privileged status of clean eaters, who were generally upper middle-class, white or white-passing, conventionally attractive women who undoubtedly benefited from both personal and structural privilege. This led to criticisms of nepotism and elitism. The majority of clean eaters attended fee-paying private schools, for example, Madeleine Shaw attended Streatham and Clapham High School and Melissa Hemsley attended Surbiton High School. Mills, the daughter of former Labour MP Shaun Woodward and Camilla Woodward, studied first at Rugby School and then the University of St Andrews, where she modelled in her spare time before her health declined. She is the granddaughter of Lord Sainsbury, owner of the supermarket chain Sainsbury's, one of the major nationwide stockists of Mills's product line. Her husband, and chief executive officer of the Deliciously Ella brand, is the son of former Labour MP Baroness Tessa Jowell and international corporate lawyer David Mills.

Even without specific connections that furthered their careers, most clean eaters benefited from financially secure backgrounds, which allowed them the time and space to develop their food knowledge and public profiles. The commercial success of their clean eating ventures extended this privilege, as they generated large incomes and became part of the mainstream food scene in Britain. Mills, for example, has published six cookbooks, including the best-selling debut cookbook of all time (over 30,000 copies sold in its first week, with an eventual bestseller award for selling over 250,000 copies).[41] Her fifth book, and the first of her books to explicitly describe itself as plant-based – in part due to the increasing popularity of veganism in Britain by the late 2010s – was the fastest-selling vegan cookbook of all time.[42] The Deliciously Ella snack

'Having been there ... I know how hard it is'   307

range, including energy balls, granola, cereal bars, frozen meals, and frozen desserts, has been hugely successful. By 2020 it was stocked 'in around 6,000 stores across the UK and Ireland', including Sainsbury's, Tesco, and Starbucks.[43]

Despite claims to ordinariness, the maintenance of a clean eating lifestyle also requires a certain level of privilege. The ability to eat clean and avoid convenience foods relies on basic cooking skills, access to kitchen equipment, having the time and energy to cook, and the ability to find and pay for sometimes hard-to-source ingredients. The assumption of accessibility is in itself indicative of privilege, especially against the backdrop of rising food insecurity and poverty in twenty-first-century Britain.[44] Likewise, clean eaters' statements about rising rates of obesity and lifestyle-related conditions do not take into account the effects of increased food poverty.[45] Critics condemned this lack of interest in and awareness of how 'ordinary' people live, as well as clean eaters' constructions of imagined readers as reflections of themselves.

Ruby Tandoh objected to implied distinctions between 'clean' and 'dirty' food. She argued that within the logic of the saying 'you are what you eat', 'junk food makes for junk people, and unfamiliar food makes for strange, "different" people'. In much of the West, 'where whiteness is seen as default, "plain" foods can come to stand for the status quo'. Therefore, the 'othering' and exoticisation of food has a dual implication. On one hand, some sorts of 'other' foods, linked to 'other' people, are seen as unappealing. They are unfamiliar, unusual, and often the object of disgust. Tandoh referred to her own experience as the 'kid who [...] got laughed at for their "weird", "smelly" packed lunch'.[46] Alternatively, the 'superfoods' that clean eaters promoted, such as chia seeds, quinoa, and acai, became understood as the 'right' kind of exotic. Mills described chia seeds as 'magic' and 'powerhouses of nutrition', quinoa as 'amazing' in both taste and 'how good it makes you feel', and acai as 'delicious' and 'unbelievably rich in antioxidants'.[47] As Tandoh argues, such descriptions fit 'into a pretty long and established tradition of white people grabbing hold of symbols of otherness while it suits them, and quickly letting go as soon as fortunes or fashions change'.[48] The obsession of predominantly white clean eaters with non-white culture expanded beyond food, with yoga and meditation espoused as parts of a 'mindful' clean lifestyle.

308 *Mass media and networks of communication*

Tandoh saw this aspect of clean eating as an explicit extension of the white upper middle-class moralising mission. Comparing the 'scavenging' of 'barbarians' with the '"whole" foods' of 'the ruling classes', Tandoh argued that 'the heart of it is that genteel, considered and aesthetically minded equate with "good", and necessary and ravenous mean "bad" [...] the moral character seems to be as much about who's eating as it is about the food itself'. The cheap, easily accessible foods of the working classes, full of processed ingredients, were by implication 'dirty' in the clean eaters' worldview. This understanding extended beyond the content of the food. Tandoh pointed out that the 'sparse, clean aesthetic' of clean eating, designed to appeal on Instagram, stood in opposition to 'the visual cacophony of supermarkets, big brands, and colourful, attention-grabbing fast food slogans'. The 'nothingness, nature and blank space' promoted by clean eaters signified class status in a world where 'having stuff' is no longer a marker of wealth.[49] By linking clean eating to a minimalist aesthetic, the claims that it was a 'lifestyle, not a diet' were confirmed in the eyes of both clean eaters and critics alike.

Tandoh also scathingly dismissed clean eating as a form of miraculous healing: 'I see your Jesus healing the blind, and I raise you Ella Mills and her postural tachycardia, the symptoms of which "all but disappeared" with the help of a vegan diet.'[50] Due to her visibility and success, Mills was the frequent target of such criticism. She therefore also took a leading role in formulating the response that became characteristic of the clean eating community: restating that clean eaters had never claimed to be scientists or medical professionals, arguing that critics had twisted the word 'clean' into something negative and unrecognisable, and even that clean eaters had never formally associated themselves with the term, but it had been pushed upon them by other people.[51]

Conclusion

On 29 September 2022 Ella Mills shared screenshots of a *Times* newspaper article to the Deliciously Ella Instagram and her personal account. The headline read 'YouGov survey portrays nation of tired, overweight layabouts', and Mills's accompanying caption lamented the lack of vegetables in British diets and how 'the public health

'*Having been there ... I know how hard it is*'   309

agenda and a focus on disease prevention appears to be rapidly slipping to the bottom of the government's agenda'.[52] Mills's framing of the story reflected the view, fundamental to clean eaters' narratives, that clean eating could improve individual health outcomes. The response to the post was almost entirely negative. With rising food and fuel prices leading to a cost of living crisis, commenters shared their disappointment in Mills's continued emphasis on the individual and seeming lack of awareness of the dire socioeconomic context. Clean eating is no longer as prominent as it once was, but posts like this indicate clean eaters' continued ability to attract attention and controversy. The episode also shows that, despite rejecting the term 'clean eating', figures like Mills maintain their emphasis on individualism, healthism, and the potential of the right diet to change the health of the nation. Criticisms of clean eating that focused on these themes therefore remain just as relevant.

In promising readers an attainable lifestyle which could cure illness, alleviate symptoms, and make the body beautiful, clean eaters emphasised relatability. They highlighted the normality of their own lives before clean eating, drawing attention to obsessions with sugar and fad dieting that led to pain, unhappiness, and physical symptoms. They invited readers to place themselves in this lifestyle, presenting the extraordinary changes to their bodies and minds as transformative but achievable through an essentially ordinary lifestyle. They claimed to eat whatever and whenever they liked, apart from processed foods, and presented this simple way of eating as offering freedom from planned and restrictive calorie-based fad diets. In holding out this heroic conversion narrative of lifestyle change, readers, as reflections of clean eaters, were encouraged to believe that they could become as happy, healthy, and beautiful as clean eaters.

Of course, this change was not that simple, but relied on a certain amount of privilege. Despite claims otherwise, clean eating took time to learn about the concept and to plan and prepare meals, and money and time to source unusual ingredients. Against the background of twenty-first-century Britain, which saw rising food poverty due to the impact of austerity measures, clean eating was ripe for criticism. Despite distancing themselves from the phrase 'clean eating', figures such as Mills continue to promote the same dietary practices and lifestyle through their social media careers as influencers and through a series of successful cookbooks. In line with religious conversion

310   *Mass media and networks of communication*

narratives, a key part of the clean eating mission was to encourage others to follow this path and take responsibility for their everyday health through making lifestyle changes, improving the lives of both individuals and society. Despite their avowedly apolitical stance, it is therefore difficult to see the difference between the stance of clean eaters and that of Conservative politicians who insist that health and happiness is within the grasp of everyone, if only they will put the effort in.

Notes

1 Tosca Reno, *The Eat-Clean Diet: Fast Fat Loss that Lasts Forever!* (Mississauga, ON: Robert Kennedy Publishing, 2007), p. v.

2 The most successful British clean eaters have all been women, perhaps because blogs and social media are generally more popular among women, but also perhaps because women are encouraged to care about their health and their bodies more than men. See: Stephanie Alice Baker and Michael James Walsh, '"Good morning fitfam": top posts, hashtags and gender display on Instagram', *New Media and Society*, 20:12 (2018); Alice E. Marwick, 'Gender, sexuality, and social media', in Jeremy Hunsinger and Theresa M. Senft (eds), *The Social Media Handbook* (New York: Taylor & Francis, 2014).

3 Anthony Warner, *The Angry Chef: Bad Science and the Truth about Healthy Eating* (London: OneWorld, 2007), p. 203.

4 Laura E. Matarese and Glenn K. Harvin, 'The Atkins diet', in Caroline Apovian, Elizabeth Brouillard, and Lorraine Young (eds), *Clinical Guide to Popular Diets* (Boca Raton, FL: CRC Press, Taylor & Francis Group, 2018); Laura Andromalos, 'The Paleo diet', in Apovian, Brouillard, and Young (eds.), *Clinical Guide to Popular Diets*.

5 Alejandro Junger, *Clean: The Revolutionary Program to Restore the Body's Natural Ability to Heal Itself* (New York: HarperOne, 2009), pp. 10–11, 164.

6 Gwyneth Paltrow, 'The power of detoxification and getting clean', *Goop* (30 October 2008): https://goop.com/wellness/detox/the-importance-of-detoxing-your-body/ (accessed 21 August 2019); Alejandro Junger, 'What people are saying', *Clean*: www.cleanprogram.com/pages/stories (accessed 28 January 2020).

7 Tosca Reno, 'My story', *Tosca Reno*: https://toscareno.com/my-story/ (accessed 20 February 2020).

8 Reno, *The Eat-Clean Diet*, p. 15.

'Having been there ... I know how hard it is'   311

9   Ella Woodward, *Deliciously Ella* (London: Yellow Kite, 2015), p. 7.
10 PoTS UK Team, 'What is PoTS?', *PoTS UK* (1 February 2015): www.potsuk.org/what_is_pots2 (accessed 28 August 2020).
11 See Lorna Nicholson, 'Important lifestyle changes – diet and fluids', *PoTS UK* (22 August 2020): www.potsuk.org/diet_and_fluids (accessed 28 August 2020); Ehlers-Danlos Support UK, 'Diet and EDS research fund', *Ehlers-Danlos Support UK*: www.ehlers-danlos.org/studies/diet-and-eds-research-fund/ (accessed 28 August 2020); The UK Mastocytosis Support Group, 'Living with mast cell disease', *UK Masto*: https://ukmasto.org/living-with-mcd/ (accessed 28 August 2020).
12 Woodward, *Deliciously Ella*, pp. 8–9.
13 Ella Mills, *Deliciously Ella with Friends* (London: Yellow Kite, 2017), p. 10.
14 Martin D. Moore, 'Food as medicine: diet, diabetes management, and the patient in twentieth century Britain', *Journal of the History of Medicine and Allied Sciences*, 73:2 (2018).
15 Michael Mosley and Mimi Spencer, *The Fast Diet: Revised and Updated* (London: Short Books Ltd, 2015), p. 1. See also *Horizon: Eat, Fast and Live Longer*, dir. Kate Dart, (BBC, 6 August 2012): www.bbc.co.uk/programmes/b01lxyzc (accessed 26 February 2020).
16 Woodward, *Deliciously Ella*, p. 9.
17 Woodward, *Deliciously Ella*, p. 10.
18 Alice Liveing, *Clean Eating Alice: Eat Well Every Day: Nutritious, Healthy Recipes for Life on the Go* (London: Thorsons, 2016), pp. 11, 17–18.
19 Adrienne Rose Bitar, *Diet and the Disease of Civilisation* (New Brunswick, NJ: Rutgers University Press, 2018), p. 4; Adrienne Rose Johnson, 'The Paleo diet and the American weight loss utopia, 1975–2014', *Utopian Studies*, 26:1 (2015).
20 Alice Liveing, *Clean Eating Alice: The Body Bible* (London: Thorsons, 2016), p. 18.
21 Bruce Hindmarsh, 'Religious conversion as narrative and autobiography', in Lewis R. Rambo and Charles E. Farhadian (eds), *The Oxford Handbook of Religious Conversion* (Oxford: Oxford University Press, 2014). Quotations at pp. 344, 352, and 361.
22 This is the alleged weight gain of first-year university students struggling to manage total control over their diet, stress, the ready availability of unhealthy food, and increased alcohol use. Jay L. Zagorsky and Patricia K. Smith, 'The freshman 15: a critical time for obesity intervention or media myth?', *Social Science Quarterly*, 92:5 (2011).
23 Woodward, *Deliciously Ella*, p. 7.
24 Woodward, *Deliciously Ella*, p. 8.

312   *Mass media and networks of communication*

25 Woodward, *Deliciously Ella*, p. 8. See also: Kris Carr, *Crazy Sexy Cancer Tips* (Lanham, MD: Rowman & Littlefield, 2007); *Crazy Sexy Cancer*, dir. Kris Carr (Red House Pictures, 2007).

26 Liveing, *Clean Eating Alice: The Body Bible*, p. 18.

27 Madeleine Shaw, *Ready Steady Glow* (London: Orion, 2016), p. 7.

28 Woodward, *Deliciously Ella*, p. 9; Liveing, *Clean Eating Alice: The Body Bible*, p. 8.

29 Ella Mills, *Deliciously Ella: The Plant-Based Cookbook* (London: Yellow Kite, 2018), p. 19.

30 Reno, *The Eat-Clean Diet*, 76.

31 Sean Redmond, 'Thin white women in advertising: deathly corporeality', *Journal of Consumer Culture*, 3:2 (2003); Frances Bozsik, Brooke L. Whisenhunt, Danae L. Hudson, et al., 'Thin is in? Think again: the rising importance of muscularity in the thin ideal female body', *Sex Roles*, 79 (2018).

32 Robert Crawford, 'Healthism and the medicalisation of everyday life', *International Journal of Health Services*, 10:3 (1980), p. 368.

33 Mills, *Deliciously Ella: The Plant-Based Cookbook*, p. 12.

34 Alice E. Marwick, 'You may know me from YouTube: (micro-)celebrity in social media', in P. David Marshall and Sean Redmond (eds), *A Companion to Celebrity* (Chichester: John Wiley & Sons, 2016), p. 334; Alice E. Marwick and danah boyd, 'I tweet honestly, I tweet passionately: Twitter users, context collapse, and the imagined audience', *New Media and Society*, 13:1 (2011).

35 Theresa M. Senft, *Camgirls: Celebrity and Community in the Age of Social Networks* (New York: Peter Lang Publishing, 2008).

36 Hindmarsh, 'Religious conversion as narrative and autobiography', p. 357.

37 Bitar, *Diet and the Disease of Civilisation*, p. 149.

38 Bee Wilson, 'Why we fell for clean eating', *Guardian*, 11 August 2017: www.theguardian.com/lifeandstyle/2017/aug/11/why-we-fell-for-clean-eating (accessed 29 September 2017).

39 Warner, *The Angry Chef*, p. 203.

40 Charlotte Cooper, *Fat Activism: A Radical Social Movement* (Bristol: HammerOn Press, 2016).

41 John Lewis, 'Food blogger Woodward sets number one record', *The Bookseller*, 4 February 2015: www.thebookseller.com/news/food-blogger-woodward-makes-number-one-record (accessed 5 September 2020); Natasha Onwuemezi, 'Ella Mills wins Nielsen Award for selling 250k copies', *The Bookseller*, 25 July 2017: www.thebookseller.com/news/ella-mills-wins-specsavers-bestseller-award-597156 (accessed 5 September 2020).

'*Having been there ... I know how hard it is*'   313

42 Keira O'Brien, 'Deliciously Ella elbows Dan Brown from the top spot', *The Bookseller*, 29 August 2018: www.thebookseller.com/news/deliciously-ella-elbows-dan-brown-top-spot-852806 (accessed 20 June 2020); Corey Lee Wren, 'The Vegan Society and social movement professionalisation, 1944–2017', *Food and Foodways: History and Culture of Human Nourishment*, 27:3 (2019).

43 Ella Mills, 'About', *Deliciously Ella*: https://deliciouslyella.com/about/ (accessed 28 August 2020).

44 Rachel Loopstra, Aaron Reeves, David Taylor-Robinson, Ben Barr, Martin McKee, and David Stuckler, 'Austerity, sanctions, and the rise of food banks in the UK', *BMJ* 350:8003 (8 April 2015).

45 NHS, 'Children from poorer backgrounds more affected by rise in childhood obesity', *NHS – Behind the Headlines* (21 March 2018): www.nhs.uk/news/obesity/children-poorer-backgrounds-more-affected-rise-childhood-obesity/ (accessed 6 April 2020).

46 Ruby Tandoh, *Eat Up!* (London: Serpent's Tail, 2018), pp. 63–4.

47 Mills, *Deliciously Ella*, pp. 17, 32, 209.

48 Tandoh, *Eat Up!*, p. 65.

49 Tandoh, *Eat Up!*, pp. 173, 195.

50 Tandoh, *Eat Up!*, p. 71.

51 See *Horizon: Clean Eating – The Dirty Truth*, dir. Tristan Quinn (BBC, 19 January 2017): www.bbc.co.uk/programmes/b08bhd29 (accessed 20 June 2020); Rachel Moss, 'Clean eating Alice on why she's keeping her name despite the trend's dark side', *The Huffington Post*, 31 January 2017: www.huffingtonpost.co.uk/entry/clean-eating-alice-on-backlash_uk_5890a8d7e4b03ab749ddaf69 (accessed 21 June 2020).

52 Ella Mills, Times Article, *Instagram* (29 September 2022): www.instagram.com/p/CjFo75Qoj1I/?hl=en (accessed 10 November 2022). For the full article, see: Andrew Ellson, 'YouGov health survey portrays nation of tired, overweight layabouts', *The Times*, 29 September 2022: www.thetimes.co.uk/article/yougov-health-survey-portrays-nation-of-tired-overweight-layabouts-g8dm97w08 (accessed 10 November 2022).

Part IV

Subjectivity and intersubjectivity

Part IV: Introduction

Kate Mahoney and Tracey Loughran

It is still too long until lunchtime. My shoulders ache a little from an early morning swim. I sit up straight to type and feel tension in my neck. Breathing in, I catch a hint of chlorine. My muscles are tired but my mind is alert. This is why I swim – to keep a clear mind, to know the power of my body, to feel active despite stationary days in front of a computer screen. Somewhere, months after I type these words, you might feel more conscious of your own body as you read them. Perhaps you are in an office much like mine, sitting at a workstation that is checked once a year to ensure that it conforms to health and safety regulations: a fixed height desk, a monitor set up to promote good posture, a chair adjustable in height with adequate support for the lumbar region, and mouse positioned so that it can be used with relaxed arm and straight wrist.[1] More likely, you are somewhere else: at a library desk, book flat down, slumped forward to read, pen at the ready in case I type something of relevance to your own research; in a coffee shop at a too-small table, wondering how long it's okay to stay after finishing your drink, unable to fully concentrate because of the noise; curled up on a chair at home, suddenly aware of your poor posture and the too-bright glare of the tablet. Wherever you are, I am writing to you, at a distance of time as well as place, and you are reading my words. A relationship, of some sort, has been established between us.

'Two persons, first person and second person: you and I, you and me.'[2] A person is a subject, a self, an individual consciousness possessed of thoughts, feelings, emotions – subjectivity. Humans live in societies, and so each person exists in relation to other subjects,

318   *Subjectivity and intersubjectivity*

selves, individual consciousnesses, and subjectivities. As we encounter others and share understandings of the world around us, we experience our identities through intersubjectivity.[3] Even if we exist to each other only as words on a page, as one felt self plus an imagined writer/reader, we are still in an intersubjective relationship. Moreover, because we are bodies as well as selves, this is an embodied relationship, felt in my chlorine-dry skin and your hunched back, in the clatter of my fingers on the keyboard, in the texture of the book jacket in your hand or the smoothness of the screen you tap. If we were in the same room, speaking, our responses to each other would modulate our relationship and our sense of our own selves within that relationship: were you wrong to tell me that secret? What have I said in response that made your eyes narrow? Is there any way you can backtrack now? Should I have tried harder to hide the surprise in my voice?

Subjectivities and intersubjectivities, made up of outlooks, emotions, and bodily sensations, constitute experiences of 'everyday health' and must form part of its history. More than this, historians are living, breathing people with our own subjectivities and health experiences, and our own relationships to our sources and our participants. We may choose not to position ourselves as part of the history, but we cannot stand outside and look upon 'everyday health' as impartial observers.[4] Of course, history is always and inevitably perspectival, no matter what the topic. But some areas of research are also likely to feel closer to the bone for more people because they relate to fundamental aspects of human experience. If we research and write about self, health, and embodiment, we are concerned with experiences close to ourselves – even if we do not share the specific experiences that we research, or include our own experiences in the text. (And, if you disagree, think about this: does it bother you that a co-written section introduction starts with a first-person experience, and you're not sure whose it is?) Part IV therefore explores ways of researching and writing about 'everyday health' that focus on subjectivity and/or intersubjectivity, highlighting the challenges that individuals in the past faced in articulating the embodied self, and those that researchers now face in negotiating their own relationships to emotive topics.

Hannah Froom (chapter 13) examines girls' experiences of menstruation in postwar Britain, arguing that within a 'culture of

Part IV: Introduction 319

concealment' that stigmatised menstruation, girls forced to use ineffective menstrual technologies became hyper-aware of their bleeding bodies. Drawing on a unique archive of women's life-writing about their youthful experiences, Froom reflects on how secrecy and shame structure women's abilities to remember, articulate, and make sense of their menstrual experiences – and how lacunae in the historical record make it even more difficult to forge experience-centred, 'everyday' understandings of menstruation that could help to challenge stigma today. Rosie Gahnstrom, Lucy Robinson, and Rachel Thomson (chapter 14) pick up this theme of young women's struggles to negotiate responses to contradictory pressures in their exploration of sexual risk, reward, and responsibility in the late 1980s. More than three decades later, they revisit a feminist research project that sought to centre young women's voices, relocate the importance of that historical moment, and reflect on the differences in what researchers saw then and what they see now. As they consider their own roles as feminist researchers, in interviewing young women and within intergenerational teams, they also make visible the figure of the researcher and the influence of her relationship to the past and present on research.

These last themes are explored in different ways in the final three chapters of the volume, which all adopt a first-person reflexive stance. Kate Mahoney (chapter 15) extends the discussion of intergenerational dynamics in research contexts, focusing on how and why oral history interviewers and participants claim belonging through positioning themselves as members of specific 'generations', and what this tells us about intersubjectivity in the interview process. Mahoney considers the unconscious identifications and projections that she brought to interviews and argues that researchers' reflection on their emotions can not only improve interview practice but is also an important element of self-care. Tracey Loughran (chapter 16) also probes oral history practice to think about the ambiguous responsibilities of the researcher for the afterlives of interviews. She proposes that oral historians seek ways to remain alive to what is at stake for interviewees when their stories are archived and describes her own experiment in trying to cultivate an emotionally engaged ethics. Finally, Carol Tulloch (chapter 17) tells the story of how the COVID-19 pandemic affected her sense of self and wellbeing, as a Black British woman and as a researcher, through unravelling the

320 *Subjectivity and intersubjectivity*

yarn of a yellow cable-knit jumper that she bought early in the first UK lockdown. This exploration of making and remaking the self at home, and of the emotional resonances of this period of emergency, invites us to reconsider how we define both the 'self' and 'everyday health', and the assumptions we make about how and where each is situated.

At issue in many of these chapters is who has the power to speak in different contexts and who is heard, and what is at stake in recording the self at (and for) different times and places.[5] Understanding 'everyday health', as the other parts of this volume have demonstrated, involves shifting from a top-down to bottom-up perspective, and subsequently reassessing who or what matters in history. When we go one step further, and centre subjectivity and intersubjectivity, we also question the ideal of 'scientific objectivity' that has traditionally governed the discipline of history. Ways of writing about subjectivity and intersubjectivity originated outside of history and took some time to infiltrate the discipline.[6] It is no accident that historians Froom, Mahoney, and Loughran invoke the methods and approaches of other disciplines in their chapters (anthropology, philosophy, psychology, and qualitative social science); that Tulloch is a design historian who is also a writer and curator, and who holds the expansive post of 'Professor of Dress, Diaspora, and Transnationalism'; and that sociologist Thomson, social researcher Gahnstrom, and historian Robinson have collaboratively produced a chapter that examines intersubjectivity within research processes.

Researching subjectivity and intersubjectivity involves working beyond the conventional boundaries of the historical discipline and finding new hearts (focal points, pulsating with emotion) for our histories.[7] As Froom suggests, this means centring different gazes. As we think about and from the perspective of neglected groups – in this section, girls, women, diasporic populations – we also open up topics that are central to the everyday and embodied experiences of millions – the home, dress, menstrual technologies – but that have been written off as unimportant and frivolous, and not the 'right' subject matter of history ... precisely because they are associated with those marginalised groups. Moreover, thinking from and about 'othered' perspectives requires different ways of researching and writing. It means seeking out and taking seriously first-person testimonies in social surveys or qualitative/life-history interviews; it

Part IV: Introduction 321

means bringing those otherwise 'hidden from history' into the archive, onto the record; it can mean bringing ourselves, as researchers, into the story.[8] As Tulloch argues, it means that we have to recognise and accommodate subjectivity because this is a crucial part of how we make meaning in our research.

This recognition of subjectivity demands understanding of different ways that people compose the self. The chapters in this section examine written, spoken, and embodied narratives as forms in which people communicate their identities and experiences. This aspect of communication is essential: it reminds us that understanding selfhood involves looking not only inwards, but outwards to both social relationships (no self exists in isolation) and culture (the crucible in which the self is forged). The psychic structure of the self is formed out of individual past and experience, but also out of elements shared within the wider culture that affect when and how people can speak, the coherence of their narratives, and how they will be heard (if at all).[9] Where Part III looked at how mass media constructs and disseminates ideas of 'everyday health', here authors focus on the effects of these discourses on audiences. Froom and Gahnstrom et al. consider how mass-market magazines expressed and shaped powerful but contradictory norms of feminine behaviour that girls and young women struggled to negotiate in their own lives. If these chapters underline that the dominant culture can silence those perceived as marginal, relegating their intimate experiences to sources of shame, then Tulloch shows that diasporic cultures, stretching across oceans, also provide symbols of belonging and connection that enable resilience in the face of oppression. These symbols travel across time as well as place and accumulate new layers of meaning as they do so; in the 1930s the Aran jumper emerged as a sign of Irish independence, in the 1960s it became part of Irish tourism, and nowadays it can act as shorthand for a certain type of authenticity that simultaneously evokes 'Irishness' but has no borders.[10]

Understanding how people compose the self also throws researchers into direct confrontation with the different temporal registers of those selves. All the chapters in this section deal with memory, the life-course, and the collision of past and present narratives of selfhood. Froom explores how women's testimonies of their menstrual lives involved new encounters with their girlhood selves that resonated in the present.[11] For Mahoney, the intersections of different models

322 *Subjectivity and intersubjectivity*

of generational experience were directly present in the research encounter, and coming to understand the reasons for an (implicit) clash of perspectives elucidates the assumptions and projections of interviewer and interviewee. That clash is a sometimes painful encounter with her own past selves for Loughran, as she revisits her own interview and the moment of that interview in the not-quite aftermath of the COVID-19 pandemic. This attention to how the moment in time affects the outcome of research is amplified in Tulloch's account of how her pandemic (and post-pandemic) self was formed out of past practices and objects, as she ricocheted between past and present in the alien temporalities of lockdown. Meanwhile, in revisiting present-centred narratives gathered in the 1980s, Gahnstrom et al. retheorise that moment in time, but also the different interpretations of researchers of different ages to young women's accounts; from this, they propose that emphasis on temporal flux is a productive way of disrupting narratives of progress that fail to illuminate the complexity of past or present and should not be carried into the future.

Gahnstrom et al. explicitly situate this concern with temporality as an outcome of their location within a feminist tradition 'that involves legacies and seeks to imagine futures'. The contributors to Part IV all identify as feminist scholars, and this is not surprising. The earliest impulses to explorations of subjectivity and intersubjectivity came from within feminist scholarship.[12] In examining from different angles the agentic capacities of girls and women (including female researchers) despite the structural constraints on their lives, these chapters tackle fundamental and still-urgent questions for feminist research. In troubling the equation of agency with empowerment and asking who is qualified to speak for and about girls' and women's lives, they demonstrate that expertise and experience in relation to 'everyday health' are complex matters in the present as well as the past. In creating forms of history that are embodied and vulnerable, they extend the feminist refusal of masculinist paradigms of knowledge and knowledge creation evident across so many chapters in Part I. In this section, the embodied self is positioned as an essential subject for history and as an essential position from which the historian speaks. The chapters in this section centre the embodied emotions, experiences, and memories of girls and women. In doing so, they cannot but provoke questions about vulnerability and

Part IV: Introduction

disclosure, whether this is in relation to respondents' difficulties in discussing taboo subjects, the injunctions to talk/confess that participants or researchers face, or the emotional costs of moving beyond the safe(r) territory of the third person. But if there are risks in this way of practising history, the rewards are even greater: we forge new connections, we speak across generations, we change what (and who) is in the archive, we transform history. We make it a place and a practice for others like us.

Notes

1 'Seating at Work', Health and Safety Executive (2002): https://www.hse.gov.uk/pubns/priced/hsg57.pdf (accessed 22 June 2023).

2 Julian Barnes, *The Only Story* (London: Vintage, 2019), p. 162.

3 The most interesting discussions of subjectivity are often in relation to particular research sources and methods: see James Hinton, *Nine Wartime Lives: Mass-Observation and the Making of the Modern Self* (Oxford: Oxford University Press, 2010), pp. 1–22; Lynn Abrams, *Oral History Theory* (Abingdon: Routledge, 2010), pp. 54–77. Historians tend not to define 'intersubjectivity'; a useful definition is given at 'Intersubjectivity', Oxford Reference: https://www.oxfordreference.com/display/10.1093/oi/authority.20110803100008603 (accessed 22 June 2023).

4 Tracey Loughran and Dawn Mannay, 'Introduction: why emotion matters', in Tracey Loughran and Dawn Mannay (eds), *Emotion and the Researcher: Sites, Subjectivities and Relationships* (Bingley: Emerald, 2018).

5 Emilie Pine writes about a departmental research day when she wanted to talk about feeling sad, but did not: 'Yes, it might have been weird for me to say I felt sad – and that's precisely why I didn't do it – but it might also have enabled us to talk about how teaching and research can give us something else, different emotions, can make us feel capable, valuable, and meaningful. That range of feeling was worth claiming, worth talking about. But I didn't claim it, and I didn't talk about it, for one reason. Because to say I felt sad would have been dangerously feminine.' Emilie Pine, *Notes to Self: Essays* (London: Penguin, 2018), pp. 190–1.

6 Andreas Boldt, 'Ranke: objectivity and history', *Rethinking History*, 18:4 (2014); Geoff Eley, *A Crooked Line: From Cultural History to the History of Society* (Ann Arbor, MI: University of Michigan Press, 2005), pp. 115–81.

7 Matt Cook, '"Archives of feeling": the AIDS crisis in Britain 1987', *History Workshop Journal*, 83 (2017).

8 Penny Summerfield, *Histories of the Self: Personal Narratives and Historical Practice* (Abingdon: Routledge, 2019); Saidiya Hartman, *Wayward Lives, Beautiful Experiments: Intimate Histories of Social Upheaval* (London: Profile Books, 2019); Leon Anderson, 'Analytic autoethnography', *Journal of Contemporary Ethnography*, 35:4 (2006); Peter Collins and Anselma Gallinat (eds), *The Ethnographic Self as Resource: Writing Memory and Experience into Ethnography* (New York and Oxford: Berghahn Books, 2010).

9 Graham Dawson, *Soldier Heroes: British Adventure, Empire, and the Imagining of Masculinities* (London and New York: Routledge, 1994), pp. 1–77; Penny Summerfield, 'Culture and composure: creating narratives of the gendered self in oral history interviews', *Cultural and Social History*, 1:1 (2004); Michael Roper, 'Slipping out of view: subjectivity and emotion in gender history', *History Workshop Journal*, 59:1 (2005).

10 Rosalind Jara, 'The Aran knit is having a pop culture renaissance – here's the mythology behind it you don't know', *British Vogue*, 15 August 2020: https://www.vogue.co.uk/fashion/article/aran-knit-renaissance (accessed 22 June 2023). The company 'Aran Islands Knitwear', established 1938, has a section in its website that references these trends and includes a photo of Taylor Swift in an Aran jumper: 'The Aran sweater – a symbol of Ireland', Aran Islands Knitwear, 7 August 2021: https://aranislandsknitwear.com/the-aran-sweater-and-its-global-audience/ (accessed 22 June 2023).

11 Penny Tinkler, Laura Fenton, and Resto Cruz, 'Introducing "resonance": revisioning the relationship between youth and later life in women born 1939–52', *Sociological Review*, Published Online First, 22 December 2022: https://journals.sagepub.com/doi/full/10.1177/00380261221140247.

12 Carolyn Steedman, *Landscape for a Good Woman* (London: Virago, 1986); Eley, *A Crooked Line*, pp. 151–81; Mary Stuart, 'You're a big girl now: subjectivities, feminism, and oral history', *Oral History*, 22:2 (1994).

13

Girlhood menstrual management and the 'culture of concealment' in postwar Britain

Hannah Froom

Introduction

In modern western culture, the widespread existence of menstrual taboos means that menstrual experiences have rarely been discussed openly and in detail. It therefore remains difficult to research the history of menstrual experience. Today, attempts to render menstruation culturally visible, to decrease stigma, and to tackle systemic factors driving period poverty are on the up, but day-to-day menstrual experience remains largely hidden.[1] This chapter draws on an extraordinary resource for historians of menstrual experience: the response of 238 cisgender women to a 1996 Mass Observation Project (MOP) Directive on 'Women's sanitary products and menstruation'.[2] The Directive (referred to as 'the Directive' or 'the Menstruation Directive' throughout this chapter) was created by Alia Al-Khalidi, a postgraduate student at Southampton Institute, in collaboration with the MOP. Different versions of the Directive were sent to women and to men. Structured as a qualitative questionnaire, the Directive sent to women asked for comments on topics including first menses, sex education, day-to-day menstrual management, advertising, Value Added Tax, menopause, and premenstrual tension. The responses to this Directive provide unique insight into girls' and women's subjective experiences of menstruation in twentieth-century Britain, shedding light on an under-researched area of 'everyday health'.

Here, I explore the responses of women born after 1950 to the Menstruation Directive, focusing particularly on women's recollections

326   *Subjectivity and intersubjectivity*

of their girlhood menstrual management practices, and the emotions, sensations, thoughts, and feelings elicited by menstruating and wearing menstrual technology. I apply a phenomenological perspective to illuminate how girls and women came to understand their menstrual bodies and experiences through sensory perceptions of dress, space, and place which were shaped by a broader 'culture of concealment' surrounding menstruation. This testimony allows us to work from the 'bottom up', to privilege the voices, perspectives, and embodied experiences of 'ordinary' women, and to explore menstruation as an 'everyday' phenomenon.[3] This approach historicises how white upper working-class and lower middle-class girls growing up in postwar Britain managed menstruation in their day-to-day lives, and the emotions this management elicited. The Directive responses reveal that it was not just stigma that made menstruation an uncomfortable experience for girls. Ill-fitting and ineffective technologies made menstruation more difficult, compounding girls' anxieties about menstrual concealment and their own menstruating bodies.

A 'culture of concealment'

Karen Houppert's phrase 'culture of concealment' encapsulates how stigma and taboos perpetuated by the menstrual technology industry have encouraged menstruation to remain hidden in the United Kingdom, Europe, and United States throughout the twentieth century, shaping menstrual experiences and perpetuating feelings of shame and secrecy among menstruators.[4] In the twentieth century, the invention, advertising, and use of modern menstrual technology entrenched concealment as a pervasive and defining facet of menstrual discourse, management, and embodiment.[5] As Andrew Shail and Gillian Howie state, advertising was, and is, the 'most explicit and loudest form of discussion of the menses'.[6] For girls growing up in postwar Britain, this 'culture of concealment' meant menstruation was rarely visible beyond advertising in women's and girls' magazines. Menstrual advertising proliferated in girls' magazines such as *Jackie*, *Honey*, and *Petticoat* in the postwar era. Menstrual technology manufacturers began to deliberately target towels and tampons at younger consumers, capitalising on the new-found spending power of teens.[7] Greater opportunities for schooling and employment, and increased disposable income, meant girls growing up in this era spent more money on themselves than their mothers had.[8] With their new-found income, girls' leisure pursuits often revolved around the purchase of dress, cosmetics, magazines, and clothes, with leisure centred on 'the department store, the cinema, the dance hall, and the mass production of newspapers, magazines and cheap books'.[9] These resources offered, in Judy Giles's words, a 'kaleidoscope of images, commodities and experiences, representing a world beyond the family, home and the locality'.[10]

Menstrual manufacturers knew that teenage girls were a lucrative market. Girls needed menstrual technologies and, if garnered early enough, brand loyalty would likely continue across the life-course. Adverts for towels and tampons tapped into postwar ideals about growing up as a process of self-actualisation, whilst also playing on adolescent awkwardness. They warned against the embarrassing spectre of stained clothes, odour, and revealing one's menstrual status, both exploiting and further entrenching ideals about secrecy and invisibility in cultural scripts about menstruation. This 'culture of concealment' ensured that menstrual experience was hidden from daily life, and, as a result, from the historical record too. As Chris Bobel notes, until recently scholarship that takes menstruation as its subject was 'relegated to the fringes' of academic study. It is still transgressive to resist menstrual concealment, and as a result subjects 'socialize this biological process – including serious inquiry into its form, function and meaning – into hiding'.[11] Histories of menstruation are sparse, and those that do exist are often 'top down'. They centre the gaze, knowledge, and perspective of individuals embedded in medical, psychiatric, political, and commercial institutions, and the discourses that emanated from these cultures, over the subjective experiences of ordinary menstruators. Furthermore, to date much of this literature has focused on North America, with much less attention to Britain in the postwar period.[12]

In producing and disseminating a Directive about menstruation, Al-Khalidi and the MOP acknowledged the blind spot that socio-cultural insistence on concealment had produced around everyday experiences of menstruation, and challenged its normalcy. The Directive provided respondents with the rare opportunity to record and relay their menstrual experiences, and to write as briefly or as extensively as they liked about an intimate aspect of their personhood

328   *Subjectivity and intersubjectivity*

and daily life. For historians interested in menstruation, the Directive responses are a rich and rare source base that provides a level of insight into 'ordinary' women's 'everyday' menstrual experiences unavailable anywhere else.

'Everyday' accounts from 'ordinary women'

Since 1981, the Mass Observation Project has sent Directives to volunteer writers at regular, typically quarterly, intervals. Seeking to understand and record everyday life in Britain, the MOP has asked for stories, anecdotes, beliefs, and observations on diverse subjects including personal hygiene, the NHS, the Falkland Islands Crisis, pocket money, Christmas cards, and dreaming. These questionnaires and responses offer a wealth of information for researchers interested in the subjectivities and everyday lives of 'ordinary' Britons both past and present. As Claire Langhamer states, the 'ordinary' and 'the everyday' are 'malleable' and 'messy' concepts, but ones closely associated with a critique of institutions and expertise.[13] Volunteers who wrote for the MOP deemed themselves 'ordinary', in opposition to identifications such as 'posh' or institutions such as 'the media', and had no 'expert' training in health or medicine. Mostly upper working- and lower middle-class, left-leaning, and white, the contributors were self-defined 'ordinary people'.[14] There are notable gaps in the archive, especially around class, race, and ethnicity, and the experiences of trans and non-binary people.[15] As this suggests, even within a project dedicated to understanding experiences that are usually unrecorded, it can be difficult to record and retrieve the experiences of the most marginalised.

In itself, MOP volunteers' commitment to recording and archiving their thoughts, experiences, and memories for a social research project marks them out as in some way extraordinary. The simultaneous typicality and atypicality of the cohort benefits historians interested in subjectivity. Writing about intimate parts of the self is a form of self-fashioning; as James Hinton explains, 'the focus is on the site of agency, where individuals are present at their own making'. Life-writing provides an opportunity to explore the 'creative moment in which an individual, struggling to make sense of him- or herself in the world, will bend, select, recombine, amend or transform sources of meaning available in the public culture'.[16]

Girlhood menstrual management 329

The Menstruation Directive asked respondents to reflect on their girlhoods, to remember their formative experiences of menstrual management, and to narrativise them. It is evident that many women thought carefully about what to write and some emphasised that they had taken time to craft their responses. Other respondents wrote spontaneously, as indicated by scribbles, crossings out, and non-linear narratives. Responses varied in length from one paragraph to ten sides of A4 paper. These responses help us to understand how subjects made and make sense of their experiences, how they articulate them, and how memory informs this process. Women's memories of their girlhood menstrual experiences, and their articulations of these memories, might not provide exact accounts of 'how it was', because people do not simply remember what happened to them. Oral historians have demonstrated that memory, shaped and reshaped by culture, is inherently unreliable. As the *History Workshop* editorial collective suggested in 1979, 'memory does not constitute pure recall: the memory of any particular event is refracted through layer upon layer of subsequent experience'.[17] Reflections on menstruation offered in Directive responses demonstrate how women's subjectivities, and memories of girlhood, were shaped by both the 'culture of concealment' and the accumulated experiences of their life-courses.

These influences can be seen in responses to the final prompt on the Directive, which encouraged writers to reflect on how they felt about menstruation, and on whether it was a suitable topic for a directive. This question implied awareness from its creators that the Directive might be viewed as unconventional, divide opinion, and elicit impassioned responses – and it did. The degree of enthusiasm and detail differed widely between responses. Some respondents stated that they had decided not to discuss their response with anyone, despite typically doing so.[18] A forty-four-year-old woman from Mirfield, who had recently experienced the menopause, refused to comment in detail. For her, menstruation had always been inconvenient and she was pleased that she no longer needed to think about it.[19] Offering only half a page of writing, a thirty-five-year-old woman living in Essex concluded that her recent hysterectomy had altered how she reflected on her girlhood menstrual experiences, resulting in 'mixed feelings' about responding.[20] A thirty-three-year-old 'part-time teacher, full-time mother' from Dorset described her visceral reaction to writing about her experiences, manifest in a 'churning

330   *Subjectivity and intersubjectivity*

stomach', whilst a seventy-seven-year-old respondent from North Yorkshire questioned whether girls now knew too much about the 'facts of life' and if this had contributed to an increased number of teenage pregnancies.[21]

Other women described the experience of responding to this Directive as 'refreshing' and affirmational, stressing that it was an important topic, worthy of study, that could make a meaningful contribution to destigmatising menstruation.[22] A thirty-two-year-old respondent from Liverpool branded the Directive 'unusual', but concluded her two pages by emphasising that she did not mind answering because increased menstrual visibility might help her nieces to avoid the 'pointless feelings of embarrassment and shame' she had experienced when growing up.[23] Respondents occasionally expressed a desire to read other responses, showing how the 'culture of concealment' had limited open discussion and understanding of other menstruators' experiences.[24] Similarly, replies expressed curiosity about the existence of the men's directive, the questions it contained, and how male Mass Observers had reacted to the Directive.[25]

As Liz Heron asserts in the introduction to her edited volume on girls growing up the 1950s, 'the past can never be disposed of, can never be cut off from our knowledge or experience of the present'.[26] Layers of subsequent life experience and cultural messaging affected the reflections women offered. The diverse array of responses demonstrates how the 'culture of concealment' maintained the contentious cultural position of menstruation from some women's mid-century girlhoods right up until the last decade of the twentieth century. These mixed reactions to rendering menstruation visible are the crucial context for understanding and interpreting women's reflections on their girlhood menstrual management, as explored in the remainder of this chapter. They show how subjects operated within a 'culture of concealment' that extended up to their time of writing, and prompt us to consider what impact this had on their subjectivities and embodied menstrual experiences.

Phenomenology, menstrual management, and dress

A phenomenological perspective can help us to interpret women's descriptions of their girlhood menstrual experiences. Phenomenology

Girlhood menstrual management   331

is concerned with understanding embodiment, and the relationship between individuals and wider societal structures. This approach can benefit historians interested in accessing and understanding the interior lives and embodied experiences of subjects in the past. This focus on subjectivity is imperative for historians interested in 'everyday health', defined as 'the emotional, psychological, and bodily state-of-being in individuals' day-to-day lives, and the strategies they pursue (or do not) to maintain equilibrium in this state-of-being'.[27] Here, I outline how phenomenological approaches might be incorporated into studies of menstrual embodiment.

Havi Carel describes phenomenology as a 'philosophical approach that focuses on phenomena (what we perceive and experience)' such as 'the experiences of thinking, perceiving, and coming into contact with the world'.[28] Many iterations of phenomenological theory presuppose that an individual's sensory perceptions influence how they interact with and interpret the world around them. The work of sociology and fashion studies scholar Joanne Entwistle on embodied dress practices provides a good example of this approach.[29] Entwistle uses phenomenology to understand what drives subjects' routine and mundane day-to-day dress practices and how these practices affect their interactions with the world, including their experiences of space and place. Entwistle does not discuss menstruation, but this chapter extrapolates from and builds upon her insights to understand embodied experiences of menstrual management, and how they relate to embodied dress practices. This, in turn, highlights the relationship between menstrual management, dress practices, and everyday menstrual experience.

Entwistle argues that sensory perceptions of dress inform the way subjects perceive, understand, and move through space. To explain the phenomenological approach to dress, she draws on Umberto Eco's account of wearing jeans a size too small. Eco notes how the jeans feel on the body, how they pinch and restrict movement, and how they elicit awareness of the lower half of the body – how they come to constitute an 'epidermic self-awareness' unfelt before:

> I lived in the knowledge that I had jeans on, whereas normally we live forgetting that we're wearing undershorts or trousers [...] as a result I assumed an exterior behaviour of one who wears jeans [...] Not only did the garment impose a demeanour on me; by focusing my attention on demeanour it obliged me to live towards the exterior world.[30]

332 *Subjectivity and intersubjectivity*

Eco records the ways that his clothing, and the feelings and sensations it elicits, mediates his experience of selfhood and how he orientates himself to the world. Using this account, Entwistle demonstrates that clothing has the potential to 'impinge upon' subjects' 'experience of the body', making them aware of its 'edges, the limits and boundaries', particularly if the clothing feels uncomfortable. This alters their comportment, and how they move through and interact with the world.[31]

A similar 'epidermic self-awareness' can be traced in experiences of menstrual management. One of the prompts in the Menstruation Directive asked respondents to describe their use of menstrual products, and to outline how and why this use had changed over time. Individuals were asked to comment on the 'availability, size, absorbency, comfort and style' of technologies. The number of references in responses to the feel of products and the bodily sensations, particularly discomfort, induced by using ill-designed and ill-fitting products suggests that these were extremely important and memorable aspects of menstrual experience that affected how girls moved through the world. A phenomenological approach to this testimony suggests that menstrual technologies made girls aware of the 'edges, limits and boundaries' of their bodies, acting as another layer of dress marked with meaning that connected them to the social world.

Entwistle asserts that while dress practices are often characterised as methods for self-expression and statements about identity, they are just as likely to be shaped by mundane factors such as a desire for comfort, or moral and social codes regarding appropriate dress. She suggests that subjects dress themselves in the knowledge that wearing clothes can be 'done' correctly or incorrectly depending on social setting, and gives examples of 'mistakes of dress', including an undone fly or a stain on a jacket.[32] Again, this point is relevant to testimony about menstrual management. Women's accounts reveal that notions of secrecy, shame, and stigma informed how they managed and dressed their menstruating bodies in girlhood, and what they deemed important to emphasise in their responses to the Menstrual Directive. The social and moral codes born from the 'culture of concealment' impinged upon day-to-day menstrual management practices. Under the guise of hygienic etiquette, these codes prioritised secrecy, invisibility, and routine care. They required girls to mask pain or discomfort, to hide menstruation and menstrual

Girlhood menstrual management

333

technology, and to limit disruption to daily practices, regardless of their feelings, in order to avoid revealing their menstrual status.

A phenomenological reading of Mass Observation testimonies

Menstrual technologies were marketed as a means for girls to manage menstruation in line with socially prescribed ideals of secrecy. They functioned as another layer of dress that enabled subjects, operating within the 'culture of concealment', to orientate themselves to the world 'correctly'. Advertising promised that the purchase and adornment of modern mass-produced menstrual technologies could meet the urgent need for invisibility within the culture of concealment, offering girls peace of mind and alleviating their shame. The 'culture of concealment' meant that blood-stained trousers, indicating a subject's status as menstruating, were regarded as a 'greater mistake of dress' than an undone fly or stain on a jacket. Testimony reveals that girls felt it to be shameful or abnormal when they inadvertently engaged in 'mistakes of dress' and rendered visible their menstrual status. Even now, the decision to ignore menstrual management and to 'free bleed' is considered transgressive, radical, disruptive, and empowering.[33] But the women who responded to the Menstruation Directive had not intended to be radical, subversive, or disruptive by not conforming to menstrual etiquette norms. Instead, girls' non-conformity was unintentional or arose from the lack of accessible facilities or technologies – a lack that itself often resulted from stigma and the culture of concealment.

Kathleen (b. 1951, first menses aged thirteen) wanted to wear miniskirts; to embody 1960s fashion trends in comfort without being restricted by her menstrual cycle.[34] Her desire to be both fashionable and comfortable, and the importance of both to her sense of self, spurred her decision to start using tampons in her later teenage years. She stated,

> My mother gave me sanitary towels, which hooked on to a belt type of thing, and I loathed this. I felt this great wedge of cotton wool or whatever it was between my legs and I felt uncomfortable [...] my friends all felt the same [...] as I got further in to my teen years, out working, wearing mini-skirts and so on, I started wearing tampons which felt less intrusive and more comfortable.[35]

334 *Subjectivity and intersubjectivity*

Whitney (b. 1970, first menses aged fifteen) also commented on the way ill-fitting menstrual technologies amplified her discomfort and changed her relationship to clothing during her teenage years. She used 'bulky standard' towels recommended by her mum for the first few years, but this meant she 'was not comfortable wearing certain clothes, especially tight ones'. The towels altered the fit and appearance of tight-fitting clothes, disrupting social codes that prioritised menstrual concealment and appropriate dress practices, whilst also hindering her ability to wear clothes comfortably.[36]

Similarly, Carol (b. 1960, first menses aged thirteen) reflected on her adolescent concerns that menstrual technologies were visible through clothing. She explained, 'it was excruciating when a towel came loose and wandered up your back [...] I was always worried that people could see a towel when I was walking along'. Carol felt 'very self-conscious' as a result of these anxieties. Her testimony implies awareness that visible menstrual technology was a 'mistake of dress' that could disrupt social codes regarding menstrual conceal-ment and appropriate dress practices. This awareness made her feel ashamed.[37] Like Carol, Billie (b. 1955, first menses aged twelve) wrote about feelings of shame and self-consciousness. She remembered after starting to menstruate feeling like she 'looked different and that everyone must be able to tell'. Her desire to conceal menstruation impacted on how she related to and interacted with other girls. She noted that she 'used to despise girls who gave away when they were menstruating'.[38] Barbara (born 1953, first menses aged twelve) also framed her response in relation to feelings of self-consciousness. She 'hated' the feel of the sanitary belt she used when she first started to menstruate. She explained, 'it dug into my puppy fat and the bulky towels were too big for me'. In contrast, 'tampons were great for an active self-conscious teenager. Nobody could tell when you were having a period, you could go swimming.'[39]

Other responses also suggest that the feel, visibility, and type of technology exacerbated feelings of shame and fear regarding menstrual concealment. Beverley (b. 1960, first menses aged thirteen) had her first period in 1973 while on holiday. At times, Beverley was unable to use over-the-counter menstrual technologies because her family could not afford them, instead using home-made 'rags'. She described what these 'rags' felt like and provided an anecdote about a situation where they had failed to conceal her period. The original syntax

Girlhood menstrual management

335

and crossings-out in Beverley's response offer insight into her psychological state at the time of writing. Beverley started to write about using 'rags', but then decided to add the clarifying information that her mother did not always have towels because they were expensive. This detail about her upbringing and her family's financial situation in turn justified Beverley's wearing of 'homemade' menstrual protection:

> I would have to whisper to my mother that I wanted a towel, I remember once or twice when she did not have any ~~she cut up~~ and could not afford to buy them – she cut up pillowcases or sheets, folded them in strips and I would have to use them with pins holding them in place, more often or not it would slop and blood would come through my jeans [...] when I was 14 and I was sitting on a washing machine with jeans on, and it had come through, all my friends – laughed and teased me, I could not go out again for weeks.[40]

By failing to conceal her period, Beverley broke social codes regarding appropriate forms of menstrual management and dress. As in the other responses discussed here, this caused her embarrassment and affected relationships with her peers.

Angela (b. 1974, first menses aged eleven) revealed, in biographical statements littered through her testimony, that she was ashamed of puberty to the point where she could not bathe, as she did not want to look at herself; that her parents were not open about sex, and that when she did learn about periods from a conversation with friends, her mum was furious. She recalled feeling like her mum wanted to protect her, but also that she had very little interest in learning about sex and periods from her mum. She wondered if this reluctance stemmed from 'terror at not being a child anymore' and said that she still felt 'immense regret' that she was no longer small. Angela described her teenage anorexia in terms of a regression to childhood and stated that after 'several years of introspection' she believed her anorexia and her shame at growing up were linked.

Angela's first period arrived during her 'top year of junior school'. She had a 'funny tummy ache' and found blood in her knickers. Angela recalled that she 'couldn't handle the physical aspects of it', because 'junior school is not really equipped for menstruating little girls!'[41] Angela described the culture surrounding menstruation at school, where the onset of a peer's first menses became the subject

336 *Subjectivity and intersubjectivity*

of gossip. She 'felt sorry for those that it happened to', but when a peer confided in her about their first period she felt 'honoured', and viewed them as 'older, and more mature'. At the same time, conveying her own feelings of shame and isolation was an important aspect of Angela's writing. She explained, 'I had heavy periods but I would have been far too embarrassed to take a change of towel with me. Once I had to ask a teacher for one, and I could have sunk through the floor I was so embarrassed.' This lack of prepared-ness, born from a sense of self-protection and self-preservation, had the opposite effect, revealing her status as menstruating and com-pounding her embarrassment.

The shame and embarrassment Angela associated with menstrua-tion and menstrual technology meant she did not want to be 'found out'. As a result, she preferred to wear six pairs of knickers to 'cope with the inevitable flooding' and to avoid 'tell-tale stains' on her clothes and the chairs she sat on. She recounted how her friend once 'wore a pink skirt once during her period and was the laughing stock of the whole school' when a bloodstain showed through. For Angela, both her clothes and the objects she interacted with, such as the chair, became potential threats that could reveal that she was menstruating. The implication that seeing menstrual blood on the chair would be deeply humiliating for her, and an invitation for others to judge and re-evaluate her, reveals how menstruation altered her sense of self, her interactions with and understandings of the objects she encountered, and how she was perceived by and interacted with her peers.

In Angela's testimony, items of dress, much like pieces of furniture, acquire symbolic dimensions intimately bound to her understand-ing and experience of her menstruating body and her interactions with people and space. Wearing multiple pairs of underwear while menstruating was an attempt to uphold the 'culture of concealment'. In linking this story to her friend's experience of leaking menstrual blood onto a pink skirt and becoming the 'laughing stock' of the whole school, she re-emphasised the role of clothing in masking or revealing menstrual status, and therefore in disrupting social codes regarding both menstrual management and dress. This story also reveals the likelihood of stigmatisation, embarrassment, and social exclusion for the girls if menstruation was not managed appropriately. Both friends 'failed' to ensure menstruation remained concealed,

Girlhood menstrual management 337

one by asking a teacher for a towel, and the other by bleeding onto her skirt.

Her friend broke social codes of dress by wearing, even unwittingly, a stained item of clothing; a doubly outrageous mistake of dress because the stain was menstrual blood. As a direct result of menstruation, Angela broke social codes of dress in multiple ways: by not wearing any menstrual technology, but also by instead wearing 'several pairs of knickers' under her school uniform in one incident and under her swimming costume in another:

> The worst time was when I went on [a] school journey to the Isle of Wight. We stayed in a small hotel, which had its own swimming pool. I had my period while I was there, and I couldn't even contemplate not going in the pool. For a start it would have singled me out from everyone else, but also, I wanted to swim, and have fun like the others. I had never heard of tampons at this stage. So I wore a sanitary towel, and several pairs of knickers underneath my swimming costume. Looking back, I can't believe I did it!

Angela tried to avoid singling herself out as menstruating to her peers by sitting at the poolside, but the multiple pairs of knickers that remained invisible under her school uniform could be seen when she was wearing the swimming costume:

> I was climbing up the slide, and a boy (who had created the name of 'Big V ...' for me already as I needed a bra) climbed up behind me and say [said] 'ugh, why have you got pants on?' The *shame* of it! I don't think he knew enough to recognise the bulge that must have been there – thank god. I discovered tampons a year or so later, at secondary school. By this stage I was no longer on my own, and periods were not so shameful.[42]

In this moment at the swimming pool, Angela's need to adhere to social codes of menstrual etiquette (ensuring her status as menstruating was not revealed to her peers) overruled the need to adhere to social codes of dress. This part of the testimony demonstrates Angela's hierarchical organisation of social codes: in this moment the social and moral imperative to keep menstruation hidden was more important and less stigmatising than adhering to dress codes. Angela used her agentic capacity to break (some of) the rules, but this was not an empowering decision. Her testimony shows that breaking

338 *Subjectivity and intersubjectivity*

social codes of dress because of menstruation caused stress and shame, even though she felt compelled to do so.

This feeling of compulsion demonstrates Angela's lack of real choices. The decision to prioritise menstrual over dress etiquette was caused by desperation and perceived necessity, as emphasised by the references to shame and embarrassment. To sit out swimming would have required conversation with teachers and revealed her status as menstruating, whilst participating in swimming lessons wearing multiple pairs of underwear at least made it possible to maintain menstrual concealment. Angela's framing of this story as 'the worst' of several implied incidents, and her retrospective disbelief that she ever made this decision, indicates its powerful place in her psyche, even at the distance of decades. This affects how we should interpret it. Angela's story illustrates the powerlessness of young girls within the 'culture of concealment', operating with limited knowledge, language, and tools for navigating the menstrual world. Agentic capacity does not equal empowerment.

For Angela, and the other women whose girlhood experiences are explored in this chapter, choices to wear certain technologies or items of clothing were shaped by their economic status, their sociocultural status (or powerlessness) as girls, and by fraught understandings of appropriate menstrual management. Whilst shame is a highly subjective emotion, felt, understood, and sometimes overcome by the individual, accounts of menstrual management reveal how larger structuring forces shaped and reshaped menstrual shame, and how these structuring forces were embodied in girls' everyday practice and experience. The 'epidermic self-awareness' girls often felt whilst menstruating demonstrates the extent to which they internalised sociocultural notions of secrecy, shame, and conceal-ment, affecting their subject positions, their relationships, and their everyday activities.

Conclusion

The accounts of menstrual experience found in the MOA privilege the narratives and voices of women without medical or professional authority or formal expertise on menstruation. They provide access to facets of menstrual experience often unexplored by histories that

Girlhood menstrual management

339

focus on institutional discourses or media representations. Evidence from the MOP enables a ground-up study of menstruation as an everyday phenomenon. Focusing on the emotions, thoughts, feelings, and sensory experiences of 'ordinary' women, these testimonies enable researchers to explore how subjects managed menstruation in their day-to-day lives, and how discourses of concealment informed these everyday menstrual management practices.

Testimony reveals that menstrual discomfort arose not only from menstrual pain and menstrual stigma, but from other aspects of embodied menstrual management. A phenomenological perspective on experiences of wearing menstrual technology reveals that while the 'culture of concealment' debilitated girls and caused feelings of shame and embarrassment, available menstrual technologies also restricted their day-to-day menstrual management. Poorly designed, ill-fitting, ineffective, or uncomfortable technologies compounded girls' uncomfortable menstrual experiences and complicated feelings about their menstruating bodies. Furthermore, this debilitation was often intensified by girls' class and economic status. Girls who used home-made 'rags' because they could not afford to purchase menstrual products experienced intensified feelings of shame and embarrassment as well as further restrictions to their comportment and day-to-day lives. These narratives show how difficult it was for girls with limited access to effective and comfortable menstrual technologies, and limited knowledge, language, and tools to navigate the menstrual world, to manage their periods in physical and psychic comfort, without shame or embarrassment. They also illuminate the complex feelings about menstruation and menstrual concealment that continued to structure women's psyches across the life-course, influencing how they felt when asked to record their experiences towards the end of the century.

In 1987, anthropologist Emily Martin called for more acknowledgement that menstruation could be described, understood, and interpreted in ways that diverged from medical explanations. She wanted an explanation focused on 'how something feels, and what you do, rather than what is happening'. Martin suggested that paying attention to women's articulations of the sensory and emotional experience of menstruation could aid understanding of the totality of menstrual experience, which in turn might help to reduce some of the disgust associated with it in popular culture.[43] In a similar

340   *Subjectivity and intersubjectivity*

vein, in 2005 the philosopher Iris Marion Young questioned the implicit assumption in much feminist literature that menstruators 'ought to have an accurate and complete understanding of the physiology of menstruation'. She stated that 'few men and women have a very accurate or complete understanding of the physiology of other internal bodily processes [...] this assumption that "menstrual knowledge" is equivalent to medical science may itself contribute to a sense of alienation women have from the process'.[44] Like Martin, Young argues that enabling subjects to focus on describing feelings and sensations associated with menstruation might be the antidote to these feelings of separation from embodied experience.[45]

These studies suggest that phenomenological approaches can complement and enhance menstruation studies in two ways. First, phenomenology sets out theoretical questions and methods that account for menstruators' assessments of what knowledge about menstruation matters to them. Second, phenomenology does not frame articulations in ways that bolster the notion that scientific explanations are the only accurate way of describing and defining menstrual experience. Indeed, it throws into question whether scientific explanations are 'accurate' in any meaningful way at all.

Amplifying embodied sensory and emotional experiences deprivileges scientific readings of menstrual experience, whilst also acknowledging that identity and politics, as well as cultural understandings of sex, gender, nature, and culture, inform how individuals understand themselves and interpret the world around them, impacting on how they are understood and treated. The phenomenological 'lived body', as Young states, offers a 'means of theorizing sexual subjectivity without danger of either biological reductionism or gender essentialism'.[46] From the perspective of a historian rather than a philosopher or anthropologist, this approach can add texture and dimension to studies of past experiences, and allow these experiences to be understood as historically and socially specific, shaped by the social mores and ideals and scientific understandings of the era in question. Avoiding biological reductionism and gender essentialism is particularly important when it comes to understanding and historicising intersectional and marginalised histories of menstruation and menstruators, but because of the culture of concealment that has surrounded menstruation, the *historical* evidence necessary to adopt this interpretive strategy is almost entirely lacking.

Girlhood menstrual management 341

The responses to the MOP's Menstruation Directive are unusual in that they allow historians to explore menstrual experience at a granular level. Analysis of these testimonies bolsters Martin's and Young's claims that describing how it feels to menstruate can contribute to ending menstrual stigma. As one woman concluded:

> I have really enjoyed this subject – a chance to reveal all those things I've never confessed to any but my best friend before [...] I feel I can write such things down now for M-O because I feel it will be met with sympathy and understanding. It's been a pleasure to get all these things off my chest, and maybe other women have felt the same too.[47]

Acknowledgements

The research on which this chapter is based was conducted during a PhD studentship funded as part of the Wellcome Trust Investigator Award in the Humanities and Social Sciences, 'Body, Self and Family: Women's Psychological, Emotional and Bodily Health in Britain, c. 1960–1990', WT 208080/Z/17/Z.

Notes

1 For more on menstruation in popular culture today see Camilla Røstvik, *Cash Flow: The Business of Menstruation* (London: UCL Press, 2022), pp. 1–3.

2 For the Directive, see '47. Spring 1996', Mass Observation Project Directives: http://www.massobs.org.uk/mass-observation-project-directives (accessed 22 March 2020). Responses to the Directive can be accessed at the Mass Observation Archive, University of Sussex. According to the biographical information all respondents were cisgender. Trans men and non-binary individuals may also menstruate, but as these Directive responses deal only with the experiences of cis girls and women, throughout this chapter I use 'girls' and 'women' in relation to this testimony. The experiences of trans and non-binary menstruators require further investigation as menstruation studies gain traction. On researching menstruation beyond the gender binary see Sarah E. Frank, 'Queering menstruation: trans and non-binary identity and body politics', *Sociological Inquiry*, 90:2 (2020), and Klara Rydstrom, 'Degendering menstruation: making trans menstruators matter', in Chris Bobel et

342   *Subjectivity and intersubjectivity*

al. (eds), *The Palgrave Handbook of Critical Menstruation Studies* (Basingstoke: Palgrave Macmillan, 2020).

3 David Bloome, Dorothy Sheridan, and Brian Street, 'Reading Mass-Observation writing: theoretical and methodological issues in researching in the Mass Observation Archive', *Mass Observation Archive Occasional Paper Series*, 1 (1996), 14, cited in Jill Kirby, *Feeling the Strain: A Cultural History of Stress in Twentieth Century Britain* (Manchester: Manchester University Press, 2019), p. 20.

4 Karen Houppert, *The Curse: Confronting the Last Unmentionable Taboo* (London: Profile Books, 1999), pp. 11–16.

5 Sharra L. Vostral, 'Masking menstruation: the emergence of menstrual hygiene products in the United States', in Andrew Shail and Gillian Howie (eds), *Menstruation: A Cultural History* (Basingstoke: Palgrave Macmillan, 2005), p. 243; Sharra L. Vostral, *Under Wraps: A History of Menstrual Hygiene Technology* (Washington, DC: Lexington Books, 2008).

6 Andrew Shail and Gillian Howie, '"Talking your body's language": the menstrual materialisations of sexed ontology', in Shail and Howie (eds), *Menstruation*, p. 1.

7 Hannah Froom, 'Menstruation, Subjectivity and Constructions of Girl-hood in Britain 1960–1980' (PhD thesis, University of Essex, 2022).

8 Penny Tinkler, 'Girlhood and growing up', in Ina Zweiniger-Bargielowska (ed.), *Women in Twentieth-Century Britain* (Harlow, Essex: Pearson Education, 2001); Penny Tinkler, '"Are you really living?" If not, "get with it!" The teenage self and lifestyle in young women's magazines, Britain 1957–70', *Cultural and Social History*, 11:4 (2015).

9 Angela Davis, *Modern Motherhood: Women and Family in England, 1945–2000* (Manchester: Manchester University Press, 2012), p. 3.

10 Judy Giles, 'Narratives of gender, class and modernity in women's memories of mid-twentieth century Britain', *Signs*, 28 (2008).

11 Chris Bobel, 'Introduction: menstruation as lens – menstruation as opportunity', in Bobel et al. (eds), *The Palgrave Handbook of Critical Menstruation Studies*, p. 1.

12 Examples include Joan Jacob Brumberg, '"Something happens to girls": menarche and the emergence of the modern American hygienic impera-tive', *Journal of the History of Sexuality*, 4:1 (1993); Janice Delaney, Mary Jane Lupton, and Emily Toth, *The Curse: A Cultural History of Menstruation* (Champaign, IL: University of Illinois Press, 1988); Røstvik, *Cash Flow*; Shail and Howie (eds), *Menstruation*; Julie-Marie Strange, 'The assault on ignorance: teaching menstrual etiquette in England, c. 1920–1960s', *Social History of Medicine*, 14:2 (2001). A recent and notable exception is Bobel et al. (eds), *The Palgrave Handbook of Critical Menstruation Studies*.

Girlhood menstrual management

343

13 Claire Langhamer, '"Who the hell are ordinary people?" Ordinariness as a category of historical analysis', *Transactions of the Royal Historical Society*, 28 (2018), 194.

14 Kirby, *Feeling the Strain*, p. 22.

15 Until the late 2010s, Directive responses were filed under 'male' or 'female', meaning that it is difficult to trace trans or non-binary experiences in the archive. In 2016, 1 per cent of MOP respondents identified as trans or non-binary. See Mass Observation Archive Annual Report, 36 (2016), p. 11: http://www.massobs.org.uk/images/Directives/MOA_Annual_Report_15–16_final.pdf (accessed 12 December 2020).

16 James Hinton, *Nine Wartime Lives: Mass Observation and the Making of the Modern Self,* (Oxford: Oxford University Press, 2010), p. 7.

17 'Editorial: Oral history', *History Workshop Journal*, 8:1 (1979) p. iii.

18 Mass Observation Archive (hereafter MOA), The Keep, University of Sussex, Menstruation (Spring 1996), SxMOA2/1/47/2, respondents P2765, W1918.

19 MOA, Menstruation, respondent S2581.

20 MOA, Menstruation, respondent L796.

21 MOA, Menstruation, respondents G2624, B736.

22 MOA, Menstruation, respondents A2212, A2685, A2751, T1843, T2713, W729, W1813.

23 MOA, Menstruation, respondent B2653.

24 MOA, Menstruation, respondents B2197, G2624.

25 MOA, Menstruation, respondents D826, H1705, H1745, L796, S2207, W1918.

26 Liz Heron, *Truth, Dare, Promise: Girls Growing Up in the Fifties* (London: Virago Press, 1985), p. 1.

27 Tracey Loughran, Kate Mahoney, and Daisy Payling, 'Women's voices, emotion, and empathy: engaging different publics with "everyday" health histories', *Medical Humanities*, 48:4 (2022), 395.

28 Havi Carel, *Phenomenology of Illness* (Oxford: Oxford University Press, 2016), p. 20.

29 Joanne Entwistle, 'Fashion and the fleshy body: dress as embodied practice', *Fashion Theory*, 4:3 (2000).

30 Umberto Eco, 'Lumbar thought', in his *Travels in Hyperreality* (San Diego, CA, New York, and London: Harcourt Brace Jovanovich, 1986), trans. William Weaver, cited in Joanne Entwistle, 'Fashion and the fleshy body', p. 334.

31 Entwistle, 'Fashion and the fleshy body', p. 334.

32 Entwistle, 'Fashion and the fleshy body', p. 337.

33 Chris Bobel, *New Blood: Third Wave Feminism and the Politics of Menstruation* (New Brunswick, NJ: Rutgers University Press, 2010).

34 MOA, Menstruation, respondent K798. 'Kathleen' is a pseudonym, as are all names of Directive respondents in the subsequent discussion. I have allocated respondents a popular name from the decade they were born that corresponds with the letter accompanying their archival reference number, for example Kathleen = K798.

35 MOA, Menstruation, respondent K798.

36 MOA, Menstruation, respondent W2731.

37 MOA, Menstruation, respondent C41.

38 MOA, Menstruation, respondent B2197.

39 MOA, Menstruation, respondent B215.

40 MOA, Menstruation, respondent B2031.

41 For more on the lack of facilities for menstruators in schools in this period see Hannah Charnock, 'Girlhood, Sexuality and Identity in England 1950–1980' (PhD thesis, University of Exeter, 2017); Angela Davis, '"Oh no, nothing, we didn't learn anything": sex education and the preparation of girls for motherhood, c. 1930–1970', *History of Education*, 37:5 (2008); Christine Farrell, *My Mother Said ... The Way Young People Learn about Sex and Birth Control* (Oxford: Routledge, 1978); Froom, 'Menstruation, Subjectivity and Constructions of Girlhood in Britain'.

42 MOA, Menstruation, respondent A2685.

43 Emily Martin, *The Woman in the Body, A Cultural Analysis of Reproduction*, rev. edn (Boston, MA: Beacon Press, 2001), p. 111.

44 Iris Marion Young, *On Female Body Experience: 'Throwing Like a Girl' and Other Essays* (Oxford: Oxford University Press, 2005), pp. 97, 102.

45 Young, *On Female Body Experience*, p. 102.

46 Young, *On Female Body Experience*, p. 410. See also Sonia Kruks, *Retrieving Experience: Subjectivity and Recognition in Feminist Politics* (Ithaca, NY: Cornell University Press, 2001), pp.1–51.

47 MOA, Menstruation, respondent P2795.

14

Is sex good for you? Risk, reward, and responsibility for young women in the late 1980s

Rosie Gahnstrom, Lucy Robinson, and Rachel Thomson

Introduction

Between 1988 and 1990, the 'Women, Risk and AIDS Project' (WRAP) interviewed 150 women aged 16–21 in London and Manchester to find out more about their sexual relationships, identities, and practices. These young women were negotiating a moment of peril (the threat of HIV and AIDS, which was still a terminal diagnosis), but also of possibility (as further and higher education and careers opened out to them). As a feminist project, WRAP utilised the space opened by official concerns around the heterosexual spread of HIV/AIDS to analyse gendered power relations by asking the question 'Is sex good for you?' WRAP was funded through a research programme concerned with risk behaviour, but the WRAP team – which included Rachel – wanted to investigate the unexamined experiences of young women. Sexual practice was a way into this.[1]

Three decades after the original project, 'Reanimating Data: Experiments with People, Places and Archives' (Figure 14.1) revisited WRAP.[2] This chapter uses the newly archived WRAP materials to map how interview participants learned and shared knowledge about sex.[3] In doing so, we engage with this moment from a new historical position, yet within a tradition of feminist scholarship. Our intention is to stage encounters between past and present, allowing both to remain visible. Inspired by scholarship on queer politics, literature, and temporalities, we look (and feel) backwards, sideways, and forwards with the WRAP materials. In these three ways of looking, our sociological and historical approaches interweave and illuminate

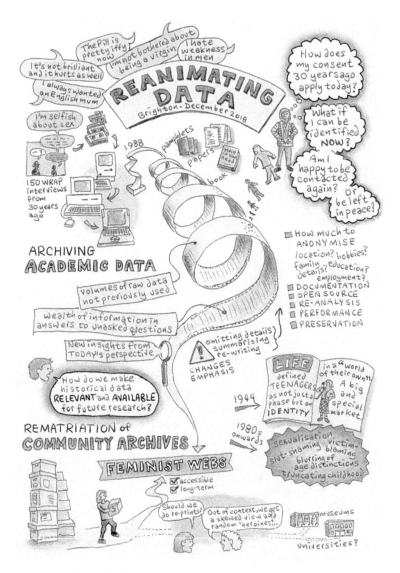

Figure 14.1 Poster for 'Reanimating Data: Experiments with People, Places and Archives' (artist Mitchi Mathias). Courtesy of Rachel Thomson. All rights reserved and permission to use the figure must be obtained from the copyright holder.

Is sex good for you? 347

each other. As researchers in the present, we learn anew from the conversations in the past, and show how knowledge moves in unexpected ways and directions.

Context: the sexual politics of the 1980s

In the late 1980s, it became possible for young women to imagine sex without marriage, love, and commitment. Contraception was available to the unmarried, further educational opportunities were opening, and popular culture was replete with representations of a new kind of pleasure-seeking girl.[4] At the same time, the sexual double standard and the valorisation of parental authority remained firmly in place.[5] This was also a moment of new sexual dangers with HIV/AIDS focusing attention on the risks of exchanging body fluids and redefining passionate fumblings in terms of safer sexual practices.

In this new politics of sex and sexuality, activists and campaigners simultaneously addressed the everyday and institutional politics of sex and gender.[6] It was a moment when forces of liberalism, feminism, and authoritarianism jousted for influence in the context of cultural, technological, and economic change.[7] Young people's sex, sexuality, and gender were debated in relation to the age of consent and competence, changes to abortion legislation, and newer contraceptive forms like Depo-Provera.[8] Single mothers, characterised as teenaged, unmarried, and welfare dependent, were at the heart of New Right sociologist Charles Murray's theorisation of 'the underclass'.[9] In such debates, questions of individual responsibility, gender roles, economic productivity, and moral codes came together.

Girls' and young women's bodies carried the weight of much social anxiety. Sexual knowledge and protection from exploitation were pitted against each other in debates on the influence on children of the media and formal education, on Section 28, new media controls over video and satellite broadcasting, Page 3, and teen-oriented advice columns.[10] Although multiple sources of formal and informal sex education existed, there was little agreement on who was qualified (or allowed) to speak of and to young people's sexuality – whether parents, schools, or medical professionals.[11] In such debates, the idea of childhood 'innocence' was composed through a series of

348   *Subjectivity and intersubjectivity*

defensive moves by parents and other authority figures, rather than speaking to children's own experiences.[12] The Gillick ruling (1985,[13] Section 28 (1988), and the Children Act (1989) all deferred to parental control rather than professional expertise to guide young people's sexual knowledge.[14] Meanwhile, increased discussion of child sexual abuse, peaking around the 1987 Cleveland child sexual abuse crisis[15] and leading to the creation of organisations like Childline and Children in Need, complicated the idea of parents as sole providers of sexual knowledge.[16]

Researchers in multiple disciplines responded to controversies around young people's sexualities by looking at the relationship between sex education and social regulation, especially in relation to pornography, new media forms and technologies, and big-budget advertising campaigns.[17] Aware of tensions between public education aimed at reducing the risks of pregnancy and HIV infection in young audiences and the leaching of 'adult' content into children's lives, researchers tried to evaluate public understanding of policy and scientific research around sex.[18] Feminist critiques also recognised how the return to 'family values' heightened the sexual double standard, made it difficult to represent women's sexualities without feeding into dominant narratives of objectification, and institutionalised abuse of vulnerable groups.[19] Understood retrospectively, this is context in which the WRAP set to work, even if it did not feel that way at the time.

Feeling backwards: the pull of bad sex and outmoded femininities

Heather Love argues that we exist within structures of feeling that connect us over time within traditions often involving difficult 'residual' feelings; this is what it means to 'feel backwards'.[20] Feeling backwards is in part a strategy for disrupting narratives of progress. It helps us notice temporal lags and generational undertows that disrupt metaphors of feminist waves. Here, feeling backwards enables us to historicise the WRAP project, locating it within a feminist critique of bad sex and outmoded femininities that framed the interviews with young women. This section considers how the original WRAP research team posed and reflected on the question 'is sex

Is sex good for you? 349

good for you' and how it enabled them to problematise the unspoken economies of heterosex, contributing to a cost-benefit analysis focused on female gratification and its failure. As researchers 'then' and 'now' have argued, where we find the traces of sexual knowledge depends on where we look, and in what context our methodologies and research questions are forged. What does it mean to ask whether sex is good for you? And who might you trust to give answers – parents, advisory agencies, magazines, teachers, the government, or even university researchers? In fact, what does the question itself even mean – what is 'sex', and what is 'good'?

In 1989 female sexuality was a focus for attention, regulation, and research. Social research commissioned around AIDS documented, measured, and storied the sexual lives of the British population.[21] WRAP addressed new concerns with the heterosexual spread of AIDS. It did so within the tradition of critical feminist thinking about women's 'sexual health' as focus on the possible transmission routes for HIV/AIDS and other sexually transmitted diseases (STDs) expanded notions of safer sex beyond pregnancy prevention. WRAP was therefore part of a feminist intervention that sought to connect the exchange of bodily fluids with questions of power, control, and consent.[22]

Reframing sex as an exchange of body fluids was part and parcel of new examinations of barrier methods, including condoms, cervical caps, and femidoms. In 1981, activist Sue O'Sullivan told how heterosexual feminists had rediscovered barrier methods ('an old fashioned method of birth control') and rejected the assumptions that they should take risks for their male sexual partners and 'pump Pills into themselves for years on end'. Although the Pill had broken the link between sex and reproduction, it had done so 'in favour of male penetration'. Heterosexual women still 'let sex happen to us' and needed to resolve 'in a pro-woman way' the contradictions in sexual relations with men. Because barrier methods 'demanded much more than passivity', they could mean more active and feminist negotiation with sex.[23]

WRAP interviews came to focus on this struggle around how to turn silent acts of 'going with the flow' into empowering communications around desires, bodies, and safety. After finding early on that 'conventional femininity' is an 'unsafe sexual identity', the team later elaborated that 'where young women adopt conventional

350 *Subjectivity and intersubjectivity*

feminine identities uncritically, their sexual safety is more likely to be at risk, since femininity requires both deference to male demands and needs, and also emotional investment in a relationship with a man'.[24]

An exchange between interviewee Rebecca (18) and interviewer Rachel (23) shows how talk within the interviews mapped sexual safety and the exchange of body fluids onto wider moral and political rationales for having sex.[25] Rebecca explained that 'when I first started sleeping with people it was something more that I did to get experience and I think just recently I have started to think it's not much of a thrill any more sleeping with these people, and I don't really know why I am doing it'. She worried that 'I will end up being like a slag which is a word I would never use about anybody'. Rachel questioned whether her partner had used this word, and Rebecca clarified, 'Nobody had called me that, it was just what I felt'.

Here, Rebecca claimed not to 'really know why' she is having sex, yet also realised that she needed (sexual) experience in order to gain understanding for herself. In seeking experiential knowledge she confronted the stigmatising categories of an old sexual politics that she rejected, yet felt implicated in ('being like a slag'). The feminist researcher noticed and focused critical attention on this space between Rebecca's aspirations and her feelings, noting that 'women think in one way they are liberating themselves to be independent, to be sexually independent, and in a way model that on men and what men do, and then it comes to the question that it doesn't feel that good'. Rebecca agreed:

> Yes I think it's like men can do that and women can't even though you wanted to [...] and men can do it but we can't anyway so it's like a conscious decision not to sleep with anyone straight away or give it a bit of time and think about it and not go straight away and leap into bed with them.

This co-produced feminist analysis can be found across the interviews, diagnosing the gendered asymmetry of the sexual double standard, and reframing the choice to step away from sexual activity as a feminist rather than simply feminine response.

Seen from the present, we recognise the negotiations needed to imagine new ways in which sex could be good for you – gaining

Is sex good for you? 351

experience and sexual knowledge, figuring things out, and working at your own pace. In 1980s Manchester it felt hard work as Rebecca struggled with the power of the category of 'slag'. Rachel noted that many other WRAP interview participants from 'the poorer areas of North Manchester' would see 'what you're saying now, the idea that you could decide to sleep with someone or not if you're going out with someone and you know this is not the person you're going to be with for the rest of your life' as 'unbelievable'. She asked Rebecca if she could explain 'how it's different for you, that you don't feel the sort of pressure that they do, which is if you're going to have a sexual relationship it's got to be very serious and long term'.

Here, a feminist account is shadowed by the presumed obsolescence of traditional working-class youth transitions. A strong distinction between choosing and being chosen is mapped onto ideas of outmoded/modern femininities that characterised the intimate cultures of the post-industrial city. In this account, freedom involves more than the saying 'yes' that the Pill made possible. It involves active self-making, revealing and challenging the sexual double standard in intimate relationships – something that can be seen as part of classed projects of the 'late-modern self characterized by emphasis on choice, fulfilment, self-discovery, self-realization and self-reflexivity'.[26]

The researcher followed up by asking if 'being able to choose who you want' was 'an important part of being liberated'. Rebecca replied:

> Yes, I think that's one of the things about sleeping with people, it's part of it, thinking I'm liberated, and I can do what I want to. I think when I was something like seventeen, I thought I want to find out about my sexuality and that's why I went out and did it, more than anything.

In the field note written shortly after the interview Rebecca and her peer group are described as 'a quite "right on" group of young people, mostly middle class, interested in sexuality and committed on a certain level to feminism. Have trouble with it all in practice.' This note framed Rebecca and her friends as an example of a category forming part of a key finding of the study, young women for whom putting feminist intentions into practice was difficult and involved multiple strategies for 'context specific empowerment', including the ability to talk about sex, willingness to deconstruct the euphemistic

352 *Subjectivity and intersubjectivity*

'sleeping with' into specific embodied practices, and privileging female sexual pleasure.[27]

Revisiting the same interview as part of the appraisal of the archive, Rachel noted, 'Interviewer makes it a political issue when it might be better to treat as a personal issue.' This suggests a lingering feeling that she did not fully hear Rebecca's account. Also remarkable is the way this conversation still resonates three decades later. Rosie, a younger researcher on the 'Reanimating Data' project, explains that Rebecca's interview stands out to her because these are questions she would have liked to be asked when she was eighteen, finding connections between her own story and one told two decades earlier. Indeed, a key finding of the revisiting project has been that contemporary young women are shocked but excited by the direct, critical, and empowering questions the original WRAP interviewers asked.[28]

So, is sex good for you? The material presented here suggests that in 1989 Britain, this was a productive question which framed the commissioning of a research study and the encounters and conversations that the study enabled. The question sits at the intersection of competing narratives about femininity: narratives of making the right choices, authenticity (the discovery of the true self), liberation (hidden sexual desires unleashed from convention and old 'rules'), and mutability (the capacity to be adaptable, reflexive, strategic, and instrumental). Feminist politics in the 1980s were recursive (as they are today), with imaginations haunted by the 'outmoded' intimacies and gendered formations of the past. Yet the past, then and now, is also available for plunder – such as reclaiming the productive awkwardness of barrier methods of contraception or the feminist questions of an earlier generation.

Feeling sideways: talking yourself into good sex

Despite the interventions of Law Lords and policy makers, girls in 1989 Britain did not passively consume sexual knowledge according to formal regulations. Before young women even got to ask or answer key questions like 'is sex good for you?' they had to navigate other obstacles: whom to ask for advice, where to look for information, and how to access knowledge. In other words, they had to work out who gets to decide the meaning and value of sex.

Is sex good for you? 353

In this second encounter we feel sideways from the WRAP study to engage with ideas about sex in contemporaneous magazines for young women. Interviewees encountered these kinds of magazines in their everyday lives as part of a wider landscape of learning about sex that also included school science lessons, parental warnings, dictionaries, porn and 'dirty books', and the trials and errors of experiential knowledge.[29] Here we connect the talk in interviews with ideas explored in magazines published at the time of the WRAP fieldwork, identifying a shared solution to the problem of bad sex – the transformative value of *talking about it*.

In 1989, a new array of guidance promised to help girls and young women to recognise and negotiate the sexual double standard. WRAP operated within a wider cultural landscape in which young women could enjoy diverse consumer goods, including print media, produced just for them. New magazines marketed at young women, like *Just Seventeen* (1983–2004) and *Mizz* (1985–2013), joined existing teen publications like *Jackie* (1964–93) and *Smash Hits* (1978–2006) on newsagents' shelves. Each combined sexuality, sociability, and pop cultural fandom in different ways.[30] In these magazines, girls' exchange of sexual knowledge was played out in public. They opened out a space for knowledge, but also invited scrutiny and critique, particularly over their suitability as a source of sexual information; *Just Seventeen*'s editors were regularly called by parents complaining about the content and detail of problem pages, especially when they covered gay or lesbian sex.[31] As the Gillick case showed, adults could endlessly compete over who had the appropriate expertise to disseminate sexual knowledge and resources to girls.[32] But, while the parent cultures argued, young women acquired and honed their sexual knowledge through magazines.[33]

If the girls' magazine market changed in the 1980s, so did the work that academic feminists did to make sense of them. As the market recognised the 'extraordinary prominence of young women in consumer culture', researchers did too.[34] Feminist scholars used these magazines as a way into analysing the interaction of class, ideology, and gender with market forces. Cultural studies of magazines like *Jackie* uncovered their valuable role in building girls' affective networks, strategies of resistive pleasure and incorporation into marketing models.[35] Arguably, in some such studies, teen readers became cyphers for scholarly debates on the possibilities of resistance

354 *Subjectivity and intersubjectivity*

within or against commercial popular culture, with the academic focus on consumption seeming to suggest that there was something 'peculiarly ideological' about girls.[36]

Organisations that promoted sexual knowledge recognised the importance of girls' magazines for shaping understandings of sex that is good for you. In magazines for adult women, such organisations pushed this message using overtly sexualised imagery. In June 1989, for example, *Cosmopolitan* featured a double page Health Education Authority advertisement which counterposed a cool monochrome image of a heterosexual couple (the woman looking into camera), echoing the aesthetics of a Calvin Klein underwear advert, with the following text:

> Condom. It's not that difficult to say is it? Well if it's not, what's stopping you? He might laugh at you for mentioning it. He might think you're easy [...] think about using one, and talk about it with your boyfriend. You never know, he might just be pleased you suggested it. Think about not having sex at all if you're not certain, or you don't really know him well enough [...] never feel shy about asking him to use a condom. AIDS. YOU'RE AS SAFE AS YOU WANT TO BE.[37]

Here, the ability to talk about sex is a gauge of whether the viewer is ready to 'do' sex.

Girls' magazines promoted the same message in their problem pages. In October 1989, a fourteen-year-old pleaded with *Just Seventeen* agony aunt Maroushka Monro: 'don't say talk it over with your boyfriend, because it's much too embarrassing. We never talk about sex or anything.' Nevertheless, after explaining the age of consent Monro advised that 'you need to talk – and take a responsible decision about this'. If the boyfriend could not cope with discussion, then 'he is not yet mature or loving enough to handle a physical relationship'. She reminded the correspondent that 'you too have a choice as to what happens to you [...] playing safe is a whole lot better than regret'.[38] Similarly, *Jackie*'s agony aunt emphasised that 'if you love and trust each other enough to start a sexual relationship, you should be able to discuss something as important as contraception too'.[39] The capacity to talk with a partner extended to the ability to negotiate with experts and professionals. One sixteen-year-old who wanted to go on the Pill but was 'too ashamed to go to the doctor' was advised to consider other

Is sex good for you? 355

methods, 'not to feel rushed or pushed into anything you don't feel ready for', and perhaps to take her boyfriend with her to the doctor: 'After all, it takes two as you say!'[40]

This emphasis on talking is aimed at empowering girls and young women. However, it risked making young women responsible for the potentially burdensome task of negotiation. There was also profit to be made from all that talking. One 1989 issue of *Just Seventeen* contained a full page advertisement for pre-recorded telephone advice lines on topics including 'who is your ideal boy', 'does he fancy you', and 'the love machine: put your passion 2 the test'. In the same year, *Cosmopolitan* offered pre-recorded messages on 'How to tell him what you like in bed', 'How to talk to a man', and 'Why can't he communicate?' alongside Tom Crabtree's regular 'On the Couch' column.[41] In both magazines, these messages were accessed via the new 0898 premium phone lines made possible by the 1984 privatisation of British Telecom.

A focus on 'communication' further complicates narratives of sexual 'liberation', especially in relation to the oral contraceptive pill. The Pill is often lauded as a turning point in women's capacity for sexual choice and agency – not only in their ability to manage their bodies and fertility, but in what new modes of 'family planning' meant for their aspirations and perceived social mobility. Some historians have decentred this narrative, pointing out the limits to women's capacity for sexual negotiation in a patriarchal culture, and looking at alternative ways of controlling fertility and reproduction.[42] WRAP interviews with young women who used the Pill point to the ways that gendered progress can be reseen as uneven. Contraception and safer sex were highly moralised, standing in for conversations that might not happen and assumptions that would not be shared.

For example, Gemma (18) cited her mother's concern that the Pill 'makes sleeping around too easy', explaining that 'she thought that I could just have sexual relationships whenever I wanted. But I wasn't going to. It was just in case I did, which I didn't plan on doing, I was prepared for it sort of thing.' For Stacey (20) the Pill became part of a set of developmental stages of a relationship signifying seriousness. She explained that among her peers 'most of the girls are on the Pill with steady boyfriends. I think they've passed the condom, casual boyfriend stage now.' Rather than talking openly

356   *Subjectivity and intersubjectivity*

and explicitly about risk, young women such as Tina (21) utilised such expectations as a way of securing safer sex, explaining that she would 'just say I'm not on the Pill [...] I don't think I'd bring the subject of safe sex up, I'd just say that I wasn't on the Pill, and sleep with them'.[43] The imperative expressed in the magazines to be open, purposeful, and transparent contrasts with the pragmatism of young women who prioritised maintaining respectability, reputation, and some form of control over their own sexual health.

There are obvious tensions between exercising choice and operating within the limits of compulsory heterosexuality. Despite expanded possibilities, in 1989, sex for girls was only really legitimised within romantic relationships. Agony aunts urged readers to talk to their partners about contraception as a shared responsibility, but in practice the status quo still meant 'letting sex happen' and appearing to be sexually unknowing. Talking about contraception was supposed to make sexual wants, needs, and desires more visible, but at the same time the Pill was meant to make intercourse more spontaneous, grown-up, and intimate. In line with the contemporaneous feminist consensus, the original WRAP analysis critiqued the ambivalence in this idea of spontaneity, arguing that it actually fostered a new kind of passivity, where it was easier to let sex happen than to engage in complex negotiations.[44]

Feeling forwards: getting sex into perspective

Revisiting sociological archives historicises social research, enabling us to encounter material from the past in new ways.[45] We sometimes discover material that appears to speak to the present, a feeling forward that might even help us to imagine the future in new ways.[46] Connecting with an interview in the archive can generate unexpected insights. For example, when we look at these interviews thirty years later, we are newly attuned to young women's reluctance to talk openly and explicitly about sexual desires, embodiment, and intentions. We stand on the other side of a debate around sexualisation that has involved, again, thinking critically about the liberatory pursuit of pleasure. We understand how sex can be mediated and marketised and why in contemporary times it could be easier to share nudes than to have a conversation or even to touch. While authenticity has never been so valued, what it now means to communicate needs and desires in romantic relationships is transposed through the rationalising logics of dating apps that allow for a pragmatic and performative signalling of intentions, motivations, and boundaries.[47]

In the final section of this chapter we feel forwards with Rosie (30), the youngest member of the 'Reanimating Data' team, who discovers an interview in the WRAP archive that helps her to illuminate the contemporary sexual landscape. The interview, conducted in 1989 by Sue Scott (then 36) reveals Jodie (17) as grappling with emergent forms of sexual understanding. In presenting key parts of her interview we gather together insights from across this chapter, historicising her account yet also hearing her questions anew in a thick present. Rosie's analysis adds a layer of futurity by reanimating this interview through the lens of current sexual politics, in ways unforeseen by the original WRAP team.[48]

Choice was at the heart of Jodie's talk in her interview. She set out the importance to her of having 'a good-looking boyfriend otherwise I will do without it'. When Sue queried whether she meant 'somebody that you find attractive or someone that everybody else thinks is good looking', Jodie explained that while other people usually found the boys she picked good looking, 'it wouldn't bother me, as long as I think he's good looking'. This desire for a 'good looking boy' might be seen as part of a wider teen culture offering boys as pin-ups in magazines such as *My Guy* and *Just Seventeen*, a starting point for a female desire that includes much more than romance.[49]

Yet having a 'hunk' was not the same as being in control. Jodie's awareness of this became apparent as she talked about how young men positioned potential partners as not being like 'other girls', and detailed her own reasons and strategies for avoiding sex even when 'in the heat of the moment you want it, you feel that you want it and everything':

> I suffer like I said from guilt and also I wouldn't like anyone to brand me easy. [...] 'you're not like any other girl'. I've heard that so many times and it's so corny that you think, you know that this person will be talking about you or discussing it with his best friend, makes me feel sick. So it's just the way I've been brought up and I know I've got to keep my name good and everything. It has been hard at times

358 *Subjectivity and intersubjectivity*

to get out of situations, but I just say, 'that's it, enough's enough', and I don't know how I have done it.

Here, Jodie used the phrase 'not like other girls' as the reported speech of boys trying to convince girls to have sex. But at other points in the interview Jodie also distinguished her trajectory from that of 'other girls' who fell pregnant at a young age. Prompted on why she had such strong feelings about not having sex without protection, she explained:

> Well mum works in a clinic for abortions and she sees girls coming in at thirteen, even fourteen, and they are expecting their second child and that has opened my eyes as well, because she has come home and she has said this girl came today, it's confidential but she only tells me because I'm her daughter and she wants to make me aware, and I don't discuss what goes on with anybody else, but that's an eye opener as well.

As a middle-class girl with ambitions, Jodie took on the assumption that the challenge was to care for one's own sexual health. She knew that young women's destinies were precarious because her mother made this clear.[50] But, despite her insistence on the importance of safe sex ('I would never have sex without protection'), her story of a recent holiday romance revealed how difficult it was to enact that commitment in practice:

> Jodie: The way I looked at it he was very health conscious, he didn't smoke, had a fabulous physique and he was down at the gym nearly every day and I thought, if he does all this for his body I don't think he is even going to allow himself to have a chance of getting AIDS, whereas he didn't know where I had been, he didn't know my history.
>
> Sue: He didn't ask you?
>
> Jodie: The only thing he asked me was, was I on the Pill. But he didn't seem to bother about wearing a condom so ever since that I have been a bit wary about it, but I think the chances of it might be very slim.
>
> Sue: It's just a matter of remembering that next time and not giving yourself that worry in the future, you just don't need to have that worry. So the time you didn't use a condom, why didn't you?
>
> Jodie: Just because there was none around at the time.

Is sex good for you? 359

Jodie picked the boy who could then pick her – she chose a partner who looked 'safe' but who was unquestioning and remained fun (no condom). She shows us that we can have sex that *looks* good, but that is not good *for* you (no condom use).

As seen already, being on the Pill meant not having to 'ruin the moment', blurring the boundaries of acceptable/respectable conduct.[51] It also involved ignoring the injunctions of agony aunts, health educators, and feminist researchers to earnestly communicate. Worried about the attention her holiday romance got from other girls, she had 'sat down and said, "look, I've not slept around, I am clean and everything"'. The boy's insistence that 'he was very health conscious and he didn't even like to talk about AIDS' reassured Jodie. However, even though 'AIDS does scare me a lot', she still took it for granted that '[w]hen you sleep with somebody you don't sit down and ask about all the previous girlfriends or boyfriends or anything like that':

> Sue: In some of the articles about AIDS it actually says that that is what you should do, but it is very difficult isn't it?
>
> Jodie: And sometimes it can be very embarrassing because you don't know how the boy is going to react. He might feel insulted in some respects.
>
> Sue: As if you are checking up on him?
>
> Jodie: Yes, as if you are checking up on him and he might not want to discuss his past life.

Forward-looking Jodie recognised sex as something exciting, the source of knowledge and experience. Yet the need to communicate (in order to get sex right) complicated its potential as a source of risk, pleasure, and status. Sue understood how Jodie might resist this responsibility, the checking-up that feels so much like a nagging pull of the past. Jodie brilliantly summed up the contradictions that she faced when she said: 'The thing I found so annoying is something that's supposed to be so romantic and intimate between two people has got so many downfalls.'

Reflecting on the WRAP interviews, Sue Scott observes that 'It did feel like you created a space where she could say something she'd not said before.'[52] These same possibilities are operational as the archives are revisited, materials reanimated, and we notice feelings

360 *Subjectivity and intersubjectivity*

and 'experiences that discourse has not yet caught up with, rather than as a legacy passed on between generations'.[53] Rosie now describes Jodie as a 'pick me' girl – a contemporary label for a girl who craves male attention and tries to attain it (to be picked) by insisting that she is not like other girls. Jodie was enthusiastic yet anxious about sex, keen to please and be pleased, uncertain about what sex is or should be. Her account vividly captures what might be involved in seeking to be the protagonist of your own romantic and sexual life in 1989. When listening to Jodie we can, in Beth Freeman's words, experience 'connections between past and present that facilitate antinarrative leaps across time'.[54]

Conclusion

Young women's sexual knowledge was a very public matter in the late 1980s, entangled with ideas of self-improvement and the competing contributions of parents, institutions, new media opportunities, and constant political discussion. This chapter has connected some of the different spaces in which sex was talked about (research, magazines) and has suggested that a popular expert consensus existed in which talking about sex was the antidote to 'bad' sex, be that unsatisfying sex, non-consensual sex, or unsafe sex. We have attempted to bring out some apparently contradictory aspects of young women's sexual identities at this moment in time. Being the one that chooses rather than the one that is chosen was important to these young women, yet agency, passivity, and control are not so easily distinguished.

Looking back at this moment now, we can see the joins and ruptures between feminist discourse and more popular and commercial articulations of choice and pleasure. Sexual communication became a focal point through which wider power relations were diagnosed and calibrated. The WRAP interviews capture candid and direct conversations between feminist researchers and young women, while also reporting back on guesswork and coded communications between sexual partners. In reanimating these interviews here, our approach has combined strategies for feeling back (noting the pull of the past within a tradition of feminist research), feeling sideways (capturing the resonances and contradictions between synchronous sources), and feeling forwards (experiencing new insights about the past

Is sex good for you? 361

through encounters with the present). In doing so we have focused attention on how in late 1980s Britain ideas of choice, agency, and self-determination were forged in the crucible of sex.

What we notice in the archive is never the same as what is there. There is an additional layer of complexity in the return to WRAP, in that it involves two intergenerational feminist research teams, working thirty years apart. Both teams are part of a tradition that involves legacies and seeks to imagine futures.[55] In this chapter we have identified tensions between what the WRAP team found in the interviews, what they thought when interviewed thirty years later, and what we find when we look again. More than this, older and younger members of the research teams past and present notice material from their own generational perspectives. This was the case in 1989, when Rachel as the youngest member of the research team challenged the more pessimistic analyses of her feminist collaborators.[56] It was the case again as Rosie brought fresh perspectives to the new research team. And it is also the case today as we share the archive with new generations of young women.[57]

Notes

1 Interview with Janet Holland (24 February 2020), *Feminist Approaches to Youth Sexualities* [Reanimating Data Project]: https://archives. reanimatingdata.co.uk/s/fays/item/1907#?c=&m=&s=&cv= (accessed 31 January 2023).

2 Economic and Social Research Council, *Reanimating Data* (ES/R009538/1), 2018–2020 (COVID extension until 2021): http://reanimatingdata.co. uk/ (accessed 31 January 2023).

3 Rachel Thomson, 'Women, Risk and AIDS Project (1989–1990)', University of Sussex Collection (2020): https://doi.org/10.25377/sussex. c.4433834 (accessed 30 May 2023).

4 Mica Nava, *Changing Cultures: Feminism, Youth and Consumerism* (London: Sage; 1992); Angela McRobbie, *Feminism and Youth Culture* (Basingstoke: Palgrave Macmillan, 1991).

5 Sue Lees, *Losing Out: Sexuality and Adolescent Girls* (London: Hutchinson, 1986); Lesley Hall, 'Birds, bees and general embarrassment: sex education in Britain, from social purity to Section 28', in Richard Aldrich (ed.), *Public or Private Education? Lessons from History* (London: Routledge, 2004).

362   *Subjectivity and intersubjectivity*

6 Sarah Crook and Charlie Jeffries, 'Introduction: thinking through the 1980s', in Sarah Crook and Charlie Jeffries (eds), *Resist, Organize, Build: Feminist and Queer Activism in Britain and the United States during the Long 1980s* (Albany, NY: State University of New York Press, 2022), p. 3.

7 Sara Scott, 'Sex and danger: feminism and AIDS', *Trouble and Strife*, 11 (Summer 1987); Rachel Thomson, 'Moral rhetoric and public health pragmatism: the recent politics of sex education', *Feminist Review*, 48 (Autumn 1994).

8 Gillian Douglas, 'Family law under the Thatcher government', *Journal of Law & Society*, 17 (1990), 411.

9 McRobbie, *Feminism and Youth Culture*, pp. 220–42; Charles Murray, *The Underclass Revisited* (Washington, DC: American Enterprise Institute, 1999).

10 Section 28, known as Clause 2a in Scotland, was a legislative act that prohibited the funding of activity involving 'the promotion of homosexuality by local authorities'. In practice, this meant that local authorities could not fund the provision of books, plays, leaflets, or films that depicted LGBTQ+ relationships positively. Page 3 refers to the tabloid practice, originating in the *Sun* but soon adopted by other newspapers, of including a photograph of a topless female glamour model on page 3 of each copy. The Sun's first Page 3 image appeared in 1970 and the last in 2015.

11 Joe Moran, 'Childhood sexuality and education: the case of Section 28', *Sexualities*, 4.1 (2001); Hannah Elizabeth, '"Private things affect other people": Grange Hill's critique of British sex education policy in the age of AIDS', *Twentieth Century British History*, 32:2 (2021).

12 Hannah Elizabeth, '"If it hadn't been for the doctor, I think I would have killed myself": ensuring adolescent knowledge and access to healthcare in the age of Gillick', in Jennifer Crane and Jane Hand (eds), *Posters, Protests, and Prescriptions: Cultural Histories of the National Health Service in Britain* (Manchester: Manchester University Press, 2022), p. 255.

13 In the early 1980s the activist Victoria Gillick, a Roman Catholic mother of ten children, launched a case against the Department of Health and Social Security (DHSS) in England and Wales. The case challenged the authority of the DHSS to enable doctors to prescribe contraception to under-16s without parental consent or to provide contraceptive advice. Although Gillick lost the case, the publicity surrounding it heightened tensions around the provision of sex education. It contributed to an atmosphere in which many people with responsibility for the wellbeing

Is sex good for you?   363

of children and adolescents felt anxious about the potential legal consequences of their actions. The guidelines set out by Lord Fraser in his judgment of the Gillick case in the House of Lords (*Gillick v West Norfolk*, 1985) apply specifically to contraceptive advice. Lord Fraser stated that a doctor should always encourage a girl aged under 16 to inform her parents or carers that she is seeking contraceptive advice (or allow the doctor to inform the parents or carers on her behalf). But if she cannot be persuaded to do so they can proceed to give contraceptive advice and treatment as long as certain conditions are met. This includes making sure it's in the girl's best interests for advice to be given and that she understands the advice. This is widely known as 'Gillick competence'.

14 Douglas, 'Family law under the Thatcher government', 418.

15 In 1987, 121 children in the administrative county of Cleveland were removed from their parents because of allegations of child sexual abuse based on controversial diagnostic tests used by paediatricians at the Middlesbrough Hospital. Ninety-four of these children were subsequently returned to their parents' care. The media coverage of the Cleveland scandal prompted intense criticism of social services.

16 Nick Basannavar, *Sexual Violence against Children in Britain since 1965: Trailing Abuse* (Basingstoke: Palgrave Macmillan, 2021), pp. 207–25.

17 Nicky Thorogood, 'Sex education as social control', *Critical Public Health*, 3 (1992); Stevi Jackson, *Childhood and Sexuality* (Oxford: Blackwell, 1982); Jane Pilcher, 'Gillick and after: children and sex in the 1980s and 1990s', in Jane Pilcher and Stephen Wagg (eds), *Thatcher's Children? Politics, Childhood and Society in the 1980s and 1990s* (London: Falmer Press, 1996), p. 77.

18 Kaye Wellings and Dominic McVey, 'Evaluation of the HEA AIDS press campaign: December 1988 to March 1989', *Health Education Journal*, 49.3 (1990); Tim Rhodes and Robert Shaughnessy, 'Compulsory screening: advertising AIDS in Britain, 1986–89', *Policy & Politics*, 18.1 (1990); Maire Messenger Davies, *Television is Good for Your Kids* (London: Shipman, 1996).

19 Lynne Segal, 'The heat in the kitchen', in Stuart Hall and Martin Jacques (eds), *The Politics of Thatcherism* (London: Lawrence and Wishart, 1983); Anna Coote and Beatrix Campbell, *Sweet Freedom: The Struggle for Women's Liberation* (London: Pan Books, 1982).

20 Heather Love, *Feeling Backwards: Love and Loss in Queer History* (Cambridge, MA: Harvard University Press, 2007).

21 See, for example, the National Survey of Sexual Attitudes and Lifestyles (Natsal), which has interviewed thousands of people every ten years

364 *Subjectivity and intersubjectivity*

since 1990: www.lshtm.ac.uk/research/centres-projects-groups/natsal (accessed 31 January 2023).

22 Interview with Janet Holland.

23 Sue O'Sullivan, 'Capping the cervix', *Spare Rib*, 105 (April 1981).

24 See Janet Holland, Caroline Ramazanoglu, Sue Scott, Sue Sharpe, and Rachel Thomson, '"Don't die of ignorance", I nearly died of embarrassment: condoms in context', *WRAP Paper* 2 (London: The Tufnell Press, 1990); Janet Holland, Caroline Ramazanoglu, Sue Sharpe, and Rachel Thomson, *The Male in the Head: Young People, Heterosexuality and Power* (London: The Tufnell Press, 1998), p. 49.

25 Interview with Rebecca (13 June 1989), *Feminist Approaches to Youth Sexualities* [WRAP]: https://archives.reanimatingdata.co.uk/s/fays/item/855#?c=&m=&s=&cv= (accessed 31 January 2023).

26 Tinkler, '"Are you really living?"', 598.

27 Janet Holland, Caroline Ramazanoglu, Sue Scott, and Rachel Thomson, 'Pressure, resistance, empowerment: young women and the negotiation of safer sex', *WRAP Paper* 6 (London: The Tufnell Press, 1991).

28 Ester McGeeney, 'Working with questions' (14 September 2020): http://reanimatingdata.co.uk/uncategorized/working-with-questions/ (accessed 31 January 2023).

29 Rachel Thomson and Sue Scott, *Learning about Sex: Young Women and the Social Construction of Sexual Identity* (London: The Tufnell Press, 1991).

30 Janice Winship, '"A girl needs to get street-wise": magazines for the 1980s', *Feminist Review*, 21.1 (1985).

31 Elizabeth, '"If it hadn't been for the doctor"'.

32 Pilcher, 'Gillick and after', p. 80.

33 Winship, '"A girl needs to get street-wise"'; McRobbie, *Feminism and Youth Culture*, pp. 135–88.

34 Angela McRobbie, 'Young women and consumer culture: an intervention', *Cultural Studies*, 22.5 (2008), 533.

35 Angela McRobbie, '*More!* New sexualities in girls', *Back to Reality? Social Experience and Cultural Studies* (Manchester: Manchester University Press, 1997), p. 190; Anna Gough-Yates, '"A shock to the system": feminist interventions in youth subculture – the adventures of *Shocking Pink*', *Contemporary British History*, 26.3 (2012).

36 Elizabeth Frazer, 'Teenage girls reading Jackie', *Media, Culture & Society*, 9.4 (1987), 407.

37 *Cosmopolitan*, June 1989.

38 *Just Seventeen*, 24 May 1989.

39 *Jackie*, 8 April 1989.

40 *Jackie*, 20 May 1989.

Is sex good for you? 365

41 *Cosmopolitan*, June 1989.

42 Hera Cook, *The Long Sexual Revolution: English Women, Sex, and Contraception 1800–1975* (Oxford: Oxford University Press, 2004); Hera Cook, 'The English sexual revolution: technology and social change', *History Workshop Journal*, 59:1 (2005); David Geiringer, *The Pope and the Pill: Sex, Catholicism and Women in Post-war England* (Manchester: Manchester University Press, 2019).

43 Holland et al., '"Don't die of ignorance"'.

44 Janet Holland, Caroline Ramazanoğlu, Sue Sharpe, and Rachel Thomson, 'Pressured pleasure: young women and the negotiation of sexual boundaries', *WRAP Paper* 7 (London: The Tufnell Press, 1992), 222.

45 Mike Savage, 'Revisiting classic qualitative studies', *Forum Qualitative Sozialforschung/Forum: Qualitative Social Research*, 6:1 (2005).

46 John Goodwin and Henrietta O'Connor, *Norbert Elias's Lost Research: Revisiting the Young Worker Project* (London: Routledge, 2015).

47 Rosalind Gill, 'The sexualisation of culture?', *Social and Personality Psychology Compass*, 6:7 (2012); Ester McGeeney and Elly Hanson, *Digital Romance: A Research Project Exploring Young People's Use of Technology in their Romantic Relationships and Love Lives* (London: National Crime Agency and Brook, 2017): www.basw.co.uk/system/files/resources/basw_85054-7.pdf (accessed 31 January 2023).

48 Interview with Jodie [pseudonym for AMD21] (9 May 1989), *Feminist Approaches to Youth Sexualities* [WRAP]: https://archives.reanimatingdata.co.uk/s/fays/item/843#?c=&m=&s=&cv= (accessed 31 January 2023).

49 Carol Dyhouse, *Heartthrobs: A History of Women and Desire* (Oxford: Oxford University Press, 2017).

50 The original WRAP analysis highlighted maternal warnings as a key site of young women's learning. See Thomson and Scott, *Learning about Sex*.

51 See also Lynne Hillier, Lyn Harrison, and Deborah Warr, '"When you carry condoms all the boys think you want it": negotiating competing discourses about safe sex', *Journal of Adolescence*, 21 (1998); Gillian Abel and Lisa Fitzgerald, '"When you come to it you feel like a dork asking a guy to put a condom on": is sex education addressing young people's understandings of risk?', *Sex Education*, 6:2 (2006).

52 Interview with Sue Scott (18 February 2020), *Reanimating Data Project* Dataset, University of Sussex: https://doi.org/10.25377/sussex.13043024.v1 (accessed 31 January 2023).

53 Elizabeth Freeman, *Time Binds: Queer Temporalities and Queer Histories* (Durham, NC: Duke University Press, 2010), p. 84.

54 Freeman, *Time Binds*, p. 126.

55 Crook and Jeffries, 'Introduction', p. 3.

56 Interview with Rachel Thomson (26 February 2020), *Reanimating Data Project* Dataset, University of Sussex: https://doi.org/10.25377/sussex.13042922.v1 (accessed 31 January 2023).

57 The archive includes material documenting how contemporary young women responded to the WRAP interviews: https://archives.reanimatingdata.co.uk (accessed 31 January 2023).

15

'What your generation probably don't understand is ...': exploring intergenerational dynamics in oral history

Kate Mahoney

Introduction

For as long as I have been conducting oral history interviews, I have been aware of the generational differences that exist between myself and my interviewees. When interviewing feminist activists for my doctoral research, my interviewees, many of whom were in their seventies, expressed surprise at my age. One interviewee jokingly suggested that I 'seemed very young to be a PhD student'. Others had strong opinions on my generation's attitude to women's rights. Some stated that women of my generation had not done the work necessary to continue the successes of the women's movement in the 1970s and 1980s. In these instances, I never felt it appropriate to offer a retort. However, I often felt a little defensive, despite being uncertain about how 'my generation' and my identification with it might be defined in the context of feminist activism.

My interviewees' reflections on my age and generation constituted intergenerational dynamics. In this context, I define intergenerational dynamics as: the interviewer or interviewee making references to their sense of generational identity; the unspoken and spoken assumptions that the interviewer and interviewee hold about their respective generations, and the way these assumptions are projected during the interview; and moments when either the interviewer or participant indicate the generational differences that exist between them. As Chandler argues, whilst oral history interviews often foster 'intergenerational talk', there remains scope to understand how 'generational and age-related dimensions of subjectivity can shape what

368   *Subjectivity and intersubjectivity*

and how material becomes available with interviews, or how that material is interpreted'.[1] This chapter therefore analyses how generational difference influences the interpersonal dynamics of oral history interviews.

The analysis in this chapter draws on my own experiences conducting oral history interviews as a postdoctoral researcher on the project 'Body, Self, and Family: Women's Psychological, Emotional, and Bodily Health in Britain, c. 1960–1990' at the University of Essex (2017–22). Whilst in this role, I carried out over thirty in-depth oral history interviews with women born between 1940 and 1970. The interviews focused on their 'everyday health' experiences across the life-course, which provides a pertinent case study for exploring intergenerational dynamics. The life-course approach encouraged women to first reflect on their childhood before documenting how their understandings and experiences of health had changed to the present day. Participants reflected on the social and cultural factors that informed their health experiences at different points in their lives. Many women suggested that particular experiences – such as the distribution of orange juice at primary school and women's current obligation to care for their children and grandchildren alongside their ageing parents – were synonymous with their generation. Our interview guide also contained a question asking participants to consider how their lives had been different to those of their mothers and grandmothers. In response, interviewees often positioned their experiences within an intergenerational framework, citing large-scale changes such as the increased numbers of women in the workplace and at university, and the introduction of the Pill, as key developments that distinguished their generation from their predecessors.

In this chapter, I first explore how interviewees defined their generational positioning in different ways. Second, I consider how and why some interviewees applied their own assumptions about my generation and its behaviours to me. I then examine the generational assumptions that I brought to interviews, focusing on the sense of familiarity I often felt when interviewing women of the same generation as my mother. Unpacking this familiarity also helps me to comprehend why interviewing women of my mother's age triggered deep emotions both during and after the interview, leading to moments of self-discovery relating to my own experiences.[2] I consider how these momentary revelations influenced the interpersonal

'*What your generation probably don't understand*'   369

dynamics of the interview. Finally, I briefly summarise how other oral historians have responded to these intergenerational dynamics, both during and after the interview. Intergenerational conversations are an intrinsic facet of oral history. As this chapter demonstrates, during the oral history encounter, 'multiple notions of intergenerationality come into play'.[3] Understanding how these different forms of intergenerational dynamics are constructed and resultantly make us feel further expands our understanding of the influence of researcher subjectivity during the oral history process.

Defining a generation

Many of the interviewees that I spoke to offered definitions of their generation and its identifying factors. Theorists of age and ageing assert that understandings of 'generation' can be broken down into three parts: 'the concept of generation in terms of life stage'; 'membership of a birth cohort (which is often ascribed particular characteristics and dispositions based on shared historical position and experience)'; and 'positions within a family structure'.[4] As Wanderbeck and Worth write, 'these three notions of generation intersect within the context of individual biographies' and are 'not necessarily experienced or understood by individuals in terms of separate dimensions'.[5] Many of the women that we interviewed for the 'Body, Self, and Family' project drew on this tripartite construction of 'generation' to define their generational identity. Exploring how women defined their generational positioning in this way provides a context for understanding how intergenerational dynamics manifested in their interviews.

Events experienced by a cohort in childhood can 'exert an important, even decisive, influence on the later attitudes and actions of its members', meaning that individuals often align their childhood experiences with their 'generational character'.[6] Our participants, born in the immediate postwar period, frequently defined their generation by the social and political developments that occurred in their childhoods, notably the emergent welfare state and its health and social benefits. Worth notes that 'the welfare state was the framework that defined the early lives of girls growing up in the post-war period'. She attributes the dominance of the welfare state

370 *Subjectivity and intersubjectivity*

in childhood recollections to the fact that it was deemed universal; its introduction affected everyone.[7]

When I interviewed Mo at her home in Witham, Essex, in January 2018, she listed a range of social developments that she had benefited from as a child and young adult. These included the success of grammar schools as a 'social mobility vehicle', the advent of the Pill, and a decline in workplace sexual harassment. Born in 1946, Mo stated that: 'I think probably my generation have had a golden era.'[8] Other interviewees born in the postwar period echoed Mo's sentiments. Born in 1944, Susan recalled that she and her brothers 'were fortunate in a sense of being babies after the war because we had a good diet'.[9] Susan attributed her healthy eating to National Dried Milk, which was introduced in 1940 as part of the Ministry of Health's National Milk Scheme. Pregnant women, and mothers with children under the age of one, were entitled to seven pints of free or subsidised milk per week on top of their normal entitlement.[10] Susan also referenced the health benefits of orange juice, which was made freely available to children in schools – another scheme introduced in response to concerns about the health of the general population in wartime Britain.[11]

Both Mo and Susan drew on popular cultural scripts that present the 1950s as a 'golden age', citing the developments in welfare, technology, and infrastructure that occurred across the decade.[12] Interviewees' employment of these 'cultural constructions in public discourse' helped to demonstrate how they constructed their identity or subject position over the course of the interview.[13] As Michael Roper argues, interviewees' choices about how they interweave 'dominant cultural forms' into their personal narratives 'can tell us something about individual subjectivity'.[14] In describing the 1950s as a 'golden age', Mo was aware that she was drawing on a popular representation of the decade that was potentially problematic, not least because she thought that women's rights and opportunities were still limited then. However, it remained important for interviewees of this generation to emphasise the benefits of being children of the welfare state, particularly because they still felt as though they were reaping the benefits. Both interviewees cited the generous pensions that they received. Mo also made an intergenerational comparison with her daughter, who had found it far harder to buy a house.

'What your generation probably don't understand'   371

As Worth argues, children born in the 1940s and 1950s were informed from a young age about the benefits of the developing welfare state. Parents told their children that the introduction of the National Health Service (NHS) transformed their access to good-quality healthcare. When interviewed by Worth, Jean, who was born in 1950 to a working-class family, recalled being told 'tales of not going to the doctors because you couldn't afford to go. My mother had two siblings that had died of diphtheria.' This form of 'intergenerational transmission' – reiterated to those born in the immediate postwar period – informed children that their experiences of health and social care were different to those of previous generations; they were the first generation to reap the benefits of the burgeoning welfare state across their life-course.[15] As Mo's and Susan's interviews demonstrate, they distinguished the beneficial effects of the welfare state on their generation not only from their predecessors' experiences, but also from those of subsequent generations.

Interviewees who were born some ten and twenty years after the end of the Second World War defined their generation's key identifiers in different ways. Whereas Mo and Susan foregrounded their childhood experiences in the 1950s, Louise believed that her current caring role within her family exemplified her generation's identity.[16] She aligned her generational identity with both her life stage and position within her family. Born in Lancashire in the mid-1960s, Louise had had children in her early forties. Both children had recently started secondary school. Alongside caring for her children, Louise also looked after her elderly parents and mother-in-law. She was aware of the cultural scripts that defined her current caring responsibilities: 'The press calls it "the sandwich generation" don't they', she stated.[17] A phrase first coined by social work and gerontology researchers in the early 1980s, 'sandwich generation' is typically used to define the 'middle-aged generation who have elderly parents and dependent children'.[18] In the 1980s, the 'sandwich generation' was deemed symptomatic of the emergence of 'four-generation modified extended families' in the mid-twentieth century onwards; a development attributed to the 'lower average age of marriage; a lower median age of parenthood; and a decrease in the number of large families, so that mothers are younger when they have their last child'.[19] Increasingly, however, the 'sandwich

372 *Subjectivity and intersubjectivity*

generation' is seen to reflect the fact that people are having children later and living longer. Contemporary definitions of the 'sandwich generation' also cite the prevalence of the 'triple-decker sandwich' – 'people in their sixties helping to care for their grandchildren, which allows their adult children to work, as well as supporting their parents in their nineties'.[20]

Despite changes in conceptualisations of the 'sandwich generation', researchers have continually emphasised the enduring stress experienced by those who fulfil multigenerational caring responsibilities. As Miller noted in 1981, those in the 'sandwich generation' are exposed to a 'unique set of unshared stressors in which giving of resources and service far outweighs giving or exchanging them'.[21] Louise reiterated the complexities of her caring role as a member of the 'sandwich generation': 'I'm aware that, that we're sort of the linchpins within the family at the moment when it comes to anything needing to happen,' she asserted. 'We're the ones that are making everything happen for the younger and older generation.'[22]

The women that I spoke to for the 'Body, Self, and Family' project therefore defined their generational identities in different ways. Their definitions typically aligned with the tripartite concept of generational identity as constructed via life-course stage, membership of a birth cohort that share specific characteristics, and position within familial structure.[23] As children of the immediate postwar period, Mo and Susan equated their generational identity with the social benefits they had reaped via the emergent welfare state. Conversely, Louise associated her generational identity with her obligation to care for both her children and her parents, a role that was both pressured and stressful. All interviewees drew on cultural scripts, such as the 1950s 'golden age' and the 'sandwich generation', to define their generational position. Their application of these scripts suggested that the interviewees did not feel alone in their experiences, but, rather, part of a collective experience that differentiated them from the lives of those in both preceding and subsequent generations.

Navigating generational assumptions

As I conducted oral history interviews for the 'Body, Self, and Family' project, I became aware that interviewees' generational

'*What your generation probably don't understand*'   373

identifications also influenced how they perceived me. Several interviewees emphasised how our generational differences ensured our contrasting experiences of life events. I found these generational differentiations interesting. Whilst I could identify with the large-scale developments – such as technological advancement – that interviewees perceived my generation to have benefited from, individual aspects of our experiences and feelings sometimes appeared comparable. My response to interviewees' assertions of generational difference perhaps elucidates the relationship between collective and individual experiences that underpin generational identities. At the same time, my role as interviewer meant that I never countered the generational assumptions that interviewees attributed to me. Consequently, they were not privy to the aspects of their experience that I deemed comparable to my own. This meant that I often became a repository for interviewees' various projections about their own generational positioning and that of succeeding generations, as well as their sense of who I was beyond the role of interviewer.

In March 2018, I interviewed Margaret at her home in Oxted, Surrey. When I originally arranged to meet Margaret via email, she stipulated that the interview would have to be organised around her work commitments as a nurse and her role as a carer for her increasingly frail mother. When I arrived at Margaret's house a month later, she took me into the kitchen and made us a cup of tea. There she calmly told me that her mother had died the week before. I was slightly taken aback by the news and offered my condolences, whilst seeking to ensure that Margaret was still happy for the interview to go ahead. She confirmed that she was. Over the course of the interview, Margaret's grief was palpable. Whilst she did not become visibly upset whilst talking about her mother, Margaret switched between past and present tense when referring to her. Describing his own experience of interviewing fathers and sons, Richard Hall refers to the 'non-fixity' of parent–child relationships. He suggests that these relationships 'remain in perpetual negotiation across the life course [...] This bubbling continuity of feeling is brought vividly to life in oral history interviews, which see men refine and recompose their memories of fatherhood and childhood in real time.'[24] Margaret's deviation between tenses appeared to reflect her own attempts to recalibrate her perception of her relationship with her mother in the face of her grief.

374   *Subjectivity and intersubjectivity*

During other parts of the interview, Margaret did become visibly upset. Early on, Margaret mentioned that her sister had died of cancer when she was eighteen and Margaret was fifteen. 'I never realised that she was actually gonna die,' Margaret remembered whilst starting to cry, 'because when you're fifteen you don't think like that, you know.'[25] As Roper writes, interviewees who have experienced past trauma have 'the capacity for their emotional states to be re-activated – voluntarily and involuntarily – at later moments'.[26] This interview reactivated Margaret's emotional state when her sister died. In using the present tense to refer to her teenage self, however, her retelling of the loss of her sister also appeared to induce an expression of her contemporary feelings of grief.

A sense of isolation pervaded Margaret's recollections of her teenage years. Her sister died during the summer holidays, and she found it incredibly difficult not being able to regularly see her friends and to talk to them about it. Margaret couched this discussion of her isolation in generational terms:

> What your generation probably don't understand is, when the school holidays came, you left the school and for six weeks [...] our school was, you know, a bus ride away, and people lived in different areas from that bus ride.[27]

Margaret's emphasis on our generational difference – as articulated through her statement 'what your generation probably don't understand is' – belied her view of the characteristics and dispositions that define my generation. Certainly, for my generation, the advent of the internet and mobile phones has been seen to ensure a greater 'sense of belonging and connectedness' amongst young people, which, as Margaret assumed, might have influenced how I engaged with my friends over the school holidays.[28] What I found striking about Margaret's use of her rural isolation to define our generational differences, however, was that her description of teenage life seemed very similar to my own. I grew up in a rural village and attended a school with a large catchment area. Many of my friends lived some distance away, which meant that I saw them less frequently over the school holidays. Even with a landline telephone and a mobile phone, it was hard not to feel isolated at times in this setting.

Margaret reiterated her sense of our contrasting generational experiences when discussing her early comprehension of health.

'*What your generation probably don't understand*'   375

During her childhood, Margaret became aware of her health because people would routinely comment on her weight. 'I was quite a chubby child, I always thought I was fat,' she stated. 'People used to say, "It's puppy fat" – you probably don't even know that.' Discourses surrounding 'puppy fat' also featured prominently in my own childhood as a concept discussed by adults around me, particularly my mother and grandmother. This is not to say that Margaret and I would have had comparable experiences of discourses surrounding 'puppy fat' whilst growing up. Our growing up in different generations, places, and families meant that our awareness of the concept would have been informed by a variety of different social and cultural influences. The comments made about Margaret's weight as a child also appeared to have a long-standing impact on her sense of self and health. When I asked her how she defined health, she related it to 'your self-esteem' and 'your appearance'.[29] I did not experience comparable comments about my weight at that age. However, it remains striking that Margaret viewed 'puppy fat' as a concept grounded in her generational experience, and not mine.

These kinds of intergenerational dynamics help to illuminate how individuals' emotions and experiences align with their generational identities. Margaret associated her childhood feelings about her body and rural isolation with her generational identity. In this way, she attributed these experiences to the specific characteristics of her birth cohort. In interviewing Margaret, I realised, however, that I did not associate my feelings relating to living in the countryside and comprehending 'puppy fat' with my generation; rather, these aspects of my individual experience felt more broadly associated with being a teenage girl and growing up in a rural area. The ways that Margaret and I constructed our respective generational identities felt at odds with one another.

This feeling of disconnect, however, was complicated. In articulating how she thought our generations differed, Margaret repeatedly brought me into the interview. By referencing 'your generation', and guessing what I did and did not know, Margaret established my presence not only as an interviewer and researcher but as an individual with my own life experiences. At the same time, the intergenerational nature of the research encounter meant that Margaret's assumptions about my generation took on an educative quality. She, as a member of an older generation, was obliged to bestow information onto me

376   *Subjectivity and intersubjectivity*

as a member of the younger generation. As the interviewer, however, I did not deem it appropriate to counter any assumptions that Margaret made about me, or to highlight where aspects of our experiences converged. In this way, I felt that I did not bring my own identity or experiences to the interview. Rather, the identity that I represented during the research encounter was as a receptacle for Margaret's projections about who I should be, based on her sense of my generation. In this way, the intergenerational dynamics present in the interview highlighted the disparity between the sense of self that interviewer and interviewee each bring to the encounter. Whilst the interviewer learns a lot about the interviewee, the interviewee remains largely unaware of the interviewer's own experiences. Margaret's use of generational signifiers to ascribe to me particular forms of knowledge and experience may have been her way of overcoming this disparity, drawing on her sense of our generational differences to bring me into the interview as an individual with my own thoughts and feelings.

Situating interviews within a familial framework

So far, I have discussed how interviewees projected their assumptions about my generation onto me as the interviewer. However, I was also responsible for projecting my own assumptions or feelings onto interviewees, based on their generational positioning. When I first started conducting interviews for the 'Body, Self, and Family' project, I was struck by the sense of familiarity and ease I felt with some participants. I have always found oral history interviewing nerve-wracking. There is the sense of trepidation in the hours leading up to the interview, fuelled by concerns about the recorder working, remembering my interview guide, ensuring that I build the necessary rapport with the interviewee so that they feel comfortable, and the hope that they will find the research encounter a valuable experience. I have typically not known what to expect before an interview. I found that when I entered the physical interview space or joined a Zoom call, I felt palpable relief when I realised I was interviewing a woman of the same generation as my mother. This relief appeared to be grounded in a perceived familiarity. I felt as though I knew how to relate to the interviewee. Micaela di Leonardo discusses

'What your generation probably don't understand'   377

comparable feelings in her exploration of kinship, class, and gender among Italian Americans in 1980s California. When di Leonardo interviewed middle-aged participants, they often perceived her as a daughter figure. The interviewees transposed di Leonardo into an 'established role'. This positioning ensured that di Leonardo built a warm rapport with her participants.[30] Yow defines this feeling as 'positive transference', citing that 'when the feelings between the narrator and interviewer are positive, the influence of this on the progress of the interview will usually be positive' too.[31]

On reflection, however, the familiarity I felt when interviewing women of the same generation as my mother was potentially problematic. First, I was placing the interviewee in the 'established role' of my mother, therefore bringing my own projections relating to my relationship with her to the research encounter. Second, I was uncertain whether this familiarity was reciprocated by my interviewees. In the interview I discuss above, Louise was of the same generation as my mother. Her children, however, were over ten years younger than me. It is therefore unlikely that Louise placed me into a comparable familial framework. Third, any perceived familiarity on the part of the researcher has the potential to cloud their capacity to critically conduct the interview. In her exploration of research encounters where she has liked the interviewee 'too much', Yow describes 'hesitating to ask some of the things of narrators for whom I felt affection lest my questions caused them discomfort'. She asserts that researchers should be aware of the effects of positive transference on their capacity to ask 'difficult questions'.[32]

As I continued to conduct interviews with women of the same generation as my mother, I came to realise that the 'established role' I placed them in also affected my emotional responses following the interview. I later came to realise that my feelings were influenced by unresolved feelings related to my mum being ill. In the final year of my doctoral degree, I moved back home to live with my parents. Shortly after, my mum was diagnosed with a serious medical condition. She had to undergo invasive surgery and extensive treatment. For a long time, we were unsure of her prognosis. During this period, I tried to avoid speculating and committed to responding only to information that we were given by my mother's consultant. 'We can only work with the information that we have,' I would repeatedly tell myself. When I started conducting interviews for the

378   *Subjectivity and intersubjectivity*

'Body, Self, and Family' project a year later, however, I was taken aback by the emotions that I experienced when I interviewed women who were the same age as my mother. By then, she was largely well again and was no longer undergoing treatment. However, my encounters with women of her generation forced me to realise that I had not fully comprehended the impact of my mother's illness, not just on myself, but on my mum too.

Louise, whom I interviewed at her home in Devon in early 2018, was a few years younger than my mother. During the interview, she described being diagnosed with a serious autoimmune condition. Louise recalled the complex emotions that accompanied her diagnosis and early treatment:

> Feeling poorly is quite, you know, there's all sorts of things that go alongside that, about how that affects us – the way we feel about our bodies – but, erm, the power relationship with the person who's providing the care, erm, and sort of the agenda, and how that's shared or dictated, erm, and I think it's very easy, as a healthcare provider, to forget the perspective of the person who's receiving the care.[33]

As Louise discussed the intricate interpersonal dynamics and emotions that accompanied her diagnosis and treatment, I was struck by the fact that my mum would have experienced a comparably complex array of feelings when she was ill. This realisation was triggered by a sudden sense of how my mum might have responded to the questions that I was asking Louise. I inadvertently visualised my mother sitting in Louise's place, discussing her own experiences with a researcher who did not share the same emotional connection with her that I did.

For Arlene Kaplan Daniels, acknowledging the 'attachments' that we develop during fieldwork can provide 'opportunities […] for self-discovery, as well as insight into the field of study'.[34] This appears to be the case for Verusca Calabria, who shares her experiences interviewing people who received and provided care at the psychiatric institution Mapperley Hospital, Nottingham during the second half the twentieth century.[35] Calabria's own mother had a breakdown when she was a child, but Calabria was 'denied access to my mother's own narrative of events until my mid-twenties'. Over the course of the interviews, Calabria realised that she had 'subconsciously been piecing together what might have happened to my mother during

'What your generation probably don't understand'   379

the worst moments of her illness [...] I was reliving some of the grief from the loss I had experienced from my past when my mother became severely ill'. As Calabria notes, oral historians might typically witness 'not only our informants' unresolved grief but also the triggering of our own unresolved emotions about past events, which may affect our responses'.[36]

When interviewing Louise, I too realised that I had unresolved feelings about my mother's illness. My perception of how my mother must have felt at the time had been eclipsed by my desire for her to be okay. I had the luxury to 'only work with the information that we had' because I was not the one who was ill. As my mother later told me, every day that she did not receive a prognosis was accompanied by the fear that she might die; a feeling that I simply could not comprehend because I did not want to lose her. Through this realisation, I also understood more readily the 'emotional residues of the past' that I unconsciously brought to interviews with women who were my mother's age.[37] These projections naturally affected my positionality as a researcher. Yet, it is only in reflecting on my positionality now that I can start to envisage how it affected my interviewing.

Barbara Erskine expresses comparable concerns in her account of conducting an interview with a man who was a pilot in the Second World War. As the interviewee described flying, Erskine was reminded of her father, who had died in a plane crash thirty years before: 'Dad's face momentarily became that of my informant. I had to ask myself, "Whose story am I listening to?"' As Erskine listened to how the interviewee lost his friends in battle, she too found herself grieving for loss. This 'sharing of feeling', she argues, was a 'springboard to better interviewing'.[38] I encountered similar feelings when I envisaged my mother telling her own story during Louise's interview. It suddenly felt as though I was listening to my mum's reflections rather than the interviewee in front of me. Whilst this visualisation helped me to uncover my unresolved feelings relating to my mother's illness, this realisation took me out of the interview encounter. It is therefore questionable whether this was a moment of 'shared feeling'. Rather, I was tuned into my own emotion and no longer focused on Louise's narrative. At the same time, Louise would not have been aware that her account triggered my own self-discovery.

380 *Subjectivity and intersubjectivity*

Yow asserts that oral historians must 'attempt to move beyond our own self-schemas, focusing the interview not on what is important in our lives, but what is important to our interviewees'.[39] The task of moving outside of ourselves during the interview, however, feels particularly difficult if the self-schemas we bring to the interview are initially unconscious. I did not appreciate how my mother's illness was affecting the interviews I conducted until I had met with several participants. I was deeply affected by the interviews that I conducted with women of my mother's generation. I would frequently drive home crying, but with little comprehension as to why I was so moved. It was not until I visualised my mother whilst interviewing Louise that I started to understand why I felt this way. However, it was difficult to understand how to respond to these emotions whilst in the thick of interviewing. It is only in unpacking these feelings through writing this chapter that I have given myself the space to consider why I felt like this and the impact of these feelings on my interviews.

The intergenerational connection that I experienced during my interview with Louise demonstrated the value in generating the space for myself, both before and after an interview, to comprehend how and why certain emotions might be triggered during the research encounter. Yow suggests a series of questions that researchers can ask themselves when an interviewer is 'too much invested in the topic, too closely identifying with a person or cause'.[40] Her questions include 'what am I feeling about this narrator?' and 'what are the effects on me as I go about this research?' It now seems obvious to me that speaking to women of a comparable age to my mum about their health experiences just months after her treatment would be emotionally triggering for me. However, despite having a strong emotional reaction after each interview, it did not occur to me to take stock and reflect on why this might be the case.

Some oral historians promote the use of research diaries, particularly for students new to oral history, to record how their project evolves, emerging ideas that they might have about their research, and their responses to each interviewee.[41] It is valuable to begin a research diary before starting a project in order to consider how particular topics and interview cohorts might affect us based on our own life experiences. Such an approach aligns with increasing efforts to factor in and foster the wellbeing of historians when

'*What your generation probably don't understand*' 381

engaging with sensitive research topics.[42] Undertaking these preliminary reflections might have helped me to envisage how my recent experiences would result in my manifestation of an intergenerational connection during the interview process; such an awareness could have both aided me to remain mindful and present during my interviews and helped me to contend with any resultant emotional impact.

Conclusion

This chapter has explored how intergenerational dynamics influence the interpersonal dynamics of oral history interviewing. It has done so by analysing my own experiences interviewing women born between 1940 and 1970 about their everyday health experiences across the life-course in late twentieth-century Britain. The women that I interviewed drew on their generational positioning to explore and define their identities. For many of the women, their sense of generational identity was predicated on the fact that the experiences endured by their generation differed to those of older and younger generations. Women born in the immediate postwar period strongly identified with the health and social care developments that they experienced as children of the welfare state and continued to benefit from across the course of their lives. Others identified with contemporary developments affecting their generation, recognising the additional caring responsibilities associated with being a member of the 'sandwich generation'.

Interviewees' generational positioning therefore influenced how they perceived me as a member of a succeeding generation. Several women whom I spoke to made assumptions about my experiences of particular life events, often as a means to imply our generational differences. Exploring where these assumptions of generational difference diverged from my own experiences provides the opportunity to examine the role of projection in the oral history process. Interviewees' suppositions about my life served to bring me into the interview narrative as a person as well as a researcher. However, they also highlighted the contrasting ways that Margaret and I had constructed our respective generational identities. My role as interviewer meant that I did not share my own experiences with

382 *Subjectivity and intersubjectivity*

Margaret but, rather, came to represent an identity predicated on her assumptions.

In recognising my own emotions in response to these assumptions, I became aware of the generational assumptions and projections that I also brought to my research encounters. When interviewing women of my mother's generation, I realised that I was situating them within a familial framework. I felt a comforting familiarity in these interviews because I was projecting onto them tenets of my relationship with my mum. Breaking down the emotions that underpinned this intergenerational connection, I came to recognise my unresolved feelings about my mother being seriously ill shortly before the interviews commenced. These encounters highlighted how intergenerational dynamics occurring during oral history interviews can trigger unresolved emotions for both the interviewer and interviewee. Comprehending these transmissions helped me to better understand my positionality as a researcher.

Acknowledgements

The research on which this chapter is based was conducted as part of the Wellcome Trust Investigator Award in the Humanities and Social Sciences, 'Body, Self and Family: Women's Psychological, Emotional and Bodily Health in Britain, c. 1960–1990', WT 208080/Z/17/Z.

Notes

1 Sally Chandler, 'Oral history across generations: age, generational identity and oral testimony', *Oral History*, 33:2 (Autumn 2005), 48–9.
2 Barbara Erskine, 'Loss and grief in oral history', paper delivered at the Annual Meeting of the Oral History Association, Milwaukee, Wisconsin (19 October 1995), quoted in Valerie Yow, '"Do I like them too much?": effects of the oral history interview on the interviewer and vice-versa', *Oral History Review*, 24:1 (Summer 1997), 75.
3 Robert M. Wanderbeck and Nancy Worth, 'Introduction', in Robert M. Wanderbeck and Nancy Worth (eds), *Intergenerational Space* (London: Routledge, 2015), p. 3.
4 Wanderbeck and Worth, 'Introduction', pp. 2–3; Robert M. Wanderbeck, 'Intergenerational geographies: age relations, segregation and

'*What your generation probably don't understand*' 383

re-engagements', *Geography Compass*, 1:2 (2007); Gunhild O. Hagestad and Peter Uhlenberg, 'The social separation of old and young: a root of ageism', *Journal of Social Issues*, 61:2 (2005).

5 Wanderbeck and Worth, 'Introduction', p. 2; Simon Biggs and Ariela Lowenstein, *Generational Intelligence: A Critical Approach to Age Relations* (London: Routledge, 2011), p. 6.

6 Howard Schuman and Jacqueline Scott, 'Generations and collective memories', *American Sociological Review*, 54:3 (June 1989), 359–60; Sean T. Lyons and Linda Schweitzer, 'A qualitative exploration of generational identity: making sense of young and old in today's workplace', *Work, Aging and Retirement*, 3:2 (2017), 210.

7 Eve Worth, *The Welfare State Generation: Women, Agency and Class in Britain Since 1945* (London: Bloomsbury, 2021), pp. 15–17.

8 Mo, interviewed by Kate Mahoney, 29 January 2018.

9 Susan, interviewed by Kate Mahoney, 25 January 2018.

10 Pam Carter, *Feminism, Breasts and Breast-feeding* (Basingstoke: Palgrave Macmillan, 1995), p. 54; Robert Mackay, *Half the Battle: Civilian Morale in Britain during the Second World War* (Manchester: Manchester University Press 2003), p. 242; Ina Zweiniger-Bargielowska, *Austerity in Britain: Rationing, Controls, and Consumption, 1939–1955* (Oxford: Oxford University Press, 2000), p. 131.

11 David Morgan and Mary Evans, *The Battle for Britain: Citizenship and Ideology in the Second World War* (London: Routledge, 1993), p. 26.

12 Nicholas Crafts, 'The British Economy', in Francesca Carnevali and Julie-Marie Strange (eds), *Twentieth-Century Britain: Economic, Cultural and Social Change*, 2nd edn (Harlow, Essex: Pearson Longman, 2007), p. 9; Roland Quinlaut, 'Britain in 1950', *History Today*, 51:4 (April 2001): www.historytoday.com/roland-quinault/britain-1950 (accessed 3 July 2022).

13 Lynn Abrams, *Oral History Theory*, 2nd edn, (London: Routledge, 2016), p. 54.

14 Abrams, *Oral History Theory*, p. 100; Michael Roper, 'Re-remembering the soldier hero: the psychic and social construction of memory in personal narratives of the Great War', *History Workshop Journal*, 50 (2000), 184.

15 Worth, *The Welfare State Generation*, p. 18.

16 Wanderbeck and Worth, 'Introduction', p. 2; Biggs and Ariela Lowenstein, *Generational Intelligence*, p. 6.

17 Louise, interviewed by Kate Mahoney, 5 February 2018.

18 Dorothy Miller, 'The "sandwich" generation: adult children of the aging', *Social Work*, 26:5 (September 1981); Elaine M. Brody, '"Women in

384 *Subjectivity and intersubjectivity*

the middle" and family help to older people', *The Gerontologist*, 21:5 (October 1981); Charles R. Pierret, 'The "sandwich generation": women caring for parents and children', *Monthly Labor Review* (September 2006), 9.

19 Miller, 'The "sandwich" generation', 419–20.

20 Christine Ro, 'Why the "sandwich generation" is so stressed out', *BBC Worklife* (29 January 2021): www.bbc.com/worklife/article/20210128-why-the-sandwich-generation-is-so-stressed-out (accessed 31 July 2022).

21 Miller, 'The "sandwich" generation', 419.

22 Louise, interviewed by Mahoney.

23 Wanderbeck and Worth, 'Introduction', pp. 2–3.

24 Richard Hall, 'Emotional histories: materiality, temporality and subjectivity in oral history interviews with fathers and sons', *Oral History*, 47:1 (2019), 62.

25 Margaret, interviewed by Kate Mahoney, 10 March 2018.

26 Michael Roper, 'Analysing the analysed: transference and counter-transference in the oral history encounter', *Oral History*, 31:2 (Autumn 2003), 21.

27 Margaret, interviewed by Mahoney.

28 Jane Burns, Michelle Blanchard and Atari Metcalf, 'Bridging the digital divide in Australia: the potential implications of the mental health of young people experiencing marginalisation', in Enico Fero et al. (eds), *Handbook of Research on Overcoming Digital Divides: Constructing an Equitable and Competitive Information Society* (Hershey, PA: Information Science Reference, 2009), p. 103.

29 Margaret, interviewed by Mahoney.

30 Micaela di Leonardo, *The Varieties of Ethnic Experience: Kindship, Class, and Gender among California Italian-Americans* (Ithaca, NY: Cornell University Press), pp. 37–8; Yow, '"Do I like them too much?"', 76.

31 Yow, '"Do I like them too much?"', 78.

32 Yow, '"Do I like them too much?"', 78.

33 Louise, interviewed by Mahoney.

34 Arlene Kaplan Daniels, 'Self-deception and self-discovery in fieldwork', *Qualitative Sociology*, 6:3 (Fall 1983), 196.

35 Verusca Calabria, 'Exploring how care has changed in mental health', *Hidden Memories of Mental Healthcare*: www.mentalhealthcarememories.co.uk/blog/expolring-how-healthcare-has-changed (accessed 29 August 2022).

36 Verusca Calabria, 'Self-reflexivity in oral history research: the role of positionality and emotions', in Peter Bray (ed.), *Voices of Illness: Negotiating Meaning and Identity* (Leiden: Brill Rodolphi, 2019), p. 282.

'*What your generation probably don't understand*'   385

37 Roper, 'Analysing the analysed', 21.
38 Erskine, 'Loss and grief in oral history', quoted in Yow, '"Do I like them too much?"', 74–5.
39 Yow, '"Do I like them too much?"', 73.
40 Yow, '"Do I like them too much?"', 79.
41 Janis Wilton, quoted in Alistair Thomson, 'Teaching oral history to undergraduate researchers', in Alan Booth and Paul Hyland (eds), *The Practice of University History Teaching* (Manchester: Manchester University Press, 2000), p. 159.
42 Jessica Hammett et al., *Researcher Wellbeing: Guidelines for History Researchers* (June 2021): https://researcherwellbeing.blogs.bristol.ac.uk (accessed 29 May 2023).

16

Cultivating vulnerability: power and the emotional ethics of oral history practice beyond the interview

Tracey Loughran

Introduction

Between 2017 and 2022 I led a project that investigated women's 'everyday health' in postwar Britain. The other members of the project team were postdoctoral researchers Daisy Payling and Kate Mahoney, and doctoral student Hannah Froom. We drew on resources including written and oral testimonies, mass-market publications, and archival materials to explore women's emotional, psychological, and bodily state-of-being in their day-to-day lives, and the strategies they pursued to maintain equilibrium in this state-of-being. The feminist and intersectional aims of the project demanded direct contact with women's voices, stories, and lives. Oral history was at the heart of the project, with plans to conduct interviews with fifty Global Majority, LGBTQ+, and working-class women born between 1940 and 1970. Our aim was always to archive these interviews as an enduring record of women's health experiences in late twentieth-century Britain.

We achieved most of these aims. In March 2018, the British Library Sound Archive agreed to archive interviews collected for the project. By May 2021, Daisy, Kate, and I had conducted eighty-seven interviews, with sixty-five of these taking place in the previous six months. Along the way, our plans hit some bumps in the road: initial difficulties in recruiting interviewees, ultimately unresolved problems in recruiting participants of diverse ethnicities and sexual orientations, learning to conduct interviews remotely because of the COVID-19 pandemic, and an unexpected spike in recruitment that generated substantial demands on the time, energy, and emotional resources of the team.[1] Despite these challenges, most interviewees expressed satisfaction or enjoyment at participating in the project. Our oral history research was therefore a 'success' in that participants deemed it worthwhile and we have created an important publicly accessible resource for future historians of postwar Britain.

Nevertheless, throughout the project the question of whether I could adequately fulfil my responsibilities to interviewees haunted me. These doubts centred on the oral historian's duty of care and respect to participants beyond the moment of the interview itself, and especially the potential consequences of archiving interviews. Standard guidelines on ethical oral history practice, and most institutional ethics review processes, focus on informed consent, avoiding harm to participants during the interview itself, copyright, and data protection. They do not say much about other concerns around how interviewees might feel about what happens to their stories afterwards, including third-party use.[2] Oral history theory explores issues of interpretive authority in publications but has less to say about the other potential afterlives of participants' stories.[3] Oral historians must continually negotiate 'personal ethical commitments' that are 'far more nuanced and contextual than the terms set out in our consent forms' with only the sketchiest of road maps.[4]

This chapter is a personal reflection on my doubts, whilst leading an oral history project, about power dynamics within the interviewer–interviewee relationship, the risks of abuse of power or paternalism, the 'ownership' of stories, and the potential consequences of the reuse of interviews in unanticipated contexts. I explore an experiment in the voluntary cultivation of vulnerability in the pursuit of an emotional engagement that insists on the constant remaking of ethics beyond the moment of the interview. This experiment was to be interviewed myself, using the same schedule used on the project to interview our participants, with the aim of archiving the interview. In doing so, I tried to make myself vulnerable and to constantly trouble my own sense of ethical practice. I remain uncertain as to whether I can fulfil my responsibilities to participants, but I now see this troubled status as necessary and even as a good.

388 *Subjectivity and intersubjectivity*

Oral history and (our) ethical practice

The project followed standard ethical procedures set out by my institution and the British Library Sound Archive. These included actions to ensure participants' informed consent (including awareness of subsequent uses of data), confidentiality, and/or anonymity; arrangements for safe storage, sharing, and archiving of personal data; and management of potential risks to participants and researchers. We provided interviewees with an information sheet about the project and required them to sign a participation agreement before the interview and a recording agreement afterwards. These forms set out terms for use of the interview in publications and other outputs, and for access to the recording and associated materials at the British Library. We reviewed information that might cause distress to third parties and discussed this with participants when sending them interview summaries or transcripts.[5] Our funding allowed the production of content summaries and transcriptions for each interview. The project therefore met major oral history organisations' criteria for best practice.[6]

It felt more chaotic on the ground. On paper, we were prepared. All team members had prior experience of conducting interviews and we undertook further training early in the project. We co-designed a semi-structured interview schedule that tried to avoid presuppositions about our participants' identities and to leave open space for unexpected responses. We agreed that our participants' emotional wellbeing was more important than our research outcomes. Aware of inevitable power differentials between interviewer and interviewee, we strove to demonstrate respect, empathy, and sensitivity in our actions before, during, and after each interview. Yet I felt in a constant state of sprawling, potentially infinite, disorganisation once the oral history research started. I had not anticipated the huge administrative burden of carrying out and preparing to archive the interviews: keeping track of correspondence, permissions paperwork, commissioning transcripts, producing interview summaries, and so on demanded constant attention.

I coped better with other forms of messiness. Conducting the interviews was never easy. Our schedule included questions on intimate topics and emotionally charged life events. Different questions provoked strong emotional responses in different women. Some narrators recounted extremely traumatic experiences. But, as a dynamic relationship, an oral history interview always requires deep responsiveness. The continual feeling of teetering on the edge of unintentionally causing distress to a person who is barely known, and whose wounds and scars therefore cannot be predicted, is unavoidably exhausting.[7] I expected this feeling, knew it would be temporary, and believed that it was in a worthwhile cause, so found little difficulty in living with it. I also believed that participants had actively chosen to tell their stories, and that once the interview started, my primary responsibility was to support this need. Buffered in these ways against the drain of interview encounters, I felt privileged to record these women's life stories.

Working within a research team also helped to transmute the unwieldiness of raw encounters into faith in the ultimate value of the project. This bolstered my confidence in our right to (unintentionally, temporarily, and with their consent) trouble our participants' emotional equilibrium. From late 2018 to mid-2020 the project team held lengthy transcript review meetings that provided opportunities to reflect on interview technique, changes to the schedule, and other practical matters. Above all, the rich understanding that emerged from our combined perspectives cheered me. This practice fell away in our intensive period of interviewing during the COVID-19 lockdown. We then encountered, separately and together, outside and within the team, different challenges.[8] Nevertheless, on my own part these meetings established lasting confidence in our shared ethos. I trusted Kate's and Daisy's capabilities as thoughtful and caring practitioners of feminist oral history at least as much as I trusted my own.

Yet from early on I felt troubled by the ethical dimensions of our oral history research. These concerns were not about the conduct of the interview or uses of the material in publications. I did feel apprehensive about how to do justice to these women's lives in print, but I also saw such concerns as business as usual. All historians face the problem of how to tread softly in the lives of others, whether our work involves deciphering the unfamiliar scripts of long-dead ancestors or sipping tea in the living rooms of women who remind us of our mothers.[9] I did not see writing about living people fairly and well as intrinsically different to other kinds of historical research. I also felt reassured by the prospect of writing about these women's lives with Daisy and Kate. I knew that we were all good historians

390   *Subjectivity and intersubjectivity*

and that together we could write a history greater than the sum of our parts.

Gradually, I realised that my sense of unease turned on what it might mean to deposit these stories, these digital ghosts of real lives, in an archive, for perpetuity, for people who had never met the participants to hear or read, for other researchers to paw and grub. What might be the afterlives of these interviews, and how much responsibility did I hold for what happened to stories that existed in this form only because I had asked to hear them? Did our participants, in giving informed consent, really understand what was at stake here? Did I?

Archiving oral history

History still worships the archive. Since the nineteenth century, archival research has been seen as fundamental to professional practice. Interrogations of the archive in recent decades have shaken but not demolished this status.[10] Oral history has a complicated relationship to the archive. For as long as history has been recorded, oral testimony has been used as source material. However, for centuries many viewed this testimony as suspicious because of its ephemerality. Sources that could not be independently verified and consulted did not meet the standard of documentary evidence. The invention of the portable tape recorder changed all that. It made interviews archivable, and this changed the status of oral history within the discipline and the profession.[11] It further promised the democratisation of history: oral history archives made of, by, and for the people, histories unspooled onto tape and then reeled back into local libraries, community centres, and archives as a resource for future generations.[12] Eventually, oral historians capitalised on the ability to return over and over to recordings of interviews to develop sophisticated theoretical approaches to memory, narrativisation, and (inter)subjectivity.[13] Oral history, then, has its own reasons to fetishise the archive.

Oral historians are nevertheless often wary about the archive in relation to their own practice. As April Gallwey notes, research on archived oral histories is often viewed as 'inferior to the practice of first-hand interviewing'.[14] This attachment to the moment of the interview echoes the long-established tenet that it is essential to listen to recordings rather than read transcripts.[15] I share many of these views, but want to pause on the strangeness of oral historians' ambivalence towards the archive, especially towards actually *using* archived oral histories. Making interviews accessible to wider audiences is often presented as an ethical imperative, an integral part of oral history's democratic mission.[16] Assumptions that archived interviews are second best sits uneasily alongside this insistence on archiving as an unambiguous good. It is an ambivalence that doubtless contributed to my hesitancy over what it meant to archive our interviews.

Certainly, I had not fully thought through the implications of archiving oral history interviews when I applied for the research grant that funded the project. I was not an experienced oral historian. Buoyed by an idealistic commitment to recording and preserving women's 'everyday' experiences and spurred on by the pragmatic aim of providing my funder with value for money, listing an archived oral history collection as an output in the bid seemed like common sense. My naivety became clear during early talks with the British Library. When the oral history curator explained that it was impracticable for participants to retain copyright of the interviews, I decided to assign copyright to myself rather than the Library (unless participants chose to opt out of this arrangement).[17] She then asked who would retain copyright of the interviews in the event of my death. I had not anticipated facing my own mortality, far less the administrative headaches it might generate, that day – though the shock may have been greater for Kate, who suddenly found herself legatee of our participants' life stories. Assigning copyright to myself felt like a heavy burden. My actions could potentially lead to misuse of someone's life story; I might unintentionally betray their trust and cause them pain or harm. I realised for the first time what a responsibility it is to bring a story into the world, and that there can be no security in promises of keeping it safe.

I did not dwell on these misgivings but at intervals they resurfaced, with greater insistence as we interviewed more women and discussed their transcripts in team meetings. I felt stilted in the first few project interviews, partly because I feared Kate and Daisy noticing deficiencies in my interview technique, but also because I was aware that unknown others would later listen to the recordings. Although I knew that

392   *Subjectivity and intersubjectivity*

an oral history interview is an organic (if semi-formal, part-structured) encounter, I worried about making mistakes or 'not doing it right' (what would 'right' have looked like?). I wanted interviews to be a safe space, but they felt very public. It did not help that, despite my best efforts to ensure informed consent, participants often seemed quite cavalier about signing the participation and recording agreements – a problem that deepened when we moved to remote interviewing. I had to accept responsibility if interviewees suffered in any way because they did not fully realise what they were getting themselves into, but I never felt certain that I had really done enough to guide this realisation.

Alongside conducting interviews, I was undertaking research with archived oral history collections. This brought home the potential disjuncture between interviewees' knowing participation in a specific and delimited project and the uses to which subsequent researchers might put their words. In the late 1980s, could any of Elizabeth Roberts' interviewees have imagined a researcher like me poring over their words to understand their body image, intergenerational relationships, and concepts of agency? Might they have spoken differently if they had? Attending conferences where speakers showed selfie-style photographs of themselves with oral history participants deepened my unease. Would people who had never attended academic conferences really want all these appraising gazes on their scaled-up faces in Lecture Theatre A? Similarly, at our project team meetings we spent hours discussing – always with care, with respect – the lives of each woman. I could not but wonder: did she imagine this, four people sitting round a table, parsing her every word, scrawling over transcripts in multicoloured pens, making connections between the different parts of her life? Would she mind?

Power, authority, and subjectivity

I had to believe that our interviewees knew what they were doing when they agreed to speak to us, and that they had actively chosen the circumstances under which they told their stories. Any other stance would be hopelessly paternalistic. But they seemed to trust too easily, and I was not sure, despite my best intentions, despite the safeguards of the consent process, despite best ethical practice,

Cultivating vulnerability 393

that either I or the process could really be trusted. I hadn't thought through what archiving the interviews meant. I hadn't realised the responsibility it entailed. I was busy, tired, sad, and often getting things wrong in my daily encounters with people I actually knew. What if I made mistakes here too?

The dynamics of power within any oral history interview depend on the collisions, often unpredictable, between its participants' multitudinous identities and histories. Likewise, material dimensions of the interview such as location, room set-up, and technology affect the extent to which each participant feels able to act and to shape the encounter in the moment.[18] The interplay of these elements constantly shifts. Within the interview context, power is skittish and capricious. Left to its own devices, however, power will skew towards interviewers, especially if they are academic historians: the interviewer determines the parameters of the project, decides what questions to ask, invites others to participate, clips on the microphones to capture voices, presses record-pause-stop, stores the recording, edits interviewees' words, and interprets their stories for wider audiences. Interviewees participate under their own volition, for their own reasons, and tell their own stories in their own ways, but once they have signed over copyright, they lose a certain amount of control. It is the historian's name on the front of the book.[19]

Oral historians have long worried about power disparities within the interviewer–interviewee relationship. From the 1970s, feminist oral historians reconceptualised the interview encounter as the melding of unique subjectivities and sought ways to rebalance power within the relationship.[20] Building on this scholarship, in 1990 Michael Frisch formulated the concept of 'shared authority' to describe practices that 'redefine and redistribute intellectual authority' and therefore empower all parties, but especially interviewees.[21] The pursuit of 'shared authority' appeals greatly to those who seek more democratic means of creating history, but even enthusiasts acknowledge that it may not be achievable.[22] Judith Stacey goes so far as to suggest that the *belief* that authority has been shared enables the interviewer to hold power in ways that are unseen, unacknowledged, and veiled by the benevolent façade of equality.[23] This is dangerous because, against the best intentions of practitioners, the result is a de facto denial of power imbalances. That denial can only ever work in favour of the person who already holds most power.

394 *Subjectivity and intersubjectivity*

Many oral historians labour in earnest to achieve 'shared authority' and/or to co-produce research and creative outputs.[24] I admire their work and I am very glad it exists, but I am unable to follow them in my own practice. It is my view that, in the end, academic oral historians are almost always able to choose, if they wish, to have the last (published) word about an interview encounter. Always and inevitably, that ability to choose is an outcome and sign of power. This power is usually exercised with great thought, care, and respect, but it is nevertheless power that participants do not possess.

As its lead, my beliefs about the operation of power shaped oral history practice on this project. We tried to make space for women to tell their own stories within the parameters of our schedule: we allowed them to decide the location, format, and pace of the encounter; during the interview itself we posed open questions, and avoided interruptions, voicing interpretations, or challenging their worldviews. But we did not take any formal measures to share authority or to co-produce outputs. In the main, this is because I could not square such measures with maintaining interpretive authority. In presenting oral history research I try to avoid overdetermined interpretations of participants' life stories, to put their own words before readers with minimal editing insofar as this is possible, and to indicate where I suspect they might disagree with my interpretation. But I do not see how I can commit both to putting forward honest interpretations based on my expertise as a professional historian and to ceding interpretive authority to others who do not hold this expertise – a failure of imagination, perhaps, and definitely hierarchical, but a stance based on unwillingness to promise participants something I *know* I cannot deliver.[25]

I am a feminist oral historian, but this blunt assertion of power may seem 'heretical' to other feminist oral historians.[26] In my research, the principle that the personal is political is expressed as a turn inwards, towards subjectivity, reflexivity, and the self, rather than outwards towards relationships with research participants.[27] This turn inwards predates my practice as an oral historian and arises out of fascination with the troubled status of the concept of 'historical objectivity' as simultaneously unobtainable and an inescapable ideal.[28] Some scholars perceive historians' autobiographical efforts as evidence of the profession's 'self-absorption'.[29] This may be true. But for me, explorations in professional selfhood create a productive uncertainty that pervades my praxis. At intervals, I return to writing autoethnographically to remind myself that historians are always present in what they see and write, to maintain a dynamic relationship with my sources, and to sharpen myself into points that prick against the temptation of complete assurance.

In the drive to reflexivity, oral history is both a powerful accelerant and a foot slammed on the brake. On the one hand, oral historians write in the first person, and usually accept that analysis of the interaction of self and other is an essential part of practising oral history, whether this reflection makes it onto the page or not.[30] On the other hand, an oral history interview is someone else's story, someone else's life. The contract is that interviewees speak and interviewers (mostly) listen. The oral historian dishonours that contract if she directs too much of the attention to herself within the interview or in her subsequent expositions of it.[31] In retrospect, a certain amount of my unease about oral history practice on this project arose because I could not reconcile the pull to explore subjectivity and the push to efface myself; the coexistence of these equally powerful impulses generated intellectual static. Gradually, I articulated the concept of cultivated vulnerability out of this white noise.

Cultivated vulnerability

In an influential set of essays, the anthropologist Ruth Behar explores what participant observation, the foundational method of social anthropology, might become in the postcolonial world. As the traditional boundaries that anthropology instituted between 'I' (white, male, western) and 'them' (racialised, feminised, other) dissolve or are kicked down, what arises in their place? Behar proposes forms of connection rather than separation; for anthropologists to become 'vulnerable observers', taking themselves as raw material and excavating similarities between their own self and other selves, and to write 'anthropology that breaks your heart', that elicits emotional identification in the effort to create a bond with readers.[32]

Behar explains that ethnography always depends on 'some form of ethnographic authority', but that she distrusts her own authority, seeing it as 'being constantly in question, constantly on the point

396   *Subjectivity and intersubjectivity*

of breaking down'. Her solution is to reject 'reigning paradigms' of 'distance, objectivity, and abstraction' and instead train her lens on herself to better understand different cultures and experiences, to stimulate new understanding in her readers, and to refashion anthropology itself.[33] Behar's success relies on her ability to expertly wield, draw out, and probe vulnerability. Her insights depend on her willingness to confront herself – but she can ask readers to meet these artful confessions with broken hearts only because her own is already pinned, sprawling and wriggling, to the page.

What does it mean to cultivate vulnerability in oral history practice beyond listening, beyond the moment of the interview?[34] As this project wore on, I came to feel that in asking participants to make themselves vulnerable through trusting another to hold their story, I had to ensure that this exchange was equitable. I had to be willing to put myself at stake, to prod my own open sores and show my scars. In oral history interviews, I listened carefully, did not impose myself, and gave little away unless directly asked. But in conference papers and published chapters, I felt compelled to push at the boundaries of bearable exposure, publicly disclosing experiences of grief, self-harm, and borderline sexual assault. I was trying to practise feminist history, but in retrospect I was also swept up in a confessional culture that makes unequal demands of women and too easily incites self-exposure as a visible mark of feminism (the #MeToo movement was at its height).[35] I agreed that autobiography was ethical practice, that 'we should not ask people to share difficult experiences and emotions with us if we are not willing to do the same'.[36] But there are limits to this commitment. I may have been ill at the time, and, eventually, I became sick of myself.

The belief that I *had* to put myself on the line because of my oral history practice was well-intentioned but ill-formed, incompletely articulated, and probably harmful. But it coalesced with a healthier desire to better understand what was at risk or on offer for interviewees. In 2018, when interviewing *Guardian* writer Annalisa Barbieri for a project on 'agony aunts', I accidentally stumbled into the role of interviewee. During our discussion, I referred to an article of Barbieri's on bereavement. Later, the interview turned to family relationships and grief. When I explained that I remembered that article because it resonated with my own experiences of grief, Barbieri – compassionate in real life as in the newspaper, but also

Cultivating vulnerability 397

a skilled journalist who was usually the person asking questions – stayed with those emotions. She led the interview for the next fifteen minutes or so. We were both aware of the recorder, and I realised at the time that my own experiences were now 'on the record', but I continued anyway – perhaps because at that time so many other people ran away from my grief, as though it had the power to drown them too, forcing me to become the flood barrier against my own pain. The moment mattered more than who might bear witness afterwards.

Over the next few months, I returned to this encounter often as I reflected on the mess of ethical issues that our interviews generated. By early 2019 I had hit on the idea of arranging to be interviewed myself, using the project schedule and archiving this interview alongside our others (but with the same option our participants held to edit or withdraw the interview). I thought this experiment might help me to negotiate an ethical stance, resting on emotional as well as intellectual understanding of the risks of misuse, towards the care of their stories. I knew it was impossible to recreate our participants' experiences of interview in this way. I am a professional historian with expertise in oral history; I had helped to design the interview schedule and had conducted interviews using it; I had already devoted a lot of thought to archival practices; and I would be able to choose my own interviewer. But in learning what it felt like to be interviewed, even under these semi-artificial conditions, I might improve my practices as an interviewer and as an interpreter of the lives of others. Aware that my own interview lived on in an archive, representing one moment among millions between my birth and death, I would be better armed against foreclosing the potential meanings of our participants' lives.

Above all, I saw living with the possible afterlives of my own archived interview as a high-wire act, one that could create a more tightly knitted safety net for our participants' stories – a way of ensuring that when I had to make decisions about what to do with these interviews, I would think once, look down at the far-off ground, think twice, and remember the consequences of losing my balance. Cultivating my own vulnerability and maintaining this state of tension through giving up (some of) my power to the archive offered a way to stay alive to that power, and to fix the indeterminacy of the present into my attempts to create a history out of these lives.

The interview and beyond

This interview was held in mid-2021, two or three months after conducting the final interview with an external participant for the project.[37] Until 2020, we had struggled to recruit oral history participants, and it looked like I had plenty of time to sort out my own interview. Then the pandemic struck, we were thrown into disarray, and an unexpected spike in recruitment meant I had little time to do anything but interview other people. Also, I didn't know who to ask to conduct the interview. As their line manager, it would be wildly inappropriate to approach Kate or Daisy. I had to find a different, skilled oral historian, generous enough to give up their time, with whom I felt able to speak freely. I toyed with the idea of asking practitioners I knew well but decided that I would probably end up feeling too constrained. For the experiment to work, I had to be committed to the same degree of honesty as our interviewees. But whereas our participants spoke to strangers who melted away after the interview encounter, whoever I asked would already be within my wider professional circle. I was likely to bump into them in other professional contexts in future years. This was a daunting prospect.

I eventually approached Amy Tooth Murphy. I did not really know Amy, though I had read her work, seen her deliver papers, and thought she was a superb oral historian. During lockdown, I interviewed her about her professional practice for a module on oral history that I convened. In that encounter I found her warm, funny, and thoughtful, and intuitively felt that I could trust her. Fortunately, Amy was enthusiastic about the possibilities of this experiment, as well as very generous with her time. I spoke so much that our interview had to be held over two sessions – the recording ran to six hours in the end.

I wanted to come to the interview schedule 'fresh', despite conducting dozens of interviews using it, so I tried not to think about the interview ahead of the first session. I wanted to leave space for our conversation to develop in unanticipated directions. Amy's personal and creative adaptations of the schedule to suit her interviewing style, as well as her sensitivity to my responses, meant that I was never in danger of finding the terrain too familiar. In fact, many of her starting assumptions and follow-up questions threw open my

Cultivating vulnerability 399

blind spots about the project. I became aware of other areas we might have probed in our oral histories, and might consider, using different sources, in our future research. At times in the interview, I did think about other participants' responses to similar questions, but not as often as I had expected. Instead, I was surprised at the prominence of certain themes (body image, depression, my passion for history) that emerged as I spoke. These are/were important parts of my present/past but I did not think the narrative of my life would take this shape. This first session was rewarding, but extremely draining – I felt more tired and exhausted than when I conducted interviews myself and realised that I may have been careless with some of our project participants.

In the week before we reconvened for the second session, I was unable to put the interview to the back of my mind. I felt, in turn, flushes of embarrassment at how I had discussed sexuality (I have been in a heterosexual relationship for nearly twenty years; my sexual identity is taken for granted in most contexts); invaded by grief at my brother's death (I had expected to talk about bereavement, but not that these feelings would stay so close to the surface); and troubled about the disclosures I might feel compelled, in the name of honesty, to make next time (but not worried that Amy might push for such admissions). These fears and feelings receded almost as soon as we started the next session. At the outset, Amy asked me to reflect on our previous encounter and this provided an opportunity to order and digest my thoughts before we went any further. This was only one of many points when I marvelled at Amy's skills as an interviewer; if the sole purpose of the experiment had been to improve my own interview technique through direct engagement with another's expertise, it would have been a worthwhile exercise.

I did not find the second session difficult, or as draining as the first. It was shorter, but knowing how it might affect me also acted as a safeguard. My dominant impression after the session was of how difficult it is to tell a life without drawing in other people. I could not speak honestly about myself without risking hurting others or giving a lopsided account of my actions. Close to the end, Amy asked how my parents might feel, knowing that I was talking about them. I had not disregarded their feelings, but I had spoken spontaneously, knowing that they would not locate or listen to an archived

Subjectivity and intersubjectivity

interview. My life as an academic is too far away from their lives. I realised that interviewees might feel similarly secure about becoming part of 'research'. Perversely, it was liberating to recognise that there could be no realistic expectation of simultaneously satisfying myself, others, and the archive. In telling my story, as in any conversation, from second to second I had to make myriad tiny calculations, conscious and unconscious, in the effort to be true to myself and neither untrue nor unkind to others. It is possible that participants felt the same. In making myself vulnerable, I discovered a certain invulnerability in myself (and perhaps in our participants?); what I felt at that moment was part, not all of me, and the telling was a moment in time, not a whole life.

Conclusion

Almost three years after the interview, I have not quite decided how to archive it. It is likely that I will withhold access for a period of at least ten years. At that distance of time, we will all be different people. The years should blunt the impact of any words that might seem sharp now. I have not listened to the interview yet and I may never do so. I read the transcript for the first time only to write this chapter. It was a surprisingly emotional experience. I felt cast back not only to the events I described, but to the moment of the interview itself: the sunlight through the window, the tiredness of the pandemic world, the hope that it was all over now, the fear that it was not. As I avoided the decision about archiving in the intervening months, I sometimes returned in my mind to specific moments of the interview and revelations that had felt far too raw and open. On reading the transcript, I was surprised to find these moments tamed on the page. I was vague, allusive, oblique. A stranger might not even fully grasp what I was talking about. In the light of day, the monsters in the dark turned out to be shadows on the wall.

Other moments hit like a ton of bricks. I found my account of adolescent depression and self-harm, facets of my past that I have written and spoken about publicly and that I believed no longer had the power to trouble me, very difficult to read. I did not find these issues challenging to talk about during the interview. If anything, I felt mildly anxious that it might be a lot for Amy to process. But it all looked so different written down; so much more concrete, so much harder to wave away. The emotional jolt of reading these passages confirmed my suspicion that it might be best to first give participants interview summaries, offering transcripts if desired rather than automatically sending them on. Not everyone wants to be confronted with visceral past words or selves, but I suspect few can resist the temptation to rifle through the pages once the transcript is there. If we do not want to overwhelm participants when we are face to face with them, we should try to avoid causing the same effect from a distance.

This jolt also forced recognition of how my narration worked overtime to play down the importance of this period in my life. In the interview, I tried very hard to claim that past pain not only doesn't *now*, but also didn't in the past, really matter that much. This tendency to minimise certain emotions reflects my own unique subjectivity, but also the cultural factors that encourage women not to recognise, dwell on, or speak about their own psychological or physical pain.[38] Reviewing other participants' transcripts, I am now often struck by moments when they work hard to efface the importance of particular events, emotions, and behaviours. More than this, I realise that as I conducted those interviews, I was sometimes unwittingly complicit in this erasure; imbricated in the same gendered culture, at the time I did not always recognise the substance of what I heard, and instead unthinkingly helped them to brush off its import.

As a result, I am now thinking again about the primacy that oral historians bestow on the act of listening to recordings rather than reading transcripts. Certainly, there are crucial aspects of conversation that no transcript can ever capture; the written word is not an adequate substitute for the speaking voice. At the same time, in listening to interviews I conducted, I am often transported back to the emotions I felt and the sense of that past moment – recall that is perhaps a false guide to what was happening both for the interviewee and under the surface of our discussion. As the voice tells us what the written word cannot, so the written word might help us to hear that voice in its fullest resonances.[39]

Did the experiment achieve what I had hoped – do I feel better equipped to hold participants' stories in trust? Yes and no. Just as participants' stories will live on in the archive, handling them ethically and well must be a living commitment. There is no possibility of

402   *Subjectivity and intersubjectivity*

resolution, only the continual remaking of this commitment.[40] In this sense, there can be no final judgement on success or failure. The purpose of the exercise is to conjure productive uncertainty, perpetual and self-conscious doubt, as the means of maintaining care of this powerful legacy. So far, it is working. As a result of making myself vulnerable, I have made and remade my understanding of participants' stories. For now, this staves off the dangers of taking their meaning for granted, taking their narration at a specific point in time as standing in for their whole lives, or failing to understand my power as legatee of their stories.

Cultivating vulnerability is a way to channel the interviewer's power within the interview relationship into operation from a similar (but not the same) position as the interviewee. This manoeuvre depends on acknowledgement of power differentials. The interviewer has no ethical obligation to be interviewed or to put her own story into the archive simply because participants have agreed to do so. Choosing to do so underlines her power. However, this acknowledgement is the starting point for a series of actions based on the simultaneous exercise and voluntary renunciation of that power. The story in the archive keeps the interviewer in a state of vulnerability, and in doing so keeps her closer to the state of nervousness and dauntedness that is 'an integral part of what it means to do oral history'.[41] Attending in this way to the afterlives of interviews creates an emotional ethics that has little to do with the paperwork submitted for institutional approval and then filed away. Instead, it is a matter of continual, reflective, and dynamic practice. An emotional ethics predicated on vulnerability is therefore imbued with the spirit of the oral history encounter itself – changing from moment to moment, as unpredictable as any human relationship, shimmering with the desire to know and to understand through connection, fixed only in its indeterminacy.

Acknowledgements

The research on which this chapter is based was conducted as part of the Wellcome Trust Investigator Award in the Humanities and Social Sciences, 'Body, Self and Family: Women's Psychological, Emotional and Bodily Health in Britain, c. 1960–1990', WT 208080/Z/17/Z.

Cultivating vulnerability

I would like to thank Amy Tooth Murphy for her generosity as a person and skill as interviewer; the experiment outlined in this chapter would not have been possible without her.

Notes

1 Tracey Loughran, Kate Mahoney, and Daisy Payling, 'Reflections on remote interviewing in a pandemic: negotiating participant and researcher emotions', *Oral History*, 50:1 (Spring 2022).
2 The kinds of issues I have in mind are not explored in the otherwise comprehensive discussions in Donald A. Ritchie, *Doing Oral History*, 3rd edn (Oxford: Oxford University Press, 2015), pp. 62–72, 186–9; Paul Thompson with Joanna Bornat, *The Voice of the Past: Oral History*, 4th edn (Oxford: Oxford University Press, 2017), pp. 332–50.
3 Katherine Borland, '"That's not what I said": interpretative conflict in oral narrative research', in Sherna Gluck and Daphne Patai (eds), *Women's Words: The Feminist Practice of Oral History* (New York: Routledge, 1991); Lynn Abrams, *Oral History Theory* (London and New York: 2010), pp. 166–9.
4 Anna Sheftel and Stacey Zembrzycki, 'Introduction', in Anna Sheftel and Stacey Zembrzycki (eds), *Oral History Off the Record: Toward an Ethnography of Practice* (New York: Palgrave Macmillan, 2013), p. 14.
5 In addition, sensitive sections are redacted and closed to public access for a set period under British Library rules.
6 Oral History Society [Rob Perks], 'Are you legal and ethical?': www.ohs.org.uk/legal-and-ethical-advice/legal-and-ethical-preparation/ (accessed 7 January 2023); Oral History Association, 'OHA principles and best practices': https://oralhistory.org/principles-and-best-practices-revised-2018/ (accessed 7 January 2023).
7 Sean Field, 'Beyond "healing": oral history, trauma, and regeneration', *Oral History*, 34:1 (2006); Liz H. Strong, 'Shifting focus: interviewers share advice on protecting themselves from harm', *Oral History Review*, 48:2 (2021).
8 Loughran, Mahoney, and Payling, 'Reflections on remote interviewing'.
9 Michael Roper, 'The unconscious work of history', *Cultural and Social History*, 11:2 (2014), 170; Katie Barclay, 'The practice and ethics of the history of emotions', in Katie Barclay, Sharon Crozier-De Rosa, and Peter N. Stearns (eds), *Sources for the History of Emotions: A Guide* (London and New York: Routledge, 2021); Jessica Meyer and Alexia Moncrieff, 'Family not to be informed? The ethical use of historical

404   *Subjectivity and intersubjectivity*

medical documentation', in Anne Hanley and Jessica Meyer (eds), *Patient Voices in Britain, 1840–1948: Historical and Policy Perspectives* (Manchester: Manchester University Press, 2021); David Wright and Renée Saucier, 'Madness in the archives: anonymity, ethics, and mental health history research', *Journal of the Canadian Historical Association/ Revue de la Société historique du Canada*, 23:2 (2012).

10 Antoinette Burton, 'Introduction: archive fever, archive stories', in Antoinette Burton (ed.), *Archive Stories: Facts, Fictions, and the Writing of History* (Durham, NC and London: Duke University Press, 2005).

11 Thompson with Bornat, *The Voice of the Past*, pp. 23–70.

12 Ronald J. Grele, 'Oral history as evidence', in Thomas L. Charlton, Lois E. Myers, and Rebecca Sharpless (eds), *Handbook of Oral History* (Lanham, MD: AltaMira Press, 2008).

13 Joanna Bornat, 'Remembering and reworking emotions: the reanalysis of emotion in an interview', *Oral History*, 38:2 (2010); Abrams, *Oral History Theory*, pp. 54–129.

14 April Gallwey, 'The rewards of using archived oral histories in research: the case of the Millennium Memory Bank', *Oral History*, 41:1 (Spring 2013), 38.

15 Raphael Samuel, 'Perils of the transcript', *History Workshop Journal*, 1:2 (1972); Alessandro Portelli, 'The peculiarities of oral history', *History Workshop Journal*, 12 (1981).

16 Oral History Society, 'Are you legal and ethical?'; Oral History Association, 'OHA principles and best practices'. The sixteen respondents to an e-survey on conducting, reusing, and archiving oral history interviews that Kate Mahoney and I conducted in mid-2020 almost all believed that interviews *should* be archived, but for different reasons (often practical, sometimes ethical) most had not consistently deposited recordings from their own projects.

17 Because copyright in words spoken lasts seventy years after the speaker dies, it is very difficult for archives and libraries to administer requests for permissions to cite from an interview (usually required for broadcast or republication of more than a paragraph or two), not least because contact details may change. The time and resource needed to recontact interviewees for permission significantly reduces the chances of the material being used in the future. We felt that if participants retained copyright, it could in practice severely restrict access to the interviews and therefore undermine the purpose of archiving them as a publicly available resource. Thanks to Mary Stewart for correspondence on this point.

18 For explorations of intersubjectivity in oral history interviews, see Carrie Hamilton, 'Sex, "silence," and audiotape: listening for female same-sex desire in Cuba', in Nan Alamilla Boyd and Horacio N. Roque

Cultivating vulnerability 405

Ramírez (eds), *Bodies of Evidence: The Practice of Queer Oral History* (Oxford and New York: Oxford University Press, 2012); Amy Tooth Murphy, 'Listening in, listening out: intersubjectivity and the impact of insider and outsider status in oral history interviews', *Oral History*, 48:1 (2020); Alan Wong, 'Listen and learn: familiarity and feeling in the oral history interview', in Sheftel and Zembrzycki (eds), *Oral History Off the Record*.

19 Alistair Thomson describes an intense and lengthy collaboration with four women 'in the making of our book' and their pleasure at 'my suggestion that their contributing role be acknowledged on the title page' – but the front cover, and so every online catalogue and bookseller, lists his name alone. Alistair Thomson, 'Moving stories, women's lives: sharing authority in oral history', *Oral History*, 39:2 (Autumn 2011), 90.

20 Kristina Minister, 'A feminist frame for the oral history interview', in Gluck and Patai (eds), *Women's Words*; for an overview of this scholarship, see Abrams, *Oral History Theory*, pp. 71–4.

21 Michael Frisch, *A Shared Authority: Essays on the Craft and Meaning of Oral and Public History* (Albany, NY: State University of New York Press, 1990), p. xx.

22 Lorraine Sitzia, 'Shared authority: an impossible goal', *Oral History Review*, 30:1 (2003).

23 Judith Stacey, 'Can there be a feminist ethnography?', in Gluck and Patai (eds), *Women's Words*.

24 See, for example, the chapters in 'Section 4: Feminists in the field: performance, political activism, and community engagement', in Katrina Srigley, Stacey Zembryzycki, and France Iavocovetta (eds), *Beyond Women's Words: Feminisms and the Practice of Oral History in the Twenty-First Century* (London and New York: Routledge, 2018), pp. 217–76; 'Part 4: Negotiating identity: sharing authority in creative practice', in Clare Summerskill, Amy Tooth Murphy, and Emma Vickers (eds), *New Directions in Queer Oral History: Archives of Disruption* (London and New York: Routledge, 2022), pp. 173–213.

25 For a short overview of alternative approaches, see Linda Shopes, 'Legal and ethical issues in oral history', in Charlton, Myers, and Sharpless (eds), *Handbook of Oral History*, p. 164. Our participants did not voice any interest in 'sharing authority' – most saw the interview as a positive but time-limited encounter.

26 Sherna Berger Gluck, 'From California to Kufr Nameh and back', in Sheftel and Zembrzycki (eds), *Oral History Off the Record*, p. 40.

27 On subjectivity, reflexivity, and women's/feminist history, see Geoff Eley, *A Crooked Line: From Cultural History to the History of Society* (Ann Arbor, MI: University of Michigan Press, 2005), pp. 155–81.

28 Tracey Loughran and Dawn Mannay, 'Introduction: why emotion matters', in Tracey Loughran and Dawn Mannay (eds), *Emotion and the Researcher: Sites, Subjectivities and Relationships* (Bingley: Emerald, 2018).

29 Richard Vinen, 'The poisoned madeleine: the autobiographical turn in historical writing', *Journal of Contemporary History*, 46:3 (2011), 537.

30 Penny Summerfield, 'Dis/composing the subject: intersubjectivities in oral history', in Tess Coslett, Celia Lury, and Penny Summerfield (eds), *Feminism and Autobiography: Texts, Theories, Methods* (London: Routledge, 2000); Juliette Pattinson, '"The thing that made me hesitate ...": re-examining gendered intersubjectivities in interviews with British secret war veterans', *Women's History Review*, 20 (2011).

31 Franca Iacovetta, 'Post-modern ethnography, historical materialism, and decentring the (male) authorial voice: a feminist conversation', *Histoire sociale/Social History*, 32:64 (November 1999); Joan Sangster, 'Politics and praxis in Canadian working-class oral history', in Sheftel and Zembrzycki (eds), *Oral History Off the Record*.

32 Ruth Behar, *The Vulnerable Observer: Anthropology that Breaks Your Heart* (Boston, MA: Beacon Press, 1996), pp. 1–33.

33 Behar, *The Vulnerable Observer*, pp. 13, 21.

34 See 'Part II: Encounters in vulnerability, familiarity, and friendship', in Sheftel and Zembrzycki (eds), *Oral History Off the Record*. Quotation Hourig Attarian, p. 78.

35 Karike Ashworth and Courtney Pedersen, 'The feminine bravery construct: the crisis of neoliberal feminine bravery in the #MeToo moment', *Feminist Media Studies*, 23:5 (2023); Amia Srinivasan, *The Right to Sex* (London: Bloomsbury, 2021), pp. 1–32.

36 Jessica Hammett, Ellie Harrison, and Laura King, 'Art, collaboration and multi-sensory approaches in public microhistory: Journey with Absent Friends', *History Workshop Journal*, 89 (2020), 265.

37 As an interim step, I was interviewed by Veronica Heney as part of her doctoral research in early 2020. This provided valuable experience of sitting on the other side of the recorder. Veronica Heney, 'Our Stories, Our Selves: Fictional Representations of Self-Harm' (PhD thesis, University of Exeter, 2022).

38 Diane E. Hoffman and Anita J. Tarzian, 'The girl who cried pain: a bias against women in the treatment of pain', *Journal of Law, Medicine & Ethics*, 29 (2001).

39 This may mean undertaking something like a simpler version of Carol Gilligan's method. See Carol Gilligan, Renée Spencer, M. Katherine Weinberg, and Tatiana Bertsch, 'On the Listening Guide: a voice-centred

relational method', in Paul M. Camic, Jean E. Rhodes, and Lucy Yardley (eds), *Qualitative Research in Psychology: Expanding Perspectives in Methodology and Design* (Washington, DC: American Psychological Association, 2003).

40 Thanks to Louise Hide for helping to clarify my thoughts on this point.

41 Sheftel and Zembryzycki, 'Introduction', p. 15.

17

... and breathe: style narratives at home, March 2020–March 2021

Carol Tulloch

For want of a yellow jumper

On 27 January 2021, during the first year of the COVID-19 global pandemic, I bought online a yellow polo-neck cable-knit wool jumper. I primarily bought it because it is yellow. I believed the colour would bring me joy, would lift my spirits. I needed that jumper.

I originally saw the jumper, physically, at the store Freight HGG, in Lewes, East Sussex before the pandemic. I returned to it time and again, as to look at it gave me so much pleasure. The colour and design of the jumper triggered the possibility of a new dimension to being me, Carol Tulloch, that I wanted to explore, to wear more colour. But I did not purchase it. I often held back from purchasing objects that I liked, that I knew would boost and enhance my sense of self. I worried that it would not fit. At the time, the jumper was categorised as menswear and I did not trust that size XL would be generous enough for my body shape. I feared the disappointment of loss if it did not fit, and I was not confident about trying it on in Freight HGG.

By January 2021, I had recalibrated my life practice within my home in the face of the coronavirus pandemic and its series of lockdowns. I now prioritised the need to 'seize the time' rather than waiting for some 'ideal' moment in the future to make life happen, make it more liveable. I decided to buy the jumper.

The way the jumper was showcased on Freight HGG's website helped this decision. It was modelled by a young, slim, white man, which reinforced how good the jumper can look on the body. I have no physical connection with this model, I am a Black woman in her sixties with a generous body shape, but I have honed the skill of seeing beyond models that do not look like me. There was a photograph of the jumper folded. Studying the cable pattern of this '100% British Wool' jumper in the website's detail window brought back haptic memories of handling the jumper at the shop. Freight HGG's reassurance about the size, and the statement that the jumpers 'are not a gender specific garment' but 'look fantastic on everyone' also helped.[1]

Buying clothes and accessories online during the first year of the pandemic also fed this 'seize the time' attitude. Retailers' generous returns policies meant I could try the jumper on in my own home, with time to really study how it worked with my body, rather than in a small changing room, where to get a good sense of how a garment looked you had to step out of the changing room into the main area of the shop where other people could see and judge you. At home I had time to be with the jumper on that first fitting. XL was the right size. The jumper worked well with my body.

What just happened?

23 March 2020, the day the UK went into its first lockdown, triggered self-reliance as a vital skill for survival. Over the next year, we experienced a series of national and local lockdowns, periods of self-isolation for those who had the virus, tier systems of lockdown severity, and phased openings of businesses, organisations, educational establishments, and mixing in groups. It sometimes seemed as if the pandemic had a levelling effect. The COVID-19 virus was indiscriminate of class, race, age, gender, and sexuality. People across the world, regardless of other differences of identity, all became less visible. Invisibility seemingly created equity between people. As the murder of George Floyd and the increase in domestic violence against women and children showed, this was not actually so. Within months of lockdown being instigated around the world, calls to helplines increased dramatically. By the first year Refuge for Women and Children of Domestic Violence reported that, in England and Wales, activity on their helpline increased by 65% each month.[2] Still, during that year of lockdowns I did not continually come face to face with

410 *Subjectivity and intersubjectivity*

'micro-racism'. I was free to just to be me, to experience what not-being-different felt like in the country of my birth.

For some of us, then, constraints offered a strange, contradictory kind of freedom. Our worlds shrank to the size of our homes. For nearly two years, coming face to face with who we *really* are was made clear within the space we called home. Inside took on expanded meaning – lockdown, shutdown, held down – 'down' is the word present in all these. But as the home moved to the forefront of who we are, the everyday – the 'mundane' acts of living day to day – provided the rhythm of meaning to lockdown life practice. Living through lockdown became about cultivating hereness in the home. Self-reliance and self-reassurance provided vital meaning to a sense of wellbeing in this new way of being. Gradually, I came to focus on taking the reins of my own life ... and to breathe.

This chapter explores the interconnections between my day-to-day living practices in lockdown and my research practice on style, dress studies, design history and critical thinking, notably on Black identities. In this chapter, as in lockdown, 'home' is the fulcrum on which everything else turns. I ask: how did we maintain our identities, developed for presentation in myriad public scenarios, but now generated in the space of wherever we called home? What did we draw on to help define our sense of self during this extraordinary time? In exploring these questions, I ricochet between my past and the present experiences, using the armature symbolism of my yellow cable-knit jumper to understand the strands of self that made/make up my being-here-now – my sense of living rather than existing. This assurance, threatened by the COVID-19 pandemic, has also led to new articulations and configurations of myself, Carol Tulloch.

The woman, Carol Tulloch, who went into the COVID-19 lockdown periods – a northern, Black British academic, maker, wife, stepmother, sister, friend, colleague – came out a different Carol Tulloch. This chapter is a starting point in charting some of those changes, and a way of working them out. My decision to pursue this text has been a struggle. I have had to return in memory to the time of COVID, re-feel the range of emotions that lockdown generated, and confront how the effects of lockdown still reverberate today (at the time of writing I have not been on a traditional two-week holiday or on an aeroplane). I have also had to tackle my anxiety about researching and writing in a new way, making sure that my

... and breathe 411

personal narrative is grounded in academic rigour and 'valid' in traditional research terms.

The chapter reflects the entanglement of the personal and the academic self, a relationship that is integral to my practice of living and my research practice. Who I am drives the research that I do. How I handled lockdown was also an issue of do I, Carol Tulloch, actually practise what I preach?

Style narratives – design history – 'I' – matter

I am a design historian who originally trained as a fashion and textiles designer. I am Black British, born in Doncaster, South Yorkshire of Jamaican parents who migrated to England in the 1950s. These biographical details have impacted on my research focus, as I use the styled Black body as the prism to explore what social, cultural, or political issues have influenced the style choices of Black people, and the contributions that Black people have made to history, society, and culture. Essentially my research is about identities, difference, and belonging, the dynamics of making (making the self or the things required to shape and maintain identities), and the different spaces where these identities operate (on the street, in the home, at the photographic studio, or at political events). What we choose to wear, and how we decide to wear it – our assemblage of garments, accessories, hairstyles, and make-up – is about styling the self, a form of autobiography.

I developed the concept of style narratives as a way to understand this making of the self through style. Style narratives is a method of reading material and visual cues to a person's sense of self as one expression of who they are, who they would like to be, their sense of being and belonging, and the context in which their styled bodies operate (this includes how others 'read' what they see people wearing). As an academic practice, style narratives is a methodology for interpreting a styled body and presenting new meanings within a particular context through analysis of style–fashion–dress, the whole system of concepts signifying the multitude of meanings and frameworks that are always 'whole-and-part' of styled self-construction. This way of seeing recognises that style is agency, a form of constructing the self and self-telling.[3]

412   *Subjectivity and intersubjectivity*

My research centres on how Black people of the African diaspora present themselves in public spaces through an aesthetic of presence, and I have used style narratives to challenge the appalling misinformation about Black history, Black lives, and their place in the world.[4] More recently, inspired by the artist-curator Lubaina Himid's work, I have extended the possibilities of style narratives to view its components as vessels that, in turn, are 'narratives on time'. The concept of garments and accessories as vessels conveys the past/present dynamic of these pieces as receptacles that carry, hold, and transport thoughts, ideas, and views of the world and how the wearer wants to respond to it. For people of the African diaspora, these vessels 'speak' through their insistence on visibility and belonging.[5] In style narratives, then, we are always making (in our own style) and seeing (in the style of ourselves and others) ways of acting in/on the world, of claiming visibility and presence, that are shaped by specific spaces and by the dynamics of history and identity in the here and now, and that offer new possibilities for being in the future.

Style narratives uses the tools of design history to articulate an individual's relationship with objects, or an object's impact on history, culture, and the individuals who design, make, or use it – to understand the individual and the object as part of each other's biography. Understanding the design/history/biography of objects extends our understanding of how people live, construct their identities, and style their bodies and homes. This approach to design history emphasises the role of people in the object's making, use, and meaning – including the researcher. Kjetil Fallan and Grace Lees-Maffei insist that design historians can 'produce *a more rational* approach' by including personal experiences in their research. If 'objects become meaningful in their encounters with subjects', then 'the meaning of things is relational: it is formed and transformed in the discursive space between object and subject'. It therefore becomes important to recognise subjectivity and to accommodate it 'as a subject of study, as constitutive of the research practitioner', as one of the factors that produces the meaning of the object in the moment of encounter.[6]

This way of practising design history leads into autoethnography and personal narrative as research methods. For Carolyn Ellis and Arthur Bochner, personal narrative is about addressing 'lived moments of struggle, resisting the intrusions of chaos, disconnection, fragmentation, marginalization, and incoherence, trying to reserve or restore the continuity and coherence of life's unity in the face of unexpected blows of fate that call one's meanings and values into question'.[7] But, like style narratives, personal narrative is never just about the self. Bryant Keith Alexander explains that it is also 'always a reflection on and excavation of the cultural contexts that give rise to experience', and that personal narratives therefore 'move from what some might presume to be an insular engagement of personal reflection, to a complex process that implicates the performative nature of cultural identity', and places 'the individual in a dialogue with history, social structure, and culture'.[8]

I have written about and from the self before, but not in ways framed as a personal narrative methodology.[9] This is new ground for me. But it makes sense to break this new ground, to blend these approaches – style narratives, design history, personal narratives – to make sense of myself in the pandemic. Style narratives is how I, as a researcher, assess lived experiences, being and belonging for different people and groups in different spaces and historical moments.[10] This is also the only way I can explore what happened to me during lockdown. Putting myself right at the centre of the narrative also means using new academic tools – different materials for a different kind of making. My relationship with the yellow jumper is one way to merge my personal and academic selves, drawing on what Sheila Fitzpatrick refers to as a 'mixture of direct (emotional) and indirect (analytical) expression' to convey the effect of the purchase, wearing, and styling it during lockdown living.[11]

This chapter is about the self in the home during lockdown, but it is also about me, a researcher with my own past, as I tried to remake the present. Because it is by and about me, it is also about style narratives: what do (did) style narratives, as a form of presentation of self to the outside world, mean in the context of lockdown? What happens to visibility and belonging when style narratives are performed in the home? What do style narratives mean when the audience is yourself, the researcher, and they are enacted so that your life will continue to have meaning in the maelstrom of the COVID-19 pandemic? Here, I use style narratives to understand the wearer's (my) identity through assessment of the cultural meaning of the genre of cable knitwear, the possible contributions of these

414   *Subjectivity and intersubjectivity*

meanings to the attachment between the jumper and the owner/ wearer (me), and the importance of the home as the arena for styling myself during lockdown.

The home as workshop of self-care and new style narratives

Lockdown disturbed space and time. Being at home ring-fenced who we are/were. Before lockdown, for so many of us home was primarily the space we passed through to go to other spaces that contributed to our sense of self. Time flickered and stuttered within the walls of the home that bounded us. We had to simultaneously negotiate acceptance of the slower pace of lockdown living, of stepping away from previous ways of engaging with the world and the trusted habits that made living possible, and, for those employed or not furloughed, speedily recalibrate our skills to learn online communication systems so that we could continue working. Again: constraint, freedom, contradiction.

Confined, the home became the mirror of who we were and how we could be. In daily, mundane acts of lockdown living, I experienced 'the use and space of ubiquitous objects' in my home and life as what Ben Highmore calls 'access to freedom'.[12] Michelle Ogundehin's statement that '[w]ithin our four walls we can dream, and work towards becoming precisely who we wish to be' resonates.[13] Ogundehin transforms Pierre Bourdieu's concept of the 'taste of necessity' – the notion that the 'taste' of those with few resources is circumscribed by what can fulfil their needs most efficiently.[14] Bourdieu had in mind those who lacked economic resources, but in lockdown we all lacked reserves, were all thrown back on what we could find around us, in our homes. There were days I just put clothes on without attention to aesthetics, and there were days where I consciously applied styling practice as action to maintain visibility that equated to still being here.

On those conscious, mindful days, I practised self-care through repurposing everyday belongings, investing them with new meaning and new life. My home became an archive out of which I remade myself. This use echoed my approach to archives in my writing and curatorial practice as radical spaces that link present, past, and future by preserving evidence of 'networks of knowledge and of a presence that is now absent', generating 'stories of lives and activities that would often be lost', and enabling 'lived experiences to be revived and reassessed time and time again'.[15] Now it was my own self, knowledge, experience, past, presence in the world at stake. Jo Melvin's vision of the house not as an archive, but as a collection of different collections, also works here. She sees these collections as perhaps attenuated archives (of a certain kind), but as even more 'like a compressed series of maps, charting territories of interaction and overlapping referents, that are recognisable outside an intersubjective familial environment to various and cross-generational communities'.[16]

In the privacy of my home, I explored the organisation of past and present, old and new ways of being, that included styling myself. In this context of ringing in the changes, I saw my home as a 'series of collections' – wardrobe, chest of drawers, storage boxes, cupboards, clothes hanging on backs of doors, hallways – that combined to form a personal archive, a unique repository for use during the pandemic. This shift in styling myself, of being more 'mindful' of what my existing clothes, accessories, make-up, perfume, and the new pieces (like my yellow cable-knit jumper) added to this collection at this time mean, provided me with a reassured sense of being-here-now, of maintaining a sense of connection between Carol Tulloch before the pandemic and Carol Tulloch in lockdown.[17]

New system to be-here-now

Wellbeing, for me, is about gaining and maintaining a sense of self in difficult circumstances. It includes caring for the self, 'composing the self', through skills learned and experiences gained over a life – bringing to the surface tacit knowledge that generates wellbeing as an intuitive act.[18] In early 2021, writing an initial version of this chapter as the keynote address for an online seminar series, a childhood memory emerged. I remembered, at the age of about ten, helping my father paint the ceiling and woodwork of our dining room in magnolia. In reality, I wasn't helping. Really, he was teaching me how to do it. The skill has stayed with me over the years. It impresses my husband, himself a very skilled DIYer.[19] It is my past, my present, a skill I will take into the future.

416 *Subjectivity and intersubjectivity*

The self in action, creation, the body doing what it knows – this is at the heart of the new system of living I created to face the period of lockdown. To connect with the outside world from inside my home, I curated core resources (magazines, newspapers, radio programmes, and Instagram posts) that chimed with my needs. I relied on their insight, honesty, care, kindness, and advice on ways to continue enjoying aspects of the life that mattered to me prior to 23 March 2020. This included making things and making myself, the twin practices that define me. Different forms of writing, stitching, cooking, designing my home, and dressing myself – the sense of who I am is embedded in these acts, experiences, and forms of tacit knowledge. These old ways of being were newly seen, felt, and understood in lockdown, and so became a new system, to be-here-now.

Lockdown enforced a pause on ways of living that the world knew. But it also enabled for me, after recalibrating to this new way of living, the agency of pause. Robert Poynton describes 'pause' as deliberately claiming time away from the pressures of life and work, carving out moments that 'give shape and texture to your experience' and can be used in different ways. It is a way 'to rest and regenerate, to become more creative, connect with other people or yourself'. Lockdown was an enforced pause of being outside the home; yet for many of us, working inside the home, the usual demarcations between work and life away from work dissolved. The actively chosen pause became even more crucial. For Poynton, a pause is 'an opening', 'a portal to other options and choices', 'a way to play around with the rhythms of your life'.[20] But where and how to take these pauses, to actively compose a life, under lockdown, within the confines of the home and whatever outdoor space is attached to it?

Choosing where you put your pauses makes an enormous difference to what your life feels like and what you do as a result. What is produced or completed (or not) during a 'pause' symbolises the possibility of gaining rather than losing time.[21] In lockdown, it became fundamental for me to claim time to make things, including to make or style myself, as a means of self-sustenance and care. This form of 'pause' enabled me to see anew, and from that to compose a life using different forms and lengths of pause. It acted as a balm against more intense aspects of life.[22] The ellipsis in the title of this chapter is the pause, the signal to stop and catch one's

... and breathe   417

breath, to realign, to regroup, to recognise needs and desires, and desires as needs.

On 7 June 2020 I wrote my 'Essentialness Manifesto' as a frame to accommodate the new paradigm of lockdown living. It listed desires that were also needs:

> Things that make my heart sing
> Sights that make my eyes hurt because of their beauty
> Anything that defines who I am now
> Things that make my journey to now
> To make
> What I NEED to include in my future journey
> Dailyness of the everyday
> 'Kindfulness'.[23]

The 'Essentialness Manifesto' pinpointed what I needed to enact to maintain self-care in this potentially psychologically and physically damaging situation. I had not bought my yellow cable-knit jumper when I wrote the manifesto, but re-reading it, I can see that the jumper fulfilled what I wanted to pursue: to make lockdown living not only about staying safe, but also an exercise in how to live, how to engage with life.

The yellow cable-knit jumper is part of me

At the time of writing in 2023, when we are now 'living with COVID', I have had my yellow cable-knit jumper for two years. My emotional attachment to it remains strong. When I view it hanging on my clothes rail or draped over the arm of the bedroom chair, it is charged with wellbeing properties. Its materiality has absorbed my hopes for it as a tool of self-care that I can wear, and that it has delivered. *My* yellow cable jumper is armature of wool, Aran aesthetic, and colour.

Aesthetic resemblance

My jumper has traits of the Aran jumper, a type of patterned knitwear characteristic of the Aran Islands off the west coast of Ireland. A typical Aran design consists of a centre panel with two side panels bordered with cable, but the knit is characterised by

418   *Subjectivity and intersubjectivity*

multiple variations on traditional stitches rather than by a particular pattern, and can therefore be quite simple or extremely complex in design.[24] The dense texture of cabled stitch patterns creates 'a visual effect that is simultaneously ornate and rustic', perhaps explaining the complex status of the Aran jumper as 'both a recurrent fashion trend and an internationally recognized symbol of Irishness'.[25]

My yellow cable knit jumper, with its 'Made in England' label, bridges these definitions. Knitted in the round on a Shima machine, a medley of cables and ribs in various sizes, basket and garter stitches symmetrically surround a centre panel of diamond cable, reaching towards side panels of basket stitch that lead into the back of the jumper.[26] There is no central panel design here. Cables dominate, interspersed with fine rib detail and a strip of garter stitch near the basket stitch side panel. The symmetry of the patterning on the back is disrupted, as the rib pattern on the right has an extra rib detail that is not mirrored on the left.

The Aran jumper emerged in the 1930s at a defining moment in Ireland's history. In late 1922 a large portion of Ireland had gained independence from the British state, leaving six counties – Northern Ireland – under rule from Westminster as part of the United Kingdom. Siún Carden shows that from the 1930s onwards, wearing Irish knitwear was a sign of separation and independence. Knitting was one means to earn a living and remain in the country during a period of high emigration rates. She argues that this scenario of reclaiming and establishing an independent Irish identity helped to fuel expanded thinking of 'the Aran jumper as an identity document'.[27] The jumper harboured and reflected Irish identity, longing, reconnection with heritage and histories beyond the Atlantic or the Irish Sea. It also became part of Irish tourism, notably in the early 1960s, when Irish Americans took to wearing Aran jumpers after the Irish folk group the Clancy Brothers and Tommy Makem appeared wearing them on the *Ed Sullivan Show*.[28]

Carden provides a way to read the past and present of Aran knitwear, showing how its 'twisting cables have been used to express evolving networks of ideas about place, belonging and cultural ownership from within and outside Ireland', and its encapsulation of 'emotionally charged ideas about nativeness and diasporic identities'.[29] In doing so, she endows the Aran jumper with research integrity – it moves from an everyday object to a symbol of loss

... and breathe 419

and longing, presence and absence, identity and power. But what do these resonances mean for the individual emotional attachment of the owner/wearer to an Aran jumper? How do they reverberate in the style narratives of a Black British woman whose research speaks to diasporic belonging and her fight, all her adult life, for recognition of belonging in England?

Armour/bandage, warmth/sun

Men's jumpers have always interested me. In my past work, they have provided insights on familial relationships, mourning and Black modernity. I saw the wool that my white working-class mother-in-law used to produce a handknitted jumper for her son, my husband, as a metaphor for the umbilical cord severed when the son chose his own design.[30] I realised that my father's pale blue jumper, hanging on my parents' wardrobe door following his sudden death, was a 'melancholy object' that symbolised loss and absence.[31] I explored how the polo-neck jumper worn by the African American artist Malvin Gray Johnson in the 1930s expressed the resonance of this symbol of Black modernity for him.[32]

Knitting has always interested me, too. I have described how the 'act of knitting represents a standpoint from which separateness and connectedness can be analysed, and [...] understood as a cohesive solution to the desire for individual needs, personal development and interaction'.[33] Hand-knitted yarn can represent a bond between the maker and wearer. The yarn of the Aran jumper could, metaphorically, be viewed as an umbilical connection to all parts of Ireland and its diaspora. For me, these meanings are important. They are part of how I, an academic researcher, seek to understand the meanings of my yellow cable-knit jumper as an object in the world. Because of who I am, they are part of (not separate from) the personal meanings of my jumper to me. They carry into my sense of the Aran jumper as equating to belonging in England, presence of being here, a personalised identity.

This personalised identity is built out of other meanings. Some are the meanings of the maker, my other self. As a maker I can see the extended meanings of materials and techniques invested in my yellow cable-knit jumper. An armature is a framework of wire or wood to build structures around, used in crafts like knitting, felting,

420 *Subjectivity and intersubjectivity*

and quilting, but it is also a form of defensive armour. The cable stitch results in a knit that is less flexible, denser, but that is also elastic and opens out the possibilities of different ways to play with surface, pattern, and texture. The rib is a structure that supports and strengthens. An Aran jumper can be a defence, a protection, a bandage.

A bandage shields so that healing can begin. I bought the yellow cable-knit jumper as a form of 'care of the self', taking control of one's self-care as a 'right to be well' as fought for and practised by feminists, Black activists, and marginalised groups since the 1960s.[34] My jumper not only protects but gives sustenance. It projects assurance of feeling and being warm. It is about physical comfort and wellbeing, but also excitement and exhilaration, enthusiasm and delight – the emotional and psychological warmth that its yellow radiates.[35] Freight HGG describes the jumper as 'ochre'. I prefer yellow. Ochre translates for me as an understated, earthy, reliable tone. The jumper may not be a 'true yellow', but next to my brown skin, and particularly on days when the winter sun lights it, the yellow sings, it diffuses a tremor of joy.

This experience of joy generated confidence when I first tried on the jumper, and it is an emotional response that has reverberated at other significant moments. Colour can be flatly defined as an 'attribute of visual experience' that has 'quantitively specifiable dimensions of hue, saturation and brightness'.[36] But it is also 'a primary sensory experience', composed of complex psychological effects, rendering its meaning subjective – colour is in the eye of the beholder.[37] Nuala Morse and Jo Volley state that 'colour is emotional: it is an immediate way in which we experience the world', and a way that we can communicate how we feel – colour matters too, to the beheld.[38] The colourist Annie Sloan believes that 'You're always learning something different with colour. It's a bit like music in that there are so many different tunes you can make that it never ends. For me, colour is fundamental to everything.'[39]

The dictionary defines colour as the effect of light reflected from a surface, but also as an attribute of forms of 'device, badge, or dress serving to distinguish or identify an individual', an aspect of outward meaning that 'serves to conceal or cloak the truth, or to give a show of justice to what is in itself unjustifiable', an 'allegeable ground or reason', a way of imbuing, charging, marking, and rendering plausible.[40] In wearing bright, joyous yellow during the solemnity of COVID, I was picking up on another dictionary definition, trying to advance life, living, and being-here-now by using colour to 'lend one's name to, represent or deal with as one's own'.[41] I also entered into systems of meaning, ways of using and understanding yellow, that were unintended or only part-realised, even if they make intuitive sense. Historically, yellow has evoked happiness, warmth, brightness, and the call to be outdoors in the sun and enjoy the day.[42] During the First World War – as for me in lockdown – it was associated with care, healing, and wellbeing. On wards for shell-shocked soldiers, walls were painted 'Sunlight Yellow', and the floor and furniture 'Sunlight Primrose'.[43]

In the present, yellow is imbued with many other meanings that make sense to me. The BBC Radio 3 series *Night Tracks* (2023), devised by Sarah Mohr-Pietsch and Hannah Peel, explored how colours are expressed through music. Mohr-Pietsch selected tracks that expressed the 'radiance and warmth', 'adoration of sunshine', and capacity for 'bearing witness to both love and pain' of yellow.[44] For me, these tracks evoked above all peace, calm, and quiet; the temporary cessation of hostilities that my jumper afforded in lockdown. I also recognise Deborah Levy's use of yellow as a marker of change in her autobiography *The Cost of Living* (2018). Following separation from her husband and moving from the family home into a smaller space with her two daughters, one of Levy's friends persuaded the writer to paint her bedroom walls yellow. She urged Levy to 'Have a go at living with colour [...] Yellow would be good for you [...] It clears up emotions and gives us a bigger sense of things.'[45] But at a time of upheaval that required all the courage she could muster, this bold design decision did not work for Levy. She could not live in yellow, and she equated this failure with her inability to live in the life she now found herself in. The courage to live in yellow is the courage to 'design' your life the way you want it to be – taking charge of the situation and shaping it, designing it to meet your needs. On reflection, that was what I was trying to do when I bought my yellow jumper. I needed the yellow to lift my confidence, spirits, and the 'joy' of life, and the wool to keep me warm. Levy's text stayed with me for some time.

422 *Subjectivity and intersubjectivity*

New love for 'dormant things'

I found during lockdown that I needed to see colour. I am surrounded by colour in my study: green walls, an orange vase, a birthday present from my stepdaughter Lucy that sits to my left on my desk, and the strips of myriad colour from the spines of books of various heights and widths on the floor-to-ceiling bookshelves that run alongside me. But I also realised that I liked to see colour at my wrist. I wore a COS jumper for an online meeting, one dormant on my clothes rail for years, primarily because of the seven-centimetre band of fluorescent pink at the end of the light grey sleeves. While I typed on my grey laptop, the twinned diagonal bands of colour that lay across the laptop, pointing towards the keyboard, soothed and enhanced the gesture of typing. I wore this top prior to buying my yellow cable-knit jumper. Lockdown meant rediscovery as well as newness.

Because of lockdown, our wardrobes have new meaning, rules have changed. I now treat mine like a unique vintage shop, rediscovering pieces not worn for some time. These pieces were 'dormant things', in Sophie Woodward's phrase – things that had accumulated in domestic spaces and were not being used, but that I had not thrown away.[46] In lockdown, dormancy took on a new role for many of us. We became reacquainted with our wardrobes and glad that we had kept things. What does it mean to wear things that hold memories specific to the wearer in the context of a global pandemic? Rediscovering garments and accessories also means rediscovering and recreating aspects of the self, invoking old skills as well as old styles in new efforts of self-care and definition.

Combining old and new pieces has led to realisation of skills that I took for granted. These older garments are still wearable due to years of attentiveness. I have had 'Big Blue', my navy blue cable-knit jumper, since around 1983–84. I bought it for a few pounds, from a sale rail of uncollected clothing, from a dry cleaner in Borough, London near where I lived. I originally wore it for warmth and as part of my individualised style statement as a fashion student. In the 1990s to early 2000s it was an essential item during the winter months during visits to France. I still wear it for warmth, but my relationship to it has evolved through my care for it, in darning holes at the elbow and its worn cuffs. This care has resulted in its

... and breathe   423

longevity of use, handwashing it to preserve its colour, shape, and texture, making it a presentable garment to wear in public for a long time. The surface of the yellow cable-knit jumper has changed a little. It has pilling from frequent use. I try to keep the pilling at bay with a clothes shaver. Care of the jumper(s) is care of me: hanging it, storing it in a garment bag, using moth repellent, and handwashing – clothes-care practice originally taught to me by my mother. Like sewing on lost buttons and restitching hems, these practices were instilled in me from childhood as looking after oneself, and to preserve clothing due to lowered household income following the death of my father. They became tacit knowledge, embodied skills, part of my armoury to survive and thrive.

Drudging clothes: no longer a definition of being 'at home'

This reacquaintance with dormant things has meant a deeper appreciation of aspects of self, but it also established other ways of being. During lockdown, clothes reserved for 'best', for work, public occasions, and statement making outside the home, were being worn in the home, as part of the supposedly 'mundane' everyday practice of being at home. Before lockdown, my new yellow cable-knit jumper, with its expanse of colour from my neck to my hip, would have been positioned in my wardrobe as statement wear, reserved for public spaces, lunch with friends, or a day out. But the shift of all meetings online made the computer or phone screen into the workplace. I gained new confidence in presenting myself to work colleagues and at meetings, notably wearing headscarves, or what I like to call a headtie.[47]

In wearing 'best' at home, I was going against cultural tenets of my Jamaican heritage of wearing 'drudging clothes' to do 'laborious work' in the home to clean, cook, or just be at home, in order to preserve one's best clothes for work, special occasions, and life beyond the home. This system of dressing, also known in Jamaica as 'yard clothes – old garments that you wear only at home' remained part of my life practice, but the shift to wearing 'best' pieces at home during lockdown reaffirmed presence, when the usual confirmation of that presence from face-to-face encounters with friends,

424 *Subjectivity and intersubjectivity*

family, colleagues, even strangers in public spaces, was not possible.[48] This was vital during COVID, as a sense of presence was profoundly needed. It was about still being alive and well.

The headtie became another symbol of working-from-home culture, as the spaces of work and home blurred. It has long been a symbol of labour, Black consciousness, and agency within the African diaspora. In my experience of wearing it during lockdown, the headtie symbolised being at and caring for the home, but also caring for the self at home in the maelstrom of COVID. This aspect of Jamaican heritage, again instilled by my mother, signified agency and became an arbiter of wellbeing. I have been wearing headties since childhood. I originally wore them as part of my drudging clothes, to protect my hair while doing domestic tasks, or used to keep preparatory hairstyles in place. In the 1970s I began to wear my headties in public spaces, as part of an individualised statement to connect with the Black activism movements.[49] In the 1980s, and up to 2020, my wearing of the headscarf changed again, as I primarily wore it with drudging clothes for domestic work, and in public spaces in leisure time or for holidays, but not for work.

I still wear the headtie for online meetings, and I have also worn it for face-to-face work meetings and public talks. Styling myself in the yellow cable-knit jumper and a New York City-map One Hundred Stars scarf, tied into a large bow at the front of my head, was not a clash of old and new references, but an example of agentic cross-time and cross-cultural referencing that has long been one of my style practices. As a fashion and textiles student in the 1980s, I wore 'Big Blue' with a red-and-white paisley voile headscarf tied at the front in a bow, an exaggerated version of the African American 'mammy' headtie.[50] I also wore this headscarf, tied in the same style, with second-hand men's suits or Second World War jodhpurs, grandad shirt, knitted slipover and argyle socks, bought at Greenwich Market, Flip in Covent Garden, or Shoreditch in east London. This style narrative at this period in my life was a deliberate act of cool, as an aesthetic of presence for a Black British woman in the 1980s. Now, it is more of an intuitive rather than deliberate style practice, as in the pairing of the yellow cable-knit jumper and the headtie. In lockdown, I produced a new style narrative of being-here-now that reverberated and expanded on my previous style narratives of becoming.

Conclusion

My yellow cable-knit jumper and headtie have long histories that incorporate colonial and postcolonial history. They make visible and material the impact of difference and simultaneously challenge that imposition of difference. The style narrative of how I wore my yellow cable-knit jumper with a headtie in my home reflects the embodied habitus of the home dweller, but in a changed context where the domestic became merged with public spaces. The personal narrative of how I styled myself at home during periods of lockdown is part of the systems of self-care I developed at this time. But it is also about the times before and beyond that moment. My research frame is informed by a past–present–future tangram: I bring into play the design, production, consumption, and use of objects to address historical, social, cultural, and political concerns, looking from the present, from an academic and personal perspective as a Black British woman at the past, distant and recent, in order to look to the future.

I first saw the yellow cable-knit jumper in a shop, but I bought it from home. Its purchase was bound up in the new system of being I devised, sometimes consciously, sometimes intuitively, during the lockdown period. I have browsed online at Freight HGG for years, but during lockdown it became one of my essential websites to visit. These websites were material comfort zones. I did not need to make a purchase. The design sites were confirmation that designers, makers, creatives were still generating new ideas, despite the possible psychological impact on them of the virus, of the isolation of lockdown, or of distance. My favourable response to designs at this time was a way of maintaining connection with the world of design that is part of who I am. It was a purchase into a sense of newness and a means to engage with the world.

I bought the jumper while writing the essay 'Epiphanies of Dress' for the 'Lubaina Himid', Tate Modern exhibition catalogue. The first time I wore the jumper was for an online meeting with Michael Wellen, editor of the catalogue and co-curator of the exhibition. Michael's first comment was on the colour of my jumper. I said something like, 'I need colour at the moment'. The incidental presence of my yellow cable-knit jumper at one of the meetings with Michael, that included viewing the garments and accessories in Lubaina Himid's

426   *Subjectivity and intersubjectivity*

works as vessels, reverberates with my research and my styled self. My yellow cable-knit jumper became a style-narrative vessel of, and about, self-care, of being-here-now during a time of crisis. The continued meaning of the jumper in my life is dependent on its constituent biographical elements – its colour, pattern, material, online purchase, and inaugural wearing during a lockdown meeting that went on to expand the meaning of style narratives through garments as vessels – as these reverberate into the era of 'living with COVID'.

In the end, this personal narrative of my relationship with my yellow cable-knit jumper is the counter-narrative I tried to invoke against the 'fragmentation of the self' that the pandemic threatened.[51] By assembling the fragments of lived experiences and skills, I tried to address what was happening beyond my control. All the elements, the fragments of my life, in my home – some visible objects, some invisible memories, some embodied skills – combined to become the collage of who I am. During that unprecedented space and time, I relied on that collage in order to be-here-now. My style narrative during lockdown was a conscious creation of what I wanted to say to myself and to people I met in work meetings online: that I am okay, coping, being-here-now. I wanted to be heard and to be seen. As a Black woman, visibility is a right I have long fought for. People saw the jumper, but the jumper also helped *me* to see me in a new light.

Lockdown released in me a need for colour. The jumper fulfilled that need. Wearing yellow was life affirming. It made me sonic. It made me beam. It made me visible.

Notes

1 'Unisex cable knit lambswool jumper', Freight HHG: https://Freight HGG HHGstore.co.uk/collections/men/products/mens-cable-knit-jumper (accessed 11 January 2023).
2 'Lockdowns around the world bring rise in domestic violence', *Guardian*, 28 March 2020: www.theguardian.com/society/2020/mar/28/lockdowns-world-rise-domestic-violence (accessed 30 May 2023); Refuge's National Domestic Abuse Helpline Service Review, 2020/21: https://refuge.org.uk/wp-content/uploads/2021/03/Refuge-Covid-Service-Report.pdf (accessed 30 May 2023).

... and breathe 427

3 Carol Tulloch, 'Style-fashion-dress: from Black to post-Black', *Fashion Theory*, 14:3 (2010), 276.

4 Carol Tulloch, *The Birth of Cool: Style Narratives of the African Diaspora* (London: Bloomsbury, 2016).

5 Tulloch, 'Epiphanies through dress', in Michael Wellen (ed.), *Lubaina Himid* (London: Tate Publishing, 2021).

6 Kjetil Fallan and Grace Lees-Maffei, 'It's personal: subjectivity in design history', *Design and Culture*, 7:1 (2015), 14, 21.

7 Carolyn Ellis and Arthur P. Bochner, 'Autoethnography, personal narrative, reflexivity: researcher as subject', in Norman K. Denzin and Yvonna S. Lincoln (eds), *Handbook of Qualitative Research*, 2nd edn (Thousand Oaks, CA, London, New Delhi: Sage, 2000), p. 744.

8 Bryant Keith Alexander, 'Performance ethnography: the reenacting and inciting of culture', in Norman K. Denzin and Yvonna S. Lincoln (eds), *The Sage Handbook of Qualitative Research*, 3rd edn (Thousand Oaks, CA, London, New Delhi: Sage, 2005), p. 424, quoting Ellis and Bochner, 'Autoethnography, personal narrative, reflexivity', p. 739.

9 See Carol Tulloch, 'Picture this, the Black curator', in Jo Littler and Roshi Naidoo (eds), *The Politics of Heritage, the Legacies of Race* (London and New York: Routledge, 2005); Sequoia Barnes and Carol Tulloch, 'Sew me a quilt. Tell you a story', The Fruitmarket Gallery, Edinburgh (25 April 2019); Carol Tulloch, 'If I don't do some couching I will burst', *European Journal of Cultural Studies*, 25:6 (2022).

10 Tulloch, *The Birth of Cool*.

11 Sheila Fitzpatrick, '"Getting personal": on subjectivity in historical practice', in Sebastian Jobs and Alf Lüdtke (eds), *Unsettling History: Archiving and Narrating in Historiography* (Frankfurt: Campus Verlag, 2010), p. 195.

12 Ben Highmore, 'Mundane tastes: ubiquitous objects and the historical sensorium', in Malcolm Quinn, David Beech, Michael Lehnert, Carol Tulloch, and Stephen Wilson (eds), *The Persistence of Taste: Art, Museums and Everyday Life after Bourdieu* (Abingdon and New York: Routledge, 2018), p. 285.

13 Michelle Ogundehin, 'Style for life', *Elle Decoration* (May 2016), 15.

14 Pierre Bourdieu, *Distinction: A Social Critique of the Judgement of Taste* (London: Routledge, 1989), p. 175; Carol Tulloch, 'The glamorous "diasporic intimacy" of "habitus": taste, migration and the practice of settlement', in Quinn et al., *The Persistence of Taste*.

15 Tulloch, *The Birth of Cool*, p. 180.

16 Email correspondence between Jo Melvin, Donald Smith, and Carol Tulloch, 22 May 2016. See Tulloch, 'The glamorous "diasporic intimacy" of "habitus"', p. 269.

428 *Subjectivity and intersubjectivity*

17 Oxford Mindfulness Foundation, 'Course Types: Introducing Mindfulness': www.oxfordmindfulness.org/learn-mindfulness/course-types/introducing-mindfulness/ (accessed 19 March 2023); Amy Twigger Holroyd, 'World 45, enactment i: invitation' (11 November 2022): https://fashionfictions.org/2022/11/11/world-45-enactment-i-material-mindfulness/ (accessed 17 January 2023).

18 Robert Poynton, *Do Pause: You are Not a To Do List* (London: The Do Book Company, 2019), p. 91.

19 Tulloch, 'Epiphanies through dress'.

20 Poynton, *Do Pause*, pp. 17–18.

21 Carol Tulloch, *Jessica Ogden: Still* (London: Chelsea College of Arts, 2017), p. 5; Carol Tulloch, 'Units of possibility: the reknit revolution', *Fashion Practice: the Journal of Design, Creative Process & the Fashion Industry*, 10:1 (January 2018), 132.

22 Poynton, *Do Pause*, p. 15; Tulloch, 'If I don't so some couching I will burst', 2.

23 Carol Tulloch, 'Essentialness Manifesto' (unpublished, 7 June 2020). 'Essentialness Manifesto', written in a personal notebook, was my way to address the impact of the COVID-19 pandemic and its lockdowns.

24 Heinz Edgar Kiewe, 'Foreword', in Shelagh Hollingworth, *Traditional Aran Knitting* (Mineola, NY: Dover Publications, 1982), p. 6; *Knitting Encyclopedia 1500 Patterns, Mon Tricot Collection* (Paris: Cie des Editions de l'Alma, 1986), p. 179.

25 Siún Carden, 'Cable crossings: the Aran jumper as myth and merchandise', *Costume*, 48:2 (2014), 260.

26 Adele Adamczewski at Freight HGG in email correspondence with Carol Tulloch, 27 September 2023.

27 Siún Carden, 'The Aran jumper', in Stuart Walker, Martyn Evans, Tom Cassidy, Jevon Jung, and Amy Twigger Holroyd (eds), *Design Roots: Culturally Significant Designs, Products, and Practices* (London, Bloomsbury, 2018), p. 70.

28 Carden, 'The Aran jumper', p. 70.

29 Carden, 'Cable crossings', 271–2; Carden, 'The Aran jumper', p. 75.

30 Carol Tulloch, 'Home knitting: culture, and counter-culture, 1953–1963', in *One-Off: A Collection of Essays by Students on the Victoria and Albert Museum/Royal College of Art Course in the History of Design* (London: V&A/RCA, 1997).

31 Margaret Gibson, 'Melancholy objects', *Mortality*, 9:4 (2004); Tulloch, *The Birth of Cool*, p. 1.

32 Tulloch, *The Birth of Cool*, pp. 75–9.

33 Tulloch, 'Home knitting', p. 211.

... and breathe   429

34 Shahida Bari, 'Radical self care', *Analysis*, Radio 4 (31 October 2020): www.bbc.co.uk/programmes/m000k7k0 (accessed 30 May 2023).

35 John Gage, *Colour and Meaning: Art, Science and Symbolism* (London: Thames & Hudson, 1999), pp. 29–30; Laurence Urdang, *The Oxford Thesaurus*, 2nd edn (Oxford: Oxford University Press, 1997), p. 575; *The Oxford English Dictionary* (hereafter *OED*), Volume XIX, 2nd edn (Oxford: Clarendon Press, 1991), pp. 918–19.

36 Peter Brunette and David Wills, *Deconstruction and the Visual Arts: Art, Media, Architecture* (Cambridge: Cambridge University Press, 1994).

37 Gage, *Colour and Meaning*, pp. 11, 53.

38 Nuala Morse and Jo Volley, 'We can use colour to communicate how we feel – here's how', *The Conversation* (22 January 2018): https://theconversation.com/we-can-use-colour-to-communicate-how-we-feel-heres-how-90157 (accessed 30 May 2023).

39 Karen Dunn, 'Annie Sloan on colour', *The Simple Things*, 38 (February 2023), 40.

40 *OED*.

41 *OED*.

42 Gage, *Colour and Meaning*, pp. 23, 30.

43 Gage, *Colour and Meaning*, p. 209.

44 Sara Mohr-Pietsch, 'Yellow', *Night Tracks*, Radio 3 (23 January 2023): www.bbc.co.uk/programmes/m001h581 (accessed 30 May 2023).

45 Deborah Levy, *The Cost of Living* (Penguin, 2018), p. 36.

46 Sophie Woodward, 'The hidden lives of domestic things', in Emma Casey and Yvette Taylor (eds), *Intimacies: Critical Consumption and Diverse Economies* (Basingstoke and New York: Palgrave Macmillan, 2015).

47 Carol Tulloch, 'That little magic touch: the headtie and issues around Black British women's identity', in Kwesi Owusu (ed.), *Black British Culture and Society: A Text Reader* (London and New York: Routledge, 2000).

48 Carolyn Cooper in email correspondence with Carol Tulloch, 18 October 2022.

49 Tulloch, 'That little magic touch'.

50 Tulloch, 'That little magic touch', p. 218.

51 Amanda Coffey, *The Ethnographic Self: Fieldwork and the Representation of Identity* (Thousand Oaks, CA, London, and New Delhi: Sage Publications, 1999), p. 35.

Index

Note: 'n.' after a page reference indicates the number of a note on that page.

19 190

3-D 278, 281

A&E department 109, 119

ableism 11, 116, 120–1, 268n.14

abortion 61, 63–5, 68–72, 74–7, 82, 88, 90–4, 96–7, 165, 177, 179–80, 183–4, 186, 191, 278, 347, 358

Abortion Act (1967) 180

Abortion Information Centre 64

abuse 66–7, 75, 94, 180, 279, 348, 363n.15, 387

activism 1–2, 4, 8–10, 15, 37, 61, 106, 119, 166, 212, 294, 306, 347

Black 120, 420, 424

disability 8, 135, 139, 144, 256

feminist 31, 33–4, 94, 138, 367

queer 199

trans 156, 165–71, 204

women's health 61, 64, 67

women's movement 34, 83–4, 87–8, 93–7

see also Black Power Movement; Disabled People's Movement; Gay Liberation Movement; movement; Women's Liberation Movement

addiction 109, 272–3, 276–8, 280, 282–3, 285

adolescence 4

advertising 1, 164, 277, 325–6, 333, 348

Africa 43, 106, 232, 412, 424

age 3–4, 12–13, 54, 131, 148, 245, 252, 367–9, 409

agony aunt 1, 46, 130, 189–91, 199–214, 354, 356, 359, 396

AIDS 9, 82, 143, 178, 185–6, 190, 222, 278, 345, 347, 349, 354, 358–9

see also HIV

AIDS Coalition To Unleash Power (ACT UP) 9

Al-Khalidi, Alia 325, 327

Alberta 64–5, 73–4, 77, 238, 245

alcohol 206, 285, 296–7, 301, 311n.22

All Party Disablement Group 188

Amsterdam 94, 102n.53

anaesthetic 70, 72, 231, 235, 238, 240, 243, 248n.21

Index

anorexia 335
anthropology 17, 42, 320, 339–40, 395–6
Arab Spring 225
Arena Three 202, 204
Ashes to Ashes 222
Association to Aid the Sexual and Personal Relationships of the Disabled (SPOD) 188
Athens 84
Atkins diet 296
Atlee, H.B. 236, 241
Attendance Allowance 134, 137
audio-visual source 286–7
austerity 295, 309
Australia 244, 277, 280, 282, 284
authoritarianism 347
autobiography 212, 300, 305, 394, 396, 411, 421
autoethnography 18, 412
Autonomous Women's Movement 84, 94
autonomy 4, 31, 61, 63, 83, 89, 96, 120, 272, 277
Avon Health Office 188
Axelrod, Julius 14

BAME 212
Bangladesh 14
Barbieri, Annalisa 396
Barnsley 14
BBC 42, 272, 278–9, 292n.55, 421
Beatles 42
Beaumont Bulletin 157–62, 211
Beaumont Society 129, 131, 155, 157–9, 161–3, 166, 170–1, 216n.20
beauty 203–5, 211, 214, 225, 278, 297, 302, 304, 417
Beauty Consumer Watchdog 278
Beckett, Elsa 253–6, 258, 260, 265, 270n.42
Being Human Festival 203
Bell, Kathryn 265
Bella 190

belonging 93, 119, 131–2, 156, 161, 319, 321, 374, 411–14, 418–19
Benjamin, Harry 163–4
Bernard, Frances 254, 260
Berners-Lee, Tim 222
biology 89, 104, 186
biomedicine 35–6, 103–4, 107, 110, 113
see also medicine
Birmingham 179, 184–5, 187, 203
birth
control 6, 65, 69–71, 94–6, 177, 179, 182, 185, 187, 193n.11, 349
see also Caesarean section; contraception; contraceptive; contraceptive pill; movement
control centre 60, 65–6
control clinic 5
rate 179, 183
reform 238, 241, 246
Birth Control and Information Centre 65
Bitar, Adrienne Rose 300
Black Beauty and Hair 202
Black Power Movement 32
see also activism, Black
Black women 8, 11, 16, 35–6, 104–6, 112, 116, 120–1, 211–12
body
Black 87, 411
building 296
female 11, 31, 89, 91, 104–5, 121, 230, 238–9, 252, 347
fluid 347, 349–50
ideal 4, 302
image/aesthetics 201–3, 298, 392, 399
impaired 252–3, 256, 258
language 283
male 11

432   *Index*

and mind 2, 17, 90, 95, 235, 238
and self 4–5, 8, 131, 317–18
wrong 154
Bodyform 1
Body, Self and Family 104–5, 198, 206, 212, 368–9, 372, 376, 378
Book/The Child, The 93
Bookwomen 93
Boots 14, 205
Boston Women's Health Collective 88
bottom-up perspective 10, 128, 238, 320
Bourdieu, Pierre 49, 414
braille 256–7
breastfeeding 94, 233
Brien, Alan 43
Brien, Joanne 183
Bristol 179, 185, 221
British Columbia 242–3
British Library 199, 268, 386, 388, 391, 403n.5
Brixton 181
Brodie, Bernard 14
Brook Advisory Centre (BAC) 129, 176–92
Brook, Helen 177–9
Brookside 221
Browne, Stella 43
Bruce, Lenny 42
Brussels 135

Caesarean section 234–5
see also birth
Calgary Birth Control Association (CBCA) 12, 15, 34–5, 60, 62–75, 77–8
see also Family Planning Clinic
California 34, 41, 377
Callaghan, James 139, 144
Calonal 14
Camden Lesbian Centre 254, 259
Canada 64, 73, 223, 231–3, 239–40, 242–4, 247n.14

cancer 273, 277–8, 280–1, 283–4, 301, 374
see also skin cancer
Cancer Research UK 277
Candice 211
capitalism 131, 137, 227
Captin 14
Caribbean 106, 116, 181
Carr, E.H. 10–11
Carr, Kris 301
celibate 264, 266
Central Council for Health Education 184
Chatelaine 10, 226, 232, 234–7, 239–40, 242–5
Chic 202, 211
child sexual abuse 348
Childbirth without Fear 230–1
Childbirth without Fear method (CWF) 232, 234, 237
childbirth 11, 94, 108, 112, 230–8
natural 223, 230–2, 234–8, 240–6
see also birth
childhood 17, 119, 208, 301, 335, 347, 368–71, 373, 375, 415, 423–4
Childline 279, 283, 348
Children Act (1989) 348
Children in Need 348
China 244
Chronically Sick and Disabled Person Act (1970) 187
Chrystal Rose Show, The 274–5
cinema 222, 327
circumcision 94
cis-normativity 156, 210
citizenship 2, 4, 15, 32, 106, 115, 119, 130
class 3, 36, 41, 86, 245–6, 252, 339, 353, 377, 409
middle class 5, 48–9, 166, 169, 232, 294, 306, 308, 326, 328, 351, 358
upper class 281, 283

Index

433

working class 5, 49, 225, 280–1, 286, 326, 328, 351, 371, 386, 419
classism 72–3
clinic 5, 17, 33, 64, 70–2, 82, 127–8, 130, 177–82, 184, 190–2, 358
Comfort, Alex 12, 33, 36, 39–42, 45–54, 56n.16
Comita, Julia 214
Commonwealth 120, 233
communication 4–5, 16, 35–6, 87–8, 93–7, 157–9, 161, 167, 222–3, 225–6, 321, 349, 355, 360, 414
condom 82, 177, 183, 186, 349, 354–5, 358–9
  see also contraception
consumer 4, 10, 31, 117, 226–7, 246, 274, 277, 279, 304–5, 326, 353
consumerism 2, 4, 32, 117
consumption 49, 273, 276, 286, 296, 354, 425
contraception 47, 61, 65, 68, 70–1, 74, 82, 88–90, 92–4, 96, 177–82, 184–7, 191, 196n.55, 278, 347, 352, 354–6, 362n.13
  see also birth, control; condom; diaphragm; intrauterine device
contraceptive 9, 42, 47–8, 61, 63, 69–70, 75, 77, 82, 90, 92, 105, 176–9, 182–4, 186–8, 190–2, 206, 347, 355, 362n.13
contraceptive pill 4, 47–8, 68, 72, 92, 163, 176–7, 182–3, 186, 190, 198, 206, 349, 351, 354–6, 358–9, 368, 370
Cook, Peter 42
cookbook 48, 224, 226, 294, 297, 299–300, 303, 306, 309

Cosmopolitan 44, 54, 202, 206, 278, 354–5
counterculture 4, 39, 41, 44
Coventry 185
COVID-19 206, 319, 322, 387, 389, 408–10, 413, 428n.23
  see also pandemic
Crabtree, Tom 355
Craggs, Charlie 204–5
culture, popular 46, 273, 339, 341n.1, 347, 354

Daily Mail 44, 278
Daily Mirror 183–4
Dalhousie University 236
Delfis Archival Center 84
Deliciously Ella 226, 294, 304, 306, 308
Delvin, David 206–7
Denmark 36, 89, 242
Department of Education 184, 186
Department of Health and Social Security (DHSS) 134–5, 138–41, 143–5, 149n.9, 184, 186, 196n.55, 362n.13
Depo-Provera 9, 105, 347
depression 143–4, 399–400
dermatology 277, 280, 282
diabetes 299
diagnosis 103–8, 110–13, 119–21, 144, 301, 345, 378
diaphragm 92, 94
Dick-Read, Grantly 223, 226, 230–40, 242–5
diet/dieting 108, 202, 225–6, 294–306, 308–9, 370
Digital Arts Festival 201–3, 212
disability 3, 114–15, 120, 139, 141–2, 146–8, 187–8, 192, 252–4, 256–8, 260, 262, 266, 269n.16, 269n.27
  benefits 16, 135–6, 144–5
  disabled women 10, 128, 131, 135, 141, 147–8, 251–5,

257–9, 262–6, 268n.12, 270n.40
learning 188
disablism 268n.14
see also activism, disability; impairment
Disability Alliance 144
Disability Discrimination Act 114
Disabled People's Movement 32, 251
Disablement Income Group 134, 137, 148
discrimination 31, 86, 114, 128, 131, 147–8, 155, 254, 266
Diva 221
divorce 4, 110, 112, 180, 243
Doctors Group 89
domestic labour 135–6, 138–40, 147–8
domestic/private sphere 62–3, 128, 189
Doncaster 161, 411
double standard 225, 347–8, 350–1, 353
Drumheller 69
Drury, Brenna 214

Eat-Clean Diet, The 294, 297
eating, clean 16, 225–6, 294–310
Eco, Umberto 331–2
Edinburgh 179, 181, 185
Education and Publication Unit 186–7
Ehrenreich, Barbara 31
emancipation 89
embodiment 3–5, 13, 18, 32, 128, 318, 326, 331, 356
emigration 418
emotion 3, 60–4, 67, 77, 86, 158, 224, 238, 320, 338, 379
empathy 53, 64, 86, 202, 287, 388
Employment and Support Allowance 134

England 35, 41–2, 118, 142–3, 159, 179, 196n.55, 237, 241, 243–4, 362n.13, 409, 411, 418–19
English, Deirdre 31
Enkin, Murray 244
entertainment 200, 202, 207, 259
equal pay 75, 136, 147
Equal Pay Act (1970) 136
Equal Rights for Disabled Women Campaign (ERDWC) 144, 147
eroticism/eroticisation 50–1, 53
Essex 201, 329
Esther 226, 272–5, 278–82, 285–7, 289n.10
ethnicity 232, 328, 386
ethnography 17–18, 395, 412
Europe 3, 35, 146, 224, 277, 326
European Council 134
European Economic Community (EEC) 16, 135, 145
exclusion 87, 116, 140, 163, 170, 212, 227, 253, 256–7, 336
exercise 54, 202, 236, 244, 301, 305
expertise, experiential 4, 31–7, 83–8, 91, 93–7, 110, 116, 119, 121, 224, 300

Falkland Islands 328
family
  life 4, 15
  planning 65–6, 73, 82, 94, 355
  planning centre 65, 178
Family Planning Act (1967) 177
Family Planning Association (FPA) 178–9, 190
Family Planning Clinic (Calgary) 73–4
  see also Calgary Birth Control Association
Fast Diet 299
Fat Liberation 9
fatherhood 373

Index

435

fatigue 104, 296, 298
femininity 89, 156, 349–50, 352
feminism 18, 61, 83, 93, 168–9,
   259, 273, 276, 347, 351,
   396
   feminist network 90, 93–4
   state 83
   see also activism, feminist
Feminist Transsexual Discussion
   Group 168
fertility 66, 105, 355
First World War 231, 421
Fisher, Nick 190
Floyd, George 409
food bank 295
Forbis, Terri 65
Foss, Chris 44
France 36, 89, 422
friendship 9, 129, 156, 162,
   166–7, 169–71, 200, 251,
   256, 262, 264
Full Personality Expression (FPE)
   157

Gavron, Hannah 5–7
Gay Liberation Movement (GLM)
   32, 251
   see also activism, queer
Gay Men's Disabled Group
   (GMDG) 260, 270n.49
Gay Pride event 224, 254–5, 261
Gaycare 260
Gemini 164–6
Gemma 141, 223, 226–7, 251–66,
   271n.66, 355
Gender and Identity Development
   Service (GIDS) 155
gender 3, 36, 41, 62, 83, 86, 106,
   120, 129, 137, 158, 171,
   200, 214, 245, 252–3,
   266, 340, 353, 377, 409
   binary 62, 341n.2
   discrimination 145, 148
   equality 147–8, 288
   genderfluid 162
   nonconformity 158

role 63, 66, 157, 164, 167,
   230, 232, 347
   transgression/non-conforming
   154, 158, 161–3, 204
general practitioner (GP) 114, 127,
   139, 182
generationality 243, 322, 348,
   361, 367–9, 372–6,
   381–2
   see also intergenerationality
genetic illness 104, 111, 113
Geneva 94
Germany 14, 242, 255
gerontology 371
Gilbert, Valerie 189
Gillick ruling 133, 190, 348, 353
Gillick, Victoria 196n.55, 362n.13
Ginsberg, Allen 42
globalisation 17
Godalming 134
Goldsmiths Queer History Fair
   206
Gove, Michael 16
Grand Prix award 1
Greater London Council 255,
   267n.6
Greece 82, 88, 90, 92
Greer, Germaine 54
Grenada 36, 107–8, 110, 115–16
grief 113, 127, 373–4, 379, 396–7,
   399
Grindr 210
Guardian 42–3, 161, 278, 396
gynaecology 11, 82, 84, 90, 186,
   239

haemoglobinopathies 104
Halifax/Nova Scotia 236
Hamilton, Evelyn 235
Hamilton/Ontario 244
happiness 2, 41, 66, 168, 264,
   300, 302–3, 305, 310,
   421
harassment 11, 114, 370
Hayman, Suzie 189–90, 202
Health Education Authority 354

436 *Index*

Health Education Council
   see Central Council for Health
     Education
health
   book 88, 92
   club 282
   emotional/ psychological 32,
     91, 198
   everyday 2–5, 8–10, 12–19, 32,
     36–7, 63, 84, 127–31,
     198, 212, 215, 221–3,
     225–7, 238, 246, 252,
     273, 286, 294–6, 298,
     310, 318, 320–2, 325,
     331, 368, 381, 386
   experience 1, 9, 33, 85, 193n.7,
     212, 233, 318, 368,
     380–1, 386
   feminist model of 61, 67
   issue 104, 148, 277–8, 285,
     296, 298, 301
   public 273–4, 278, 280, 282,
     284, 308
   reproductive 67, 94, 177–8,
     180, 182, 188, 190–2,
     193n.7, 206, 230, 233,
     239, 243
   service 63–5, 70–2, 74–5, 116,
     120, 178
   sexual 60, 66, 68, 75, 94,
     177–83, 187–8, 190–2,
     193n.7, 349, 356, 358
   studies 84–6, 95
   women's 60–1, 64–5, 77, 89,
     94, 98n.1, 234, 273, 278,
     386
healthcare 34, 63–9, 72–4, 76,
     85–6, 104, 106, 127, 144,
     155, 252, 295, 371
   policy 64, 72
   professional 35, 109, 114, 116,
     118
   provider 109, 378
   system 15, 32, 35, 66, 77–8,
     88, 90, 92, 130, 245,
     249n.50

   sexual 63, 69, 72, 76–7
   women's 60–1
healthiness 40–1
healthism 295, 303, 309
Healthwatch Essex Young Mental
     Health Ambassador
     212–14
Heath, Edward 144
Heeswyk, Dorothy van 181
Hemsley, Melissa 306
Henderson, Jane 41
heteronormativity 33, 157–8,
     210–11
heterosexism 212
heterosexuality 40–1, 50–1, 157–8,
     202, 210–12, 345, 349,
     354, 356, 399
Hilliard, Marion 239–40, 246n.3
Himid, Lubaina 412, 425
Hinge 210
History and Archives Conference
     205
history
   Black 412
   democratisation of 390–1,
     393
   design 320, 410–13
   disability 252
   of medicine 103, 206, 233
   oral 35, 65, 103, 106–7, 131,
     141, 178, 199, 205,
     212, 214, 319, 367–9,
     372–3, 376, 380–2,
     386–98, 402, 404n.16,
     404n.18
     ethical practice 387–9,
      391–2, 396–7, 401–2
   postcolonial 425
   trans 129, 154–5
   women's 10, 253
HIV 82, 345, 347–9
   see also AIDS
Holbrook, David 45
homophobia 11, 203, 259
homosexuality 158, 214, 217n.35,
     221, 271n.51, 362n.10

Index

Honey 191, 326
hospital 64, 71–2, 105, 108–9, 114, 117–18, 127–8, 165, 234, 237, 242, 245, 246n.3, 249n.51, 259
Housewife's Non-Contributory Invalidity Pension (HNCIP) 128–9, 134–48
Hoxton 108
humour 43, 156, 159, 169–71, 202
Hutchinson, Fay 180, 190
hypervisibility 5, 11, 13–14
hypnosis 237, 241
hysterectomy 329

identity
  Black 410
  female 273, 350
  gender 3, 155–7, 162
  generational 367, 369, 371–3, 375, 381
    see also intergenerationality; generationality
  lesbian 262–3
  medical 253, 256
  migrant 104–6
  national 16, 115–16
  queer 155, 160, 210
  sexual 349, 360, 399
  trans 129, 154–6, 158, 160, 162, 164–8, 170, 210
imagined communities 4
immigration 14, 115–16
impairment 137–41, 146, 256–8, 269n.27
  see also disability
impotence 180
Incapacity Benefit 134, 137, 145
inclusion 51, 72, 253, 262, 265
India 14, 42, 48, 243–4, 296
Indigenous people 65, 73–4
individualism 2, 300, 309
Industrial Injuries 146
inequality 8, 26n.53, 34, 136, 187, 252

infertility 11
infrastructure 65, 370
injustice 8, 143, 257
Instagram 16, 201–2, 227, 294, 308, 416
intergenerationality 13, 156, 186, 208, 319, 361, 367–71, 375–6, 380–1, 392, 415
  see also generationality; identity, generational
International Tribunal and Meeting on Reproductive Rights 94
internet 4, 15, 127, 154, 202, 222, 295, 304, 374
  see also social media
intersubjectivity 5, 318–20, 322, 404n.18
intrauterine device (IUD) 70–2, 91, 176, 186
  see also contraception; contraceptive
invisibility 5, 11–14, 211–12, 327, 332–3, 409
Ireland 181, 307, 417–19
Israel 255
Italy 244

Jackie 202, 221, 326, 353–4
Jamaica 107, 411, 423–4
Japan 14, 48
Johannesburg 232
Johnson, Barbara 39, 47
Johnson, Malvin Gray 419
Jones, Hattie 242
Jowell, Tessa 306
Junger, Alejandro 296–7
junk food 301, 307
Just Seventeen 190, 353–5, 357

Keeping, Dorothy 188
Kennedy, Robert 297
KENRIC 260, 270n.45
King, Rosemary 162
Kinsey, Alfred 39–40, 164
kinship 32, 35, 70, 104–6, 377

438 *Index*

knowledge
  experiential 83–4, 116, 350, 353
  expert/specialist 46, 48
  medical 88, 96, 108, 113, 121
  scientific 66, 84, 86, 91, 95
  sexual 51, 92, 176–7, 184–7, 192, 347–9, 351–4, 360
Krafft-Ebing, Richard von 51
Kreitman, Tricia 190
Kurtz, Irma 52

Labour Party 144, 147, 306
Lagos 110
Lamaze method 230, 232, 236–7, 244
Lamaze, Fernand 223
Lambeth Sickle Cell and Thalassaemia Centre 103
Late Show with Joan Rivers, The 274
Lawson, Nigella 306
Leeds 161, 164, 269n.27
Leontidou, Eftychia 84
Lesbian Custody Project 262
Lethbridge/Alberta 65
Levy, Deborah 17, 421
Lewis, Peter 44–5, 54
LGBTQ+ 4, 8, 16, 82, 160, 199, 203, 205, 208–12, 214–15, 217n.35, 271n.51, 362n.10, 386
liberalism 40, 347
liberation 8, 12, 61, 65–8, 75–7, 88–90, 96–7, 123n.21, 258–9, 266, 352, 355
Liberation Network of People with Disabilities 252
life expectancy 4, 285, 301
lifestyle 211, 225, 273, 276, 286, 295, 298–9, 301–5, 308–10
  change 298, 301, 309–10
  clean 294, 303, 307
  sexual 40, 49
Lil-lets 1

Liverpool 179, 182, 330
Liverpool Daily Post 45
lockdown 10, 127, 206, 320, 322, 389, 398, 408–11, 413–17, 421–6, 428n.23
London Hospital 231
London School of Economics 6
Lorde, Audre 87
Lovell, Anne 190

magazine
  teenage 177–8, 188–92, 205, 207
  women's 6, 44, 51, 190, 199–200, 202, 204–5, 211–12, 223, 225, 232–3, 278
malaria 104
Manchester 143, 164, 345, 351
Mapperley Hospital Nottingham 378
marginalisation 199, 268n.10, 413
Marie Stopes UK 130
Marketing Week's Masters Awards 1
marriage 4–5, 42, 47, 71, 75, 82, 110–12, 117, 123n.21, 138, 177, 180, 347, 371
Martin, Emily 339–41
Maslow, Abraham 50
mass communication 4, 222–3, 225, 228n.4
mass media 5, 15, 35, 128, 222–3, 225–7, 228n.4, 273, 295, 321
Mass Observation Project (MOP) 141, 214, 325, 327–8, 330, 338–9, 341, 343n.15
Masters, William 39, 47
masturbation 92
materialism 2
McFadyean, Melanie 190
McKee, Glen 260
Medical Care Act (Canada) 73
medical
  authority 10, 32, 234
  discourse 33

Index

establishment 61–4, 67–8, 77, 139, 235, 244
humanities 13, 16, 26n.51
intervention 115, 154–5, 231, 237–8, 246
professional 3, 66, 69–70, 72, 206, 303, 308, 347
system 2, 31, 66, 96, 104, 119, 121
medicalisation 35, 105, 154, 227, 231, 234, 252, 254, 266
Medicare (Canada) 72, 249n.50
medicine 3, 14, 34, 36, 46, 64, 103–5, 108, 120, 128, 140, 171, 206, 226, 274, 328
alternative 296, 301
genetic 104, 120
natural 94
see also biomedicine
Mediterranean 105
Melvin, Jo 415
memory 104, 106, 112, 115–16, 207, 214, 242, 321–2, 328–9, 332, 373, 390, 409–10, 415, 422, 426
menarche 176
menopause 89, 94, 222, 234, 325, 329
Menstruation Directive 325–33, 341, 341n.2, 343n.15, 344n.34
menstruation 1, 234, 318–19, 325–40, 341n.1–2
menstrual cycle 11, 90, 94, 333
menstrual experience 90, 318
menstrual product 1–2, 332, 339
menstrual taboo 1, 325
menstrual technology 326, 334, 336–7, 339
see also tampon
menstrual towel 326–7, 333–7
Mering, Joseph von 14
Metapolitefsi period 82–4, 88
Middle East 224

Middlesbrough Hospital 363n.15
midwifery 237, 242–3, 249n.44
migration 4, 35, 104–6, 120
Mills, David 306
Mills, Ella 226–7, 294–5, 298–9, 301–4, 306–9
misogyny 11, 69, 72–3
mistreatment 91
Mitchell Beazley 41
Mitchell, James 41
Mizz 190, 353
Mobility Allowance 134, 137
Mohr-Pietsch, Sarah 421
monogamy 278
Monro, Maroushka 354
Montreal 244
morality 33, 40, 42, 76, 177, 191, 275
Morris, Joan 244
Morse, Harmon Northrup 14
mortality 277, 391
infant/childhood 110, 112, 119, 242
Mosley, Michael 299
motherhood 5–6, 66, 106, 112, 232–3, 238, 270n.40, 273, 275, 278, 284, 286
Movement for the Liberation of Women (MLW) 88, 91
movement
activist 8–9, 15, 166
anti-fluoride 9
anti-vaccination 9
birth control 34, 82–5, 87, 93, 95, 97
body-positive 294, 306
boundary 84–5, 95
disability 135
ecological 82
feminist 82, 84, 90
health 15, 88
liberation 32, 252–3, 266
MeToo 221, 396
natural childbirth 231, 233, 235, 238

440 *Index*

peace 267n.4
women's 15, 34, 83–4, 87–8, 93–7, 253, 367
see also activism
Mukti 202
Multinational Women's Liberation Group 94
Mungan, Gunilla 68
My Guy 357

Napa 14
National Assistance Board 137
National Co-ordinating Centre for Public Engagement 198
National Health Service (NHS) 48, 104–5, 155, 243, 285, 371
National Insurance 128, 137–8, 145, 147–8
National Trust 210
neoliberalism 31
New York 14, 163, 296, 424
New York Times 39, 42, 297
New Zealand 242
Nigeria 106, 110–12, 117, 119
Non-Contributory Invalidity Pension (NCIP) 134–5, 138, 144
North America 3, 16, 35–6, 60, 224, 255, 296, 327
Northern T.V. Newsletter 159
Nottingham 14, 378
Nova 51–2, 191, 202

O'Sullivan, Sue 349
obesity 302, 307
objectification 348
objectivity 36, 62, 64, 67, 86, 320, 394, 396
see also subjectivity
Observer 45, 49
Okotoks 65
Oni, Lola 103, 117
Oparah, Julia Chinyere 106
Oprah Winfrey Show, The 274, 279

otherness 86, 307
Ottawa/Ontario 243–5
Out on Tuesday 224, 263
ovulation 92
Oxygen 297

paediatrics 109, 363n.15
pain 51, 70, 90–1, 97, 103–4, 107–9, 114–16, 119, 123n.19, 231–2, 235–7, 239, 245, 258, 298, 309, 322, 332, 339, 391, 397, 401, 421
Paleo diet 296
Paltrow, Gwyneth 297
pandemic 206, 319, 322, 387, 398, 400, 408–10, 413, 415, 422, 426, 428n.23
see also COVID-19
paracetamol 14
paternalism 62, 117, 387
patient
consumerism 4, 32, 117
experience 110, 118
group 4, 8, 32, 35, 116
patriarchy 6, 11, 31, 33, 61–3, 66–7, 75, 77, 88–90, 92, 96, 112, 355
Pearce, K.I. 71
Peel, Hannah 421
Pelican Original 42
Personal Independence Payment 134
Personal, Social, Health, and Economic education (PSHE) 214
Petticoat 189, 326
phenomenology 18, 326, 330–2, 339–40
Phillips, Jean 60, 69, 74
philosophy 10, 61, 66, 83, 109, 320, 331, 340
physiotherapy 17, 244
Poland 14, 244
population control 94
pornography 45, 188, 263, 348

Index

poverty 94, 134–5, 137, 145, 187, 276, 295, 307, 309, 325
Powell, Enoch 115
pregnancy 11, 47–8, 53, 60–1, 63, 66, 68, 71–2, 82, 90, 92, 94, 107–8, 120, 177–80, 182–3, 189, 191, 206, 230–1, 233–4, 238–41, 246, 330, 348–9
property law 75
psychiatry 46, 165, 327, 378
psychology 2–3, 15, 32, 39, 43, 50, 54, 144, 238, 248n.21, 269n.27, 276, 278, 280, 284, 320, 331, 335, 386, 401, 417, 420, 425
psychoprophylaxis 232, 244
psychotherapy 191, 223, 232, 275
puberty 335
public engagement 13, 132, 198–200, 206
public sphere 2, 83, 128, 178
Purnell, Alice 157–8

queer
experience 172n.9, 203, 208, 210–11
people 13, 131–2, 172n.9, 204–5, 208–11, 214, 224
politics 18, 345
public history 132
queerness 209–11
theory 18

race 3, 36, 86, 115, 120, 131, 232, 245–6, 252, 328, 409
racism 11, 94, 104–5, 109, 115–16, 120–1, 212, 245, 410
radio 222, 259, 294, 416
Radio Times 279, 282
Rantzen, Ester 272, 275, 279–88
rape crisis centre 75
Raymond, Charles 44, 48

Rayner, Claire 1
Refuge for Women and Children of Domestic Violence 409
religion 43, 46, 70, 94, 222, 274, 300, 305, 309
Reno, Tosca 294, 296–9
reproduction 32, 47, 61, 64–6, 82, 89, 104, 110, 238, 349, 355
reproductive rights 65, 75, 93–4
Research Exercise Framework 14
resistance 5–6, 8–10, 19, 67, 70, 85, 106, 119–20, 131–2, 147, 208, 223, 227, 261, 353
Responsible Society 187
retirement 136
Roberts, Elizabeth 392
Robins, Denise 189, 206
Rombauer, Irma 49
Royal Academy of Dramatic Arts 5
Royal Army 231
Royal College of Nursing 199, 206

Sally Jessy Raphael Show, The 274
Salmon, Julian 260
Sappho 202, 204, 222, 254, 260
Saunders, Adele 234
Scandinavia 93
School Publication Advisory panel 186
science and technology studies (STS) 18, 84–6, 95
Scotland 142, 181, 217n.35, 271n.51, 362n.10
Scott, Sue 357, 359
Second World War 2–3, 31, 35, 115–16, 184, 273, 371, 379, 424
Section 28, 208, 214, 217n.35, 261–2, 271n.51, 347–8, 362n.10
self-care 2, 10, 204, 319, 414, 417, 420, 422, 425–6

442 *Index*

self-determination 82, 120, 361
self-harm 396, 400
Self-Help Association For
　　Transsexuals (SHAFT)
　　169–70
selfhood 3–5, 18, 32, 128, 132,
　　223, 321–2, 394
Senegal 104, 123n.19
Sequel 260, 270n.45
Severe Disablement Allowance
　　(SDA) 145–6
sex
　advice 33, 43
　education 96, 176–8, 184–9,
　　191–2, 196n.55, 214–15,
　　222, 325, 347–8, 362n.13
　life 15, 40–1, 54, 163, 182–3,
　　360
　orgasm 40, 43, 50–1, 90, 180
　permissiveness 31, 33, 40, 42,
　　48, 129, 177
　premarital sex 176
　promiscuity 177, 183
　safe/safer sex 185–7, 347, 349,
　　355–6, 358
　sexual behaviour 39, 42, 51,
　　164, 178–9
　sexual experience 47, 185, 189,
　　350
　sexual freedom 40, 54
　sexual hygiene 63
　sexual liberalisation 40–1, 46,
　　82
　sexually transmitted disease
　　(STD) 60, 71, 73–5, 77,
　　177, 179, 224, 349
Sex Education Resources Centre
　188
Sex Orientation Scale 164
sexism 31, 67, 116, 120–1, 166,
　　174n.52, 245
sexology/sexologist 12, 16, 33, 35,
　　46–7, 51, 164
sexualisation 356
sexuality 3, 32, 39, 45, 48, 50,
　　55n.5, 61, 66, 88–9, 94,

　　96, 130, 177–8, 182, 187,
　　192, 252–3, 347, 351,
　　353, 399, 409
　asexuality 262, 265
　bisexuality 155, 202–5, 208,
　　263, 266
　lesbian 265
　non-binary people 13, 162,
　　214, 328, 341, 343n.15
　sex research 39
　sexual 'abnormality' 40
　sexual assault 114, 221, 396
　sexual 'normality' 40, 47, 50,
　　55n.9
　sexual politics 36, 350, 357
　sexual radicalism 43
　sexual revolution 33, 39, 41,
　　43, 49
　theory of 39
　women's 239, 265, 349
Shaw, Madeleine 306
She 189, 202, 206
sickle cell disease (SCD) 8–9,
　　35–6, 103–21, 123n.19,
　　123n.21
Sickle Cell Society 107
Simkin, Ruth 70
Sisters Against Disablement 252
skin cancer 273, 277–8, 280–1,
　　283–6
　see also cancer
Sloan, Annie 420
Smash Hits 353
social media 5, 16, 107, 154,
　　221–3, 225–6, 294, 300,
　　304–5, 309, 310n.2
　see also internet
social science 320
social security 128, 134–8, 140,
　　145–7, 259
social services 135, 143, 363n.15
sociology 5–6, 25n.46, 42, 154,
　　256, 320, 331, 345, 347,
　　356
South Asia 105, 141, 202
Southampton Institute 325

Index

Spastics Society 188
Spectator, The 45
Spock, Benjamin 42
Sporcle 202–3
stereotype 204, 265, 281
sterilisation 71, 94
stigma 66, 110, 120, 238, 262–3, 276, 282, 288, 319, 325–6, 332–3, 339, 341
stigmatisation 115, 226, 237, 277, 281, 286, 336
Stopes, Marie 43, 130, 178–9
stress 4, 92, 111, 127, 157, 162, 241, 301, 303, 311n.22, 338, 372
subjectivity 3, 5, 8, 18–19, 317–18, 320–2, 328, 331, 340, 367, 369–70, 390, 394, 401, 410, 412
  see also objectivity
subordination 89, 91
Suffolk 231
sunbed 272–3, 277–8, 281–8
Sunbed Association, The (TSA) 281–2, 285
Sunday Times 43, 165
Supplementary Benefits Commission 137
Surgery and Emotion project 206
sweaty concept 34, 85, 87, 95–7
Sweden 242, 244, 255
Switzerland 242

tabloid 130, 225, 294, 362n.10
taboo 1, 42, 239, 323, 325–6
talk show 16, 223–4, 272–80, 286–8, 290n.21
tampon 1, 8, 326–7, 333–4, 337
  see also menstrual technology
Tandoh, Ruby 306–8
tanorexia 224–5, 273, 278, 280, 283, 285–7
Tavistock Clinic 155
teenager 2, 4, 68, 177, 179, 183–4, 188, 190–1, 200–2, 208, 334

television 1, 4–5, 10, 16, 18, 42, 176, 221–7, 259, 267n.4, 273–9, 281–2, 286–7, 292n.55, 294
thalidomide 144
That's Life! 279
Thatcher, Margaret 135
Therapeutic Abortion Committee (TAC) 71–2
therapy 2, 275, 279
  alternative 108, 123n.19
  sexual 42
  see also chemotherapy; physiotherapy; psychotherapy
This Nation Tomorrow 42
Time Out 257
Times, The 39, 42, 308
Titmuss, Richard 6
top-down perspective 3, 8–9, 32, 127–8, 131, 226, 320
  see also bottom-up perspective
Toronto/Ontario 237, 239, 244
Tory Party 16, 131, 135, 145, 310
trans
  community 129, 154–6, 164, 169, 171
  cross-dressing 156–8, 161, 204
  people 9, 13, 154–5, 157, 164, 166, 170, 216n.20
  sex change 154, 163, 165
  sex reassignment surgery 155, 165
  transfemininity 129, 155–6, 162, 164, 166–7, 169–71, 204
  transgender 155–6, 162–3, 204–5
  transitioning 154–5, 164, 351
  transmisogyny 168, 174n.52
  transness 154, 164
  transphobia 204
  transsexual/transsexualism 156, 158, 161, 163–4, 166, 169, 204
  transvestite 156–8, 161–4

444 *Index*

Transsexual Action Group (TAG)
129, 155, 166, 168–70
trauma 83, 97, 155, 169, 170–1,
374, 389
Trisha 274
Tsuuit'ina 65
TV/TS Group 129, 155, 163–6,
170, 173n.31
Tweedie, Jill 43, 45, 49, 54
Twickenham 257
Tylenol 14

unhappiness 5, 54, 309
Union of the Physically Impaired
Against Segregation 139,
256
University of Essex 201, 368
University of Roehampton 206
University of St Andrews 306
Uruguay 296
USA 14, 42, 123n.19, 224, 233,
244, 274, 326

Vaccine Damage Payments Scheme
144, 146
Valentine's Day Late 199, 206,
208–10
van de Velde, Theodoor 43
Vancouver/British Columbia 240
Vanessa Show, The 274, 278–9,
281, 285–7
vasectomy 71
veganism 299, 306, 308
Vel'vovskii, I.Z. 223, 232
venereal disease
see sex; sexually transmitted
disease
victimhood 212, 252
vulnerability 97, 208, 322, 387,
395–7, 400, 402

Wales 179, 196n.55, 221,
362n.13, 409
Walgreens 14
Wanham 65
War Pensions 146

Warner, Anthony 295, 305–6
Waugh, Auberon 45, 51–2
weight loss 202, 297–9, 301, 306
welfare state 2–3, 15, 32, 113,
115, 128, 130–1, 135–6,
140–2, 145, 147–8, 295,
369–72, 381
welfarism 2, 4
wellbeing 2–4, 41, 61, 63, 77,
197n.55, 198, 201, 212,
223, 226, 262, 265, 273,
275, 286, 297, 303, 319,
380, 410, 415, 417,
420–1, 424
children's 279, 283–4, 362n.13
cultural 75
emotional/mental 253, 264,
296, 388
social 68, 75
women's 70, 276, 278
Wellcome Library for the History
of Medicine 131, 233
Wellcome Trust 16, 131, 198
Wellen, Michael 425
wellness 2, 303
West Africa 35–6, 103, 105
West Indies 116
Whitechapel 231
Whitehouse, Mary 42
Wiley, Elizabeth 242–3
Winnipeg/Manitoba 240
Woman 207
Woman's Own 6, 202
Women, Risk and AIDS Project
(WRAP) 345, 348–9,
351–3, 355–7, 359–61,
365n.50, 366n.57
Women's Bookstore 84, 93
Women's College Hospital
(Toronto) 239
Women's Day 224, 259
Women's Group in Denmark
(WGD) 89
Women's Health Movement
(WHM) 9, 31, 34, 36,
60

Index 445

Women's International Information
and Communication
Service 94
Women's Liberation Movement
(WLM) 9, 31–2, 89, 166,
251, 253–4, 256
see also feminism; movement;
women's
Women's Reproductive Rights
Campaign (WRRC) 93

women's shelter 75
Woodward, Camilla 306
Woodward, Shaun 306
World Health Organization
(WHO) 66

yoga 94, 296, 305, 307

Printed in the USA
CPSIA information can be obtained
at www.ICGtesting.com
JSHW012012240924
70430JS00003B/11